50 Challenging Spinal Pain Syndrome Cases

For Butterworth-Heinemann:

Commissioning Editor: Heidi Allen
Project Development Manager: Robert Edwards
Project Manager: Andrea Hill
Designer: George Ajayi

50 Challenging Spinal Pain Syndrome Cases

Lynton G.F. Giles MSc, DC(C), PhD (WAust)

Adjunct Associate Professor, School of Public Health and Tropical Medicine,
Faculty of Medicine, Health and Molecular Sciences,
James Cook University, Townsville, Queensland, Australia

Director, Multidisciplinary Spinal Pain Unit, The University of Queensland,
Townsville Health Service District's Kirwan Campus,
Kirwan, Queensland, Australia

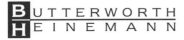

BUTTERWORTH-HEINEMANN
An imprint of Elsevier Science Limited

First published 2003

ISBN 0 7506 4008 1

British Library Cataloguing in Publication Data
A catalogue record for this book is available from the British Library

Library of Congress Cataloging in Publication Data
A catalog record for this book is available from the Library of
Congress

Note
Medical knowledge is constantly changing. As new information
becomes available, changes in treatment, procedures, equipment, and
the use of drugs become necessary. The author and the publishers
have taken care to ensure that the information given in this text is
accurate and up to date. However, readers are strongly advised to
confirm that the information, especially with regard to drug usage,
complies with the latest legislation and standards of practice.

 your source for books,
journals and multimedia
in the health sciences

www.elsevierhealth.com

The
publisher's
policy is to use
**paper manufactured
from sustainable forests**

Printed in China by RDC Group Limited

Contents

Preface

Conditions causing spinal pain syndromes are many and varied. During the last 30 years different interesting and challenging cases have been collected, 50 of which are presented in this text.

Knowledge is ever increasing on spinal anatomy and the possible mechanisms by which pain may be experienced. Therefore, an introductory chapter summarizes current possible pain mechanisms, based on known anatomical principles. Because spinal pain syndromes can be complex, there is often a tendency for clinicians to label patients as being 'neurotic' or, when patients are involved in litigation, as having litigation 'neuroses' as motives. However, it should be remembered that it is not always possible to diagnose a patient's spinal pain condition because of many factors such as the limitations of imaging procedures and the specificity and sensitivity of laboratory tests; so patients should not be considered as malingerers unless there are very strong grounds for doing so. Imaging frequently only provides shadows of the truth and laboratory tests can be misleading, so it is imperative to take a careful history and to perform a thorough physical examination followed, as indicated, by appropriate imaging and laboratory procedures.

In some of the cases presented in this text, gross anatomy and pathology, as well as histopathology specimens obtained from postmortem material, with changes similar to the clinical cases presented, are used to illustrate how such findings in patients may cause spinal pain syndromes and provide a basis upon which to recommend treatment options.

The cases begin with the most frequent spinal level of involvement (lumbar spine) and conclude with the least frequent spinal level of involvement (thoracic spine).

L.G.F. Giles

General introduction

INTRODUCTION

The diagnosis of spinal pain syndromes is often difficult, as the anatomy of the spine and its adjacent soft tissue structures is complex. For details of spinal anatomy and histology see Rickenbacher et al (1982), Moore (1992), Cramer (1995), Giles (1997, 1999) and Giles and Baker (1998) as the purpose of this introductory chapter is to provide a synopsis of diagnoses based on a sound anatomical foundation as well as on clinical and physical findings. In addition, it should be noted that the neurophysiology of pain is not fully understood at this time. For example, when Slipman et al (1998) studied the mechanical stimulation of cervical nerve roots C4 to C8 in patients with cervical radicular symptoms who were undergoing diagnostic selective nerve block, to document the distribution of pain and paraesthesiae that result from stimulation of specific cervical nerve roots, and to compare that distribution to documented sensory dermatomal maps, they demonstrated a distinct difference between *dynatomal* and *dermatomal* maps. A dynatome is the distribution of referred symptoms from root irritation and this is different to the sensory deficit outlined by dermatomal maps. Slipman et al (1998) suggest that cervical dermatomal mapping is inaccurate, as the distribution of referred symptoms from cervical root irritation (dynatome) is different than the sensory deficit outlined by dermatomal maps. Therefore, it is reasonable to suggest that a similar neurophysiological finding may occur

at other spinal nerve root levels. Thus when considering neurological tests such as pinprick or light touch, summarized later in this text, it would be prudent to remember the work of Slipman et al (1998).

Low back pain is experienced by 80–90% of the population (Deen 1996), while 34–40% of the population experience neck and arm pain (Hardin & Halla 1995) compared to 7–14% of the population that experience thoracic spine pain (Pedersen 1994, Hinkley & Drysdale 1995). Therefore, musculoskeletal spinal pain can be a significant health problem.

Spinal pain syndromes must be viewed in the context of (i) clearly defined pathological conditions, and (ii) the less well-defined, but much more prevalent, condition of spinal pain of mechanical origin (Stoddard 1969, Kenna & Murtagh 1989). It is imperative to distinguish mechanical causes of spinal pain from other causes, as patients with mechanical disorders of the spine are likely to respond dramatically to manual treatment (Kenna & Murtagh 1989).

A major difficulty involved in evaluating a patient with spinal pain of mechanical origin, with or without root symptoms, is that many causes of pain are possible. Because the painful structure, or structures, are not amenable to direct scrutiny, a tentative diagnosis is usually arrived at for an individual case by taking a careful case history and employing a thorough physical examination, with imaging and laboratory procedures as indicated. There are four main approaches to patient evaluation: (i) history;

(ii) assessment of pain (using subjective self-report measures estimating pain severity, quality and location); (iii) investigation of personality structure, including the use of appropriate subjective questionnaires; and (iv) clinical identification of signs and symptoms, including spinal joint motion palpation, and signs and symptoms deemed excessively, or inappropriately, abnormal (Main & Waddell 1982). However, caution has to be exercised when making judgements on an individual's behavioural responses to examination as serious misuse and misinterpretation of behavioural signs has occurred in medicolegal contexts using such signs (Main and Waddell 1998).

There is still little consensus, either within or among specialties, on the use of diagnostic tests for patients with spinal pain syndromes, and the underlying pathology responsible for various spinal pain problems remains elusive (Videman et al 1998). Furthermore, in spite of following a thorough examination procedure, one often merely eliminates overt pathologies and the precise cause of spinal pain syndromes of mechanical origin often remains obscure (Turner et al 1998).

Specifically, diagnostic problems relate to: (a) the limitations of many diagnostic procedures, including plain film radiography, computerized tomography (CT), magnetic resonance imaging (MRI), myelography, discography and bone scans; (b) some diagnostic and therapeutic chemical agents being harmful, as can be the case when such chemicals injected into intervertebral discs extravasate into the epidural space (Weitz 1984, Adams et al 1986, MacMillan et al 1991) causing complications due to contact between them and neural structures (Dyck 1985, Merz 1986, Watts & Dickhaus 1986); (c) inadequacies in the precise anatomical knowledge of the spine including its nociceptive tissues; (d) anatomical complexity of the spine often making roentgenographic interpretation difficult (Le-Breton et al 1993); and (e) there sometimes being multifactorial causes of pain at a given level of the spine (Haldeman 1977, Gross 1979), e.g. injury to the intervertebral disc, the zygapophysial facet joints or to the segmental

soft tissue structures. A further important point to remember is that a *central* disc herniation may cause spinal pain alone without radiculopathy (Postacchini & Gumina 1999) whereas a posterolateral or far lateral disc herniation will cause radicular pain (Keim & Kirkaldy-Willis 1987).

Also, there is often disagreement on which imaging procedures have diagnostic validity for mechanical spinal pain, although it is generally agreed that, for plain film X-ray examinations, two views of the same anatomical region at right angles is the minimum requirement (Henderson et al 1994), and that erect posture radiography (Giles & Taylor 1981) and functional views (Jackson 1977) are more useful. Furthermore, Buirski and Silberstein (1993) correctly noted that MRI can only be used as an assessment of nuclear anatomy and not for symptomatology, and Schellhas et al (1996) showed that significant cervical disc anular tears often escape MRI detection. In addition, Osti and Fraser (1992) concluded that lumbar discography is more accurate than MRI for the detection of anular pathology. However, according to Shalen (1989), lumbar discography is a controversial examination that is regarded by some radiologists and spine surgeons as barbaric and non-efficacious (Wiley et al 1968, Clifford 1986, Shapiro 1986). For lumbar spine CT and MR imaging, Willen et al (1997) showed that the diagnostic specificity of spinal stenosis will increase considerably when the patient is subjected to an axial load, and Danielson et al (1998) concluded that, for an adequate evaluation of the cross-sectional area, CT or MR studies should be performed with axial loading in patients who have symptoms of lumbar spinal stenosis.

In the thoracic spine, with its particular combination of intervertebral and various synovial joints, the most common cause of thoracic spine pain syndromes is dysfunction and degeneration of spinal intervertebral joints and the associated rib articulations (Kenna & Murtagh 1989). Root compression due to posterolateral disc protrusion, with resulting signs and symptoms of intercostal radiculopathy, such as pain, paraesthesiae and sensory disturbances, has to be differentiated from overt pathological conditions such as neoplasms. Thoracic disc protrusion has long been a difficult clinical entity to diagnose (Brown et al 1992) as symptoms can vary dramatically from none at all to motor and sensory deficits resulting from spinal cord compression (myelopathy) – pain, muscle weakness, and spinal cord dysfunction are the most common clinical symptoms (Cramer 1995). On the other hand, thoracic disc protrusion can produce spinal cord compression with bladder incontinence and signs of an upper motor neuron lesion (Kenna & Murtagh 1989) and occasionally paraplegia. As the thoracic cord is immobilized by the dentate ligaments, the anterior spinal artery may be significantly compressed by a relatively small central disk protrusion (Pate & Jaeger 1996) and, because there is little extradural space in the thoracic spinal canal, a comparatively small disc protrusion may have pronounced effects on the neurology (Hoppenfeld 1977). Thoracic cord compression can also be caused by ossified ligamenta flava in caucasians (van Oostenbrugge et al 1999) as well as in Japanese people (Otani et al 1986, Yonenobu et al 1987, Kojima et al 1992).

It is still only rarely possible to validate a diagnosis in cases where pain arises from the spine (White & Gordon 1982) and, because it is not possible to establish the pathological basis of spinal pain in 80–90% of cases (Chila et al 1990, Spratt et al 1990, Pope & Novotny 1993), this leads to diagnostic uncertainty and suspicion that some patients have a 'compensation neurosis' or other psychological problem. It is also appropriate at this time to recognize the role of psychosocial factors in spinal pain. Although the complex interaction of psyche and soma in the aetiology of spinal pain is not well understood, a psychogenic component may be primary (conversion disorder), secondary (depression caused by chronic pain), contributory (myofascial dysfunction), or absent (Keim & Kirkaldy-Willis 1987).

It is reasonable to broadly classify acute spinal pain as being of 7–28 days or less duration, which may be followed by a sub-acute stage of up to 12 weeks; after this the pain can be considered chronic (Skoven et al 2002).

HISTORY OF SPINAL PAIN

The importance of an exhaustive case history cannot be overemphasized and it should take into account facts such as the patient's age, occupation, onset of pain, previous injuries, medication, recreational activities, pain aggravation and characteristics, location, distribution, and any related neurological symptoms (numbness, paraesthesiae, muscle weakness). Some conditions provide reasonably characteristic patterns, while others do not. For example, pain that occurs at night, and which is relieved by aspirin, may be associated with an osteoid osteoma that is a benign tumour of bone (Keim & Kirkaldy-Willis 1987). Night pain *per se* should be considered as being of probable serious pathological change.

Taking into consideration the issue of dermatomes and dynatomes (Slipman et al 1998), an important neurological concept that has been recognized for anatomically normal spines, and which needs to be considered during the examination is that the distribution of cutaneous areas supplied with afferent nerve fibres by single posterior spinal nerve roots i.e., dermatomes of the human body (Dorland's *Illustrated Medical Dictionary* 1974, Barr and Kiernan 1983), has been fairly well established (Fig. i).

According to Keim and Kirkaldy-Willis (1987), this enables deficits of a specific nerve root to be accurately localized during sensory examination. However, it is important to note that Jinkins (1993) and Slipman et al (1998) question this concept and suggest that there is, in fact, some overlap of sensation.

Thus, until a thorough history has been taken and a complete physical examination and any appropriate imaging or laboratory tests have been performed, as considered necessary, to rule out organic disease, it is not wise to label a patient as being neurotic or a malingerer, particularly as it is thought that such patients form only a small minority of cases (Teasell 1997). Furthermore, there has long been a misconception

Figure i Dermatomes on the anterior and posterior surfaces of the body. Axial lines, where there is numerical discontinuity, are drawn thickly. (Modified from Wilkinson, JL (1986) Neuroanatomy for medical students. John Wright and Sons, Bristol, p 29.)

that *all* injuries should heal after 6 weeks; however, clinical experience and follow-up studies (Mendelson 1982, Radanov et al 1994) clearly demonstrate that not *all* patients necessarily get better and that there is a significant subset who continue to suffer from chronic symptoms (Teasell 1997).

It is worth noting the sobering comment of Professor Ruth Jackson in her classic textbook *The Cervical Syndrome* (1977) in which she wrote:

When one who is not completely versed in the symptomatology of disorders of the cervical spine has completed… the examination, he may have drawn the conclusion that the patient is psychoneurotic. However, to draw such a conclusion is a reflection on the examiner's diagnostic ability and not on the patient, until proven otherwise.

This comment applies equally well to all regions of the complex human spine.

BRIEF SUMMARY OF SPINAL INNERVATION

The innervation of the lumbar, cervical and thoracic spines is extremely complex as partly shown in Figs ii, iii and iv, respectively. Although part of the innervation of the anterior and posterior elements of the lumbar spine is shown schematically in Fig. ii, the innervation shown for the cervical and thoracic spines is less detailed in order to simplify the diagrams. However, the basic neuroanatomical principles shown for the lumbar spine are largely the same for each spinal level, bearing in mind the different osteological and soft tissue structures for the three levels of the spine; full details of spinal innervation can be found in standard textbooks such as *Gray's Anatomy* and *Moore's Clinically Oriented Anatomy*, or in anatomy texts specifically related to the spine (Rickenbacher et al 1982, Cramer & Darby 1995).

IMAGING

Routine radiographs of the spine, and when indicated by the history and symptoms, the chest, should be taken to establish a baseline and to rule out metabolic, inflammatory, and malignant conditions (Keim & Kirkaldy-Willis 1987). As long as proper coning of the X-ray beam is used in conjunction with high speed screens and films, and appropriate filtration of the X-ray beam, there is minimal X-radiation to the patient while obtaining maximum quality X-ray films. These radiographs should be taken in the erect

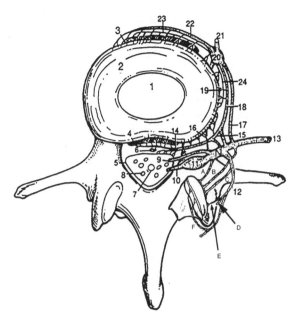

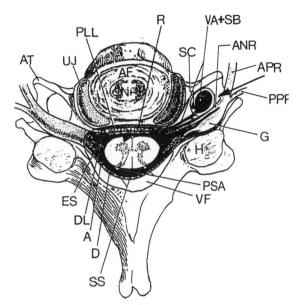

Figure ii A schematic diagram showing basic lumbar vertebral anatomy and part of the innervation of the anterior and posterior structures of the vertebral column: 1 = nucleus pulposus; 2 = anulus fibrosus; 3 = anterior longitudinal ligament/periosteum; 4 = posterior longitudinal ligament/periosteum; 5 = dural tube/thecal sac; 6 = epidural vasculature; 7 = filum terminale; 8 = intrathecal lumbosacral nerve root; 9 = ventral (anterior) root; 10 = dorsal (posterior) root; 11 = dorsal root ganglion (spinal ganglion); 12 = dorsal ramus of spinal nerve; 13 = ventral ramus of spinal nerve; 14 = recurrent meningeal nerve (sinuvertebral nerve of von Luschka); 15 = autonomic (sympathetic) branch to recurrent meningeal nerve; 16 = direct somatic branch from ventral ramus of spinal nerve to lateral disc; 17 = white ramus communicans (not found caudal to L2); 18 = grey ramus communicans (multilevel irregular lumbosacral distribution); 19 = lateral sympathetic efferent branches projecting from grey ramus communicans; 20 = paraspinal sympathetic ganglion (PSG); 21 = paraspinal sympathetic chain; 22 = anterior paraspinal afferent sympathetic ramus projecting to PSG; 23 = anterior sympathetic efferent branches projecting from PSG; 24 = lateral paraspinal afferent sympathetic ramus projecting to PSG. (Note: Afferent and efferent sympathetic paraspinous branches/rami may be partially combined *in vivo*.) A = neural fibres from main trunk of spinal nerve (N); B = neural fibres from ventral ramus (13) of spinal nerve; C = neural fibres from dorsal ramus (12) of spinal nerve; E = neural fibres from medial branch (D) of dorsal ramus (12); F = neural fibres from lateral branch of dorsal ramus (12) of the spinal nerve. (Modified from: Jinkins JR et al American Journal of Neuroradiology 1989 10: 219–251; American Journal of Roentgenology 1989 152: 1277–1279 and Jinkins JR 1997 Clinical anatomy and management of low back pain, pp. 255–272; Auteroche P Anatomia Clinica 1983 5: 17–28.)

Figure iii A schematic diagram of a typical cervical vertebra showing basic cervical vertebral anatomy and part of the neuroanatomy within the spinal and intervertebral foramen canals. The arrow points to the origin of the recurrent meningeal nerve and the arrow head shows the anterior spinal artery. A = arachnoid; AF = anulus fibrosus; ANR = anterior nerve root; APR = anterior primary ramus; AT = anterior tubercle; D = dura; DL = dentate ligament; ES = epidural space; G = spinal ganglion; H = hyaline articular cartilage on the superior articular facet; NP = nucleus pulposus; PLL = posterior longitudinal ligament; PPR = posterior primary ramus; PSA = posterior spinal arteries; R = recurrent meningeal nerve; SC = sympathetic chain; SS = subdural space; UJ = uncovertebral joint; VA+SB = vertebral artery and spinal branch; VF = vertebral foramen. The diagram does not show the innervation of the intervertebral disc or the zygapophysial (facet) joints and other structures. (Modified from: Jackson R 1977 The cervical syndrome. Charles C Thomas, Springfield.)

posture, using carefully standardized procedures; for example, to accurately determine whether possibly significant leg length inequality is present with corresponding pelvic obliquity causing postural (compensatory) scoliosis in the spine (Giles & Taylor 1981, Giles 1984, 1989). In the cervical spine, functional flexion and extension views may show instability; sagittal plane displacement between two cervical vertebrae of more than 3.5 mm, or relative sagittal plane angulation greater than 11°, is considered to represent cervical segmental instability

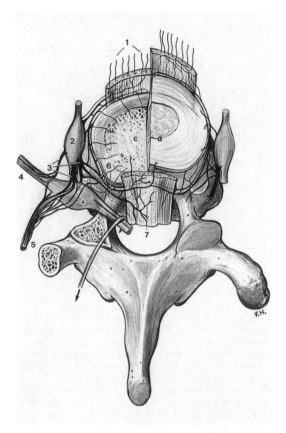

Figure iv   A schematic diagram showing basic thoracic vertebral anatomy and the nerve supply of the thoracic ventral compartment at the level of the vertebral body (c) and at the level of the intervertebral disc (d). The ventral and dorsal roots of the spinal nerve are retracted dorsally (arrow). Bundles of nerve fibres originating from rami communicantes (3) pass cranial and caudal to the spinal nerve and the dorsal root ganglion (G) towards the dorsal ramus of the spinal nerve (5). Large and small sinuvertebral nerves (6) derive from the rami communicantes. 1= anterior longitudinal ligament nerve plexus; 2 = paraspinal sympathetic ganglion; 3 = rami communicantes; 4 = ventral ramus of the spinal nerve; 5 = dorsal ramus of the spinal nerve; 6 = sinuvertebral nerves; 7 = posterior longitudinal ligament nerve plexus. The diagram does not show the innervation of the intervertebral disc or the zygapophysial (facet) joints and other structures. (From Groen GJ et al 1990 American Journal of Anatomy 188: 282–296.)

(White et a1 1975) – that is, horizontal or angular instability (Dai 1998).

Bogduk's (1999) 'modified criteria for the use of plain films in low back pain' that are based on the work of Deyo and Diehl (1986) are of concern when viewed in the light of some of the following cases on over 30 years experience in the diagnosis of spinal pain syndromes. Bogduk (1999) states 'plain films may be used as a screening test for "red flag" conditions if a patient presents with any of the following features': history of cancer, significant trauma, weight loss, temperature >37.6 °C, risk factors for infection, neurological deficit, minor trauma in patients (over 50 years of age, known to be osteoporotic or taking corticosteroids), no improvement over 1 month. Clearly, it is better for a patient to undergo plain film radiography when indicated by the history (unless there is a contraindication such as pregnancy) at the onset of symptoms, rather than to risk misdiagnosis and mismanagement, both of which would be disadvantageous to patients. This is particularly important when treatment by spinal manipulation is considered as the application of mechanical forces to a spine that may have degenerative changes, or overt pathological changes, could be dangerous.

Further imaging procedures may be necessary: such as (i) magnetic resonance imaging, which can provide very good detail of soft tissue structures in and about the spinal column without the need of radiation or of contrast, (ii) CT scans which are particularly good at showing bony structures and are useful for some neural problems, (iii) myelography or post myelography CT scans for demonstrating lesions of the spinal cord and canal such as neoplasm and disc herniation, and (iv) bone scans when tumour, infection or small fracture(s) are suspected, and (v) when indicated, discography to show tears in the intervertebral disc and internal disc disruption. Possible complications of an invasive procedure should always be considered.

Unfortunately, all the preceding procedures have some limitations, for example plain film radiographs will not show an osseous erosion until approximately 40% decrease in bone density has occurred (Michel et al 1990, Perry 1995) and Schellhas et al (1996) and Osti and Fraser (1992) found that discography is more accurate than MRI for the detection of anular pathology in the cervical and lumbar spines, respectively. Therefore, these limitations show, as stated above, that imaging procedures may only give a 'shadow of the truth' and this important fact should be remembered. This is particularly true when a patient's physical examination and imaging studies are not remarkable and do not pinpoint the cause of symptoms, as imaging cannot show all tissue injuries (Giles & Crawford 1997). The limitations of present diagnostic imaging procedures in not being able to show all soft tissues are an unfortunate but obvious fact.

It is known that a high prevalence (20–70%) of lumbar disc abnormalities has been detected in asymptomatic individuals by MRI (Boden et al 1990, Jensen 1994, Boos et al 1995), a finding that raises questions about the morphology-based understanding of pain pathogenesis in patients with disc abnormalities (Boos et al 2000). Furthermore, Karppinen et al (2001) found that MRI scans from 180 patients with unilateral sciatic pain suggested that a discogenic pain mechanism other than nerve root entrapment generates the subjective symptoms among sciatic patients.

A further difficulty is that the nomenclature and classification of lumbar disc pathology is not standardized (Fardon et al 2001), although Pfirrmann et al (2001) have suggested a method for grading disc degeneration on T2-weighted MRI.

When nerve root dysfunction is suspected, electromyography (EMG) and nerve root conduction studies can be helpful (Hoppenfeld 1977).

It is important to note the following comments regarding imaging shown in this text:

- Plain film anteroposterior radiographic images of the spine are printed as if the clinician were looking at the patient's back; i.e. a marker showing 'R' indicates the patient's right side.
- Spinal CT scans are viewed, as usual, from 'below'; i.e. remember that the clinician 'looks up' the patient's spinal canal with the patient supine, so the patient's right side is marked 'R' on the left side of the axial CT scan figure(s).
- MRI studies may show both sagittal and axial images. The same principle as for CT scans is applied to MRI axial images; i.e. the patient's right side is on the left of the figure(s).

- MRI T1-weighted images produce essentially a *fat image* in which structures containing fat (bone marrow, subcutaneous fat) appear bright, while structures containing water (oedema, neoplasm, inflammation, cerebrospinal fluid, sclerosis) appear dark (Yochum & Barry 1996).
- MRI T2-weighted images produce essentially a *water image* in which structures containing predominantly free or loosely bound water molecules (oedema, neoplasm, inflammation, cerebrospinal fluid, healthy nucleus pulposus) appear bright, while substances with tightly bound water (ligaments, menisci, tendons, calcification, sclerosis) appear dark (hypointense) (Yochum & Barry 1996).
- Patient identification details have been blacked out to maintain patient confidentiality.

LABORATORY TESTS

When bony pathology is suspected, serum calcium, phosphorus, alkaline phosphatase (particularly alkaline phosphatase isoenzyme determination by electrophoresis, which differentiates alkaline phosphatase of osteoblastic origin from alkaline phosphatase from other sources (Brown 1975)), and acid phosphatase may be helpful in detecting bone disease. Early inflammatory changes may be detected by an increase in C-reactive protein (CRP) and/or an increase in the erythrocyte sedimentation rate (ESR). A full blood count can be helpful, for example, in cases where there is suspicion of primary haematological disorders and for some infections (Henderson et al 1994). Immunoelectrophoresis of serum and urinary proteins may also be useful diagnostic procedures in the diagnosis of multiple myeloma (Brown 1975). Other tests that should be considered, when indicated, are blood culture and sensitivity, and for genitourinary tract infections urine culture and sensitivity, as well as latex flocculation for rheumatoid spondylitis, and serum and urine amylase and lipase for chronic pancreatitis (Collins 1968, Schroeder et al 1992). In addition, it may be necessary to assess bone density using a dual energy X-ray absorption (DEXA) bone desitometer in osteoporotic patients. In males, prostate-specific antigen (PSA) should be considered if there is any suspicion of prostate malignancy.

In this book it is not necessary to list every spine-related condition with its possible abnormalities in serology, haematology, urinalysis and other laboratory tests, as these have been well documented in numerous clinical diagnosis texts. In some publications, particular reference to spinal pathological conditions and related pathology tests have been summarised (Haldeman et al 1993, Henderson et al 1994).

Laboratory evaluations are important when the clinician suspects metabolic disturbance, malignancy, infection or one of the arthritides such as ankylosing spondylitis or rheumatoid arthritis. Nonetheless, it should be noted that various tests have different levels of *accuracy*, as calculated from their *sensitivity* (proportion of individuals with the condition whose tests are positive) and *specificity* (proportion of individuals without the condition whose tests are negative (Bloch 1987, Nachemson 1992, Henderson et al 1994)).

A summary of the chief conditions causing spinal tenderness is shown in Table i.

TREATMENT

Having considered the above issues of anatomy and careful diagnosis, the clinician will be faced with deciding upon the most appropriate form of treatment. If one adheres to the principle of 'do no harm' and of taking the 'least invasive treatment approach', patients will benefit. Unfortunately, there has been an unreasonable and ongoing struggle between certain groups of clinicians in health care to dominate other groups in spite of evidence of one form of conservative treatment achieving greater success, for example in the case of low back pain (Meade et al 1990, 1995). A conservative approach to spinal pain treatment, such as spinal manipulation, should always be considered as the first option when there are no contraindications to such treatment.

There are several treatment options for dealing with spinal pain syndromes of mechanical

Table i Summary of chief conditions causing spinal tenderness

1. Diseases of the overlying skin and subcutaneous tissue
    These are usually clinically obvious and include potentially serious conditions such as melanoma.

2. Diseases of the vertebral column
    Inflammatory
        Pott's disease
        Staphylococcal spondylitis
        Typhoid spine
        Spondylitis ankylopoietica
        Actinomycosis
        Hydatid cyst
        Paget's disease

    Degenerative
        Spondylosis
        Osteochondritis (rare)
        Nucleus pulposus herniation

    Neoplastic
        Primary tumour
        Secondary deposit
        Myelomatosis
        Leukaemic deposits

    Traumatic
        Fracture
        Dislocation
        Nucleus pulposus herniation

    Erosion by aortic aneurysm

3. Diseases of the spinal cord and meninges
    Metastatic epidural abscess or tumour
    Meningioma
    Neurofibroma
    Herpes zoster
    Meningitis serosa circumscripta
    Tumour of the spinal cord
    Syringomyelia

4. Hysteria and malingering: compensation neurosis

5. Metabolic disorders: osteoporosis, osteomalacia, hyperparathyroidism

Modified from Mackenzie, I (1985) Spine, tenderness of. In: Hart FD (ed.) French's index of differential diagnosis. 12th edn. Butterworth & Co. Ltd, p 788.

origin, for example, acupuncture, medication and spinal manipulation. Patients should be given the opportunity to try whichever of these options they would prefer, in consultation with their clinician, as not one discipline has 'all the answers' for every patient. The ideal situation for diagnosing and treating acute and chronic spinal pain syndrome patients is to have a multidisciplinary team of individuals who specialize in different diagnostic and treatment modalities.

Table ii Some possible causes of spinal pain of mechanical origin with or without radicular pain

Nerve root conditions

- Adhesions between dural sleeves and (a) the joint capsule with nerve root fibrosis (Sunderland 1968, Jackson 1977, Wilkinson 1986) and (b) intervertebral disc herniation (Wilkinson 1986).
- Intervertebral disc degeneration and fragmentation (Schiotz & Cyriax 1975), or nucleus pulposus extrusion (Mixter & Ayer 1935) causing nerve root compression, or nerve root 'chemical radiculitis' (Marshall & Trethewie 1973).

Zygapophysial joint conditions

- Joint derangement (subluxation) due to ligamentous and capsular instability (Hadley 1964, Cailliet 1968, Jackson 1977, Macnab 1977, van Norel & Verhagen 1996).
- Joint capsule tension with encroachment upon the intervertebral foramen lumen (Jackson 1977).
- Joint degenerative changes, e.g. 'meniscal' incarceration (Schmorl & Junghanns 1971), traumatic synovitis due to 'pinching' of synovial folds (Giles 1986), synovial fold tractioning against the pain-sensitive joint capsule (Hadley 1964), and osteoarthrosis (Jackson 1977).
- Joint effusion with capsular distension which may (a) exert pressure on a nerve root (Jackson 1977), (b) cause capsular pain (Jackson 1966), or (c) cause nerve root pain by direct diffusion (Haldeman 1977).
- Joint capsule adhesions (Jackson 1977, Farfan 1980, Giles 1989).

Intervertebral disc conditions

- Disc herniation into the spinal and intervertebral canals.
- Spondylosis (Young 1967, Jackson 1977).

Miscellaneous conditions

- Spinal and intervertebral canal (foramen) stenosis (Young 1967, Jackson 1977, Epstein & Epstein 1987, Rauschning 1992).
- Intervertebral canal (foramen) venous stasis (Giles 1973, Sunderland 1975).
- Myofascial genesis of pain (trigger areas) (Travell & Rinzler 1952, Bonica 1957, Simons & Travell 1983).
- Baastrup's syndrome (Bland 1987).
- Osseous spinal anomalies, e.g. bilateral cervical ribs, block vertebra (Jackson 1977).

At the beginning of the lumbar, cervical and thoracic spine sections, respectively, a detailed list of possible pathological causes of pain will be presented. In addition it is necessary to list the possible causes of spinal pain of mechanical origin as briefly summarized in Table ii which provides a summary of some literature references over the years in order to provide a historical background to this complex issue of spinal pain of mechanical origin.

REFERENCES

Adams M A, Dolan P, Hutton W C 1986 The stages of disc degeneration as revealed by discogram. Journal of Bone and Joint Surgery 68B: 36.
Auteroche P 1983 Innervation of the zygapophysial joints of the lumbar spine. Anatomia Clinica 5: 17–28.
Barr M L, Kiernan J A 1983 The human nervous system. An anatomical viewpoint, 4th edn. Harper and Row, Philadelphia.
Bland J H 1987 Disorders of the cervical spine. Diagnosis and medical management. WB Saunders, Philadelphia.
Bloch R 1987 Methodology in clinical back pain trials. Spine 12: 430.
Boden S D, Davis D O, Dina T S, Patronas N J, Wiesel S W 1990 Abnormal magnetic-resonance scans of the lumbar spine in asymptomatic subjects: A prospective investigation. Journal of Bone and Joint Surgery (America) 72: 403–408.
Bogduk N 1999 Evidence-based clinical guidelines for the management of acute low back pain. National Medical Research Council, Canberra, Australia, November 1999.
Bonica J J 1957 Management of myofascial pain syndromes in general practice. Journal of the American Medical Association 164: 732–738.
Boos N, Rieder R, Schade V, Spratt K, Semmer N, Aebi M 1995 Volvo Award in Clinical Sciences. The diagnostic accuracy of magnetic resonance imaging, work perception and psychosocial factors in identifying symptomatic disc herniations. Spine 20: 2613–2625.
Boos N, Semmer N, Elfering A, Schade V, Gal I, Zanetti M, Kissling R, Buchegger N, Hodler J, Main C J 2000 Natural history of individuals with asymptomatic disc abnormalities in magnetic resonance imaging. Spine 25: 1484–1492.
Brown M D 1975 Diagnosis of pain syndromes of the spine. Orthopedic Clinics of North America 6: 233–248.

Brown C W, Deffer P A, Akmakjian J et al 1992 The natural history of thoracic disc herniation. Spine 17: S97–S102.

Buirski G, Silberstein M 1993 The symptomatic lumbar disc in patients with low back pain: magnetic resonance imaging appearances in both a symptomatic and control population. Spine 18: 1808–1811.

Cailliet R 1968 Low back pain syndrome, 2nd edn. FA Davis, Philadelphia.

Chila A G, Jeffries R R, Levin S M 1990 Is manipulation for your practice? Patient Care 15 May: 77–92.

Clifford J R 1986 Lumbar discography: An outdated procedure (letter). Journal of Neurosurgery 64: 686.

Collins R D 1968 Illustrated manual of laboratory diagnosis. JB Lippincott Co., Philadelphia.

Cramer G D 1995 The thoracic region. In: Cramer GD, Darby SA (eds) Basic and clinical anatomy of the spine, spinal cord, and ANS. Mosby, Baltimore.

Cramer G D, Darby S A (eds) 1995 Basic and clinical anatomy of the spine, spinal cord, and ANS. Mosby, Baltimore.

Dai L 1998 Disc degeneration and cervical instability. Spine 23: 1734–1738.

Danielson B I, Willen J, Gaulitz A, Niklason T, Hansson T H 1998 Axial loading of the spine during CT and MR in patients with suspected lumbar spinal stenosis. Acta Radiologica 39: 604–611.

Deen H G 1996 Concise review for primary-care physicians. Diagnosis and management of lumbar disk disease. Mayo Clinic Proceedings 71: 283–287.

Deyo R A, Diehl A K 1986 Lumbar spine films in primary care: current use and effects of selective ordering criteria. Journal of General Internal Medicine 1: 20–25.

Dorland's illustrated medical dictionary, 25th edn. 1974 WB Saunders, Philadelphia.

Dyck P 1985 Paraplegia following chemonucleolysis. Spine 10: 359.

Epstein N E, Epstein J A 1987 Individual and coexistant lumbar and cervical spinal stenosis. In: Hopp E (ed.) Spinal stenosis. Spine: State of the Art Reviews 1: 401–420.

Fardon D F, Milette P C 2001 Nomenclature and classification of lumbar disc pathology. Spine 26: E93–113.

Farfan H F 1980 The scientific basis of manipulative procedures. Clinics in Rheumatic Diseases 6: 159–178.

Giles L G F 1973 Spinal fixation and viscera. Journal of Clinical Chiropractic Archives 3: 144–165.

Giles L G F 1984 Letter to the Editor. Spine 9: 842.

Giles L G F 1986 Lumbo-sacral and cervical zygapophysial joint inclusions. Man Med 2: 89–92.

Giles L G F 1989 Anatomical basis of low back pain. Williams & Wilkins, Baltimore.

Giles L G F 1997 Introductory graphic anatomy of the lumbosacral spine. In: Giles LGF, Singer KP (eds) Clinical anatomy and management of low back pain. Butterworth-Heinemann, Oxford, p 40.

Giles L G F 1999 Diagnosis of thoracic spine pain and contraindications to spinal mobilisation and manipulation. In: Giles LGF, Singer KP (eds) Clinical anatomy and management of thoracic spine pain. Butterworth-Heinemann, Oxford.

Giles L G F, Baker P G 1998 Introduction. In: Giles LGF, Singer KP (eds) Clinical anatomy and management of cervical spine pain. Butterworth-Heinemann, Oxford, p 15.

Giles L G F, Crawford C M 1997 Shadows of the truth in patients with spinal pain: A review. Canadian Journal of Psychiatry 42: 44–48.

Giles LGF, Taylor J R 1981 Low back pain associated with leg length inequality. Spine 6: 510–521.

Groen G J, Baljet B, Drukker J 1990 Nerves and nerve plexuses of the human vertebral column. American Journal of Anatomy 188: 282–296.

Gross D 1979 Multifactorial diagnosis and therapy for low back pain. In: Bonica JJ, et al (eds) Advances in pain research and therapy, Vol 3. Raven Press, New York, pp 671–683.

Hadley L A 1964 Anatomico-roentgenographic studies of the spine. Charles C. Thomas, Springfield, IL.

Haldeman S 1977 Why one cause of back pain? In: Buerger AA, Tobis TS (eds) Approaches to the validation of manipulation therapy. Charles C. Thomas, Springfield, IL, pp 187–197.

Haldeman S, Chapman-Smith D, Paterson D M 1993 Guidelines for chiropractic quality assurance and practice parameters. Aspen, Gaithersburg, pp 55–80.

Hardin J G, Halla J T 1995 Cervical spine and radicular pain syndromes. Current Opinion in Rheumatology 7: 136–140.

Henderson D, Chapman-Smith D, Mior S, et al 1994 Clinical guidelines for chiropractic practice in Canada. Journal of the Canadian Chiropractic Association (Suppl.) 38.

Hinkley H J, Drysdale I P 1995 Audit of 1000 patients attending the clinic of the British College of Naturopathy and Osteopathy. British Osteopathy Journal 16: 17–22.

Hoppenfeld S 1977 Orthopaedic neurology: A diagnostic guide to neurologic levels. JB Lippincott, Philadelphia.

Jackson R 1966 The cervical syndrome, 3rd edn. Charles C. Thomas, Springfield, IL.

Jackson R 1977 The cervical syndrome, 4th edn. Charles C. Thomas, Springfield, IL.

Jensen M D, Brant-Zawadzki M N, Obuchowski N, Modic M T, Malkasian D, Ross J S 1994 Magnetic resonance imaging of the lumbar spine in people without back pain. New England Journal of Medicine 331: 69–73.

Jinkins J R 1993 The pathoanatomic basis of somatic and autonomic syndromes originating in the lumbosacral spine. Neuroimaging Clinics of North America 3: 443–463.

Jinkins J R 1997 The pathoanatomic basis of somatic, autonomic and neurogenic syndromes originating in the lumbosacral spine. In: Giles LGF, Singer KP (eds) Clinical anatomy and management of low back pain. Butterworth-Heinemann, Oxford, pp 255–272.

Jinkins J R, Whittemore A R, Bradley W G 1989 The anatomic basis of vertebrogenic pain and the autonomic syndrome associated with lumbar disk extrusion. American Journal of Neuroradiology 10: 219–251, American Journal of Roentgenology 152: 1277–1289.

Karppinen J, Malmivaara A, Tervonen O, Paakko E, Kurunlahti M, Syrjaala P, Vasari P, Vanharanta H 2001 Severity of symptoms and signs in relation to magnetic resonance imaging findings among sciatic patients. Spine 26: E149–E154.

Keim H A, Kirkaldy-Willis W H 1987 Clinical symposia. Low back pain, Vol 39. Ciba-Geigy, Jersey.

Kenna C, Murtagh J 1989 Back pain and spinal manipulation. Butterworths, Sydney, pp 165, 166, 171, 173.

Kojima T, Oonishi I, Kurokawa T. Ossification of the ligamentum flavum in the thoracolumbar spine of young adults report of two cases. International Orthopaedics 1992; 16: 75–79.

Le-Breton C, Meziou M, Laredo J D 1993 Sarcomes pagetiques rechidiens. A propos de huit observations. Revue du Rhumatisme (ed Française) 60: 16–22.

Mackenzie I 1985 Spine, tenderness of. In: Hart FD (ed.) French's index of differential diagnosis, 12th edn. Butterworth & Co. Ltd, Oxford, p 788.

MacMillan J, Schaffer J L, Kambiry P 1991 Routes and incidence of communication of lumbar discs with surrounding neural structures. Spine 16: 167–171.

Macnab I 1977 Backache. Williams & Wilkins, Baltimore.

Main C J, Waddell G 1982 Chronic pain, distress and illness behaviour. In: Main CJ (ed.) Clinical psychology and medicine: a behavioural perspective. Plenum Publishing Corp., New York, pp 1–62.

Main C J, Waddell G 1998 Behavioural responses to examination. A reappraisal of the interpretation of 'nonorganic signs'. Spine 23: 2367–2371.

Marshall L L, Trethewie E R 1973 Chemical irritation of nerve root in disc prolapse. Lancet 2: 320.

Meade T W, Dyer S, Browne W, Townsend J, Frank A O 1990 Low back pain of mechanical origin: randomised comparison of chiropractic and hospital outpatient treatment. British Medical Journal 6737: 1431–1436.

Meade T M, Dyer S, Brown W, Frank A O 1995 Randomised comparison of chiropractic and hospital outpatient management for low back pain: results from extended follow up. British Medical Journal 7001: 349–350.

Mendelson G 1982 Not 'cured by a verdict'. Effect of a legal settlement on compensation claimants. Medical Journal of Australia 2: 219–230.

Merz B 1986 The honeymoon is over: Spinal surgeons begin to divorce themselves from chemonucleolysis. Journal of the American Medical Association 256: 317.

Michel B A, Lane N E, Jones H H, et al 1990 Plain radiographs can be used in estimating lumbar bone density. Journal of Rheumatology 17: 528–531.

Mixter W J, Ayer J B 1935 Herniation or rupture of the intervertebral disc into the spinal canal. New England Journal of Medicine 213: 385–393.

Moore K L 1992 Clinically Oriented Anatomy, 3rd edn. Williams & Wilkins, Baltimore.

Nachemson A L 1992 Newest knowledge of low back pain. A critical look. Clinical Orthopedics and Related Research 279: 8–20.

Osti O L, Fraser R D 1992 MRI and discography of annular tears and intervertebral disc degeneration. A prospective clinical comparison. Journal of Bone and Joint Surgery 74-B: 431–435.

Otan K, Aihara T, Tanaka A, Shibasaki K 1986 Ossification of the ligamentum flavum of the thoracic spine in adult kyphosis. International Orthopaedics 10: 135–139.

Pate D M, Jaeger S A 1996 Thoracic spine. In: Lawrence DJ (ed.) Advances in chiropractic, Vol 3: 111–145.

Patten J 1996 Neurological differential diagnosis, 2nd edn. Springer-Verlag, Berlin, p 282.

Pedersen P 1994 A survey of chiropractic practice in Europe. European Journal of Chiropractic 42: 3–28.

Perry W 1995 Measurement of bone density in osteoporosis (letter). British Medical Journal 311: 952.

Pfirrmann C W A, Metzdorf A, Zanetti M, Hodler J, Boos N 2001 Magnetic resonance classification of lumbar intervertebral disc degeneration. Spine 26: 1873–1878.

Pope M H, Novotny J E 1993 Spinal biomechanics. Journal of Biomechanical Engineering 115: 569–574.

Postacchini F, Gumina S 1999 Clinical features. In: Postacchini F (ed.) Lumbar disc herniation. Springer-Verlag, New York, p 207.

Radanov B P, Sturzenegger M, DeStefano G, Schindrig A 1994 A relationship between early somatic, radiological, cognitive and psychosocial findings and outcome during a one-year follow-up in 117 patients suffering from common whiplash. British Journal of Rheumatology 33: 442–448.

Rauschning W 1992 Spinal anatomy: the relationship of structures. In: Haldeman S (ed.) Principles and practice of chiropractic, 2nd edn. Appleton & Lange, Norwalk, pp 63–72.

Rickenbacher J, Landolt A M, Theiler K 1982 Applied anatomy of the back. Springer-Verlag, Berlin.

Schellhas K P, Smith M D, Gundry C R, Pollei S R 1996 Cervical discogenic pain. Prospective correlation of magnetic resonance imaging and discography in asymptomatic subjects and pain sufferers. Spine 21: 300–312.

Schiotz E H, Cyriax J 1975 Manipulation past and present. William Heinemann Medical Books, London.

Schmorl G, Junghanns H 1971 The human spine in health and disease, 2nd edn. Grune and Stratton, New York.

Schroeder S A, Tierney L M, McPhee S J, et al 1992 Current medical diagnosis and treatment. Appleton & Lange, Norwalk.

Shalen P R 1998 Radiological techniques for diagnosis of lumbar disc degeneration. SPINE: State of the Art Reviews 3: 27–48.

Shapiro R 1986 Current status of lumbar discography (letter). Radiology 159: 815.

Simons D G, Travell J 1983 Common myofascial origins of low back pain. Postgraduate Medicine 73: 55–108.

Skoven J S, Grasdal A L, Haldorsen E M H 2002 Relative cost-effectiveness of extensive and light multidisciplinary treatment programs versus treatment as usual for patients with chronic low back pain on long-term sick leave. Spine 27: 901–910.

Slipman C W, Plastaras C T, Palmitier R A, Huston C W, Sterenfeld E B 1998 Symptom provocation of fluoroscopically guided cervical nerve root stimulation. Are dynatomal maps identical to dermatomal maps? Spine 23(20): 2235–2242.

Spratt K F, Lehmann T R, Weinstein J N 1990 A new approach to the low-back physical examination. Behavioural assessment of mechanical signs. Spine 15: 96–102.

Stoddard A 1969 Manual of osteopathic practice. Hutchinson, London.

Sunderland S 1968 Nerves and nerve injuries. E.S. Livingstone, Edinburgh.

Sunderland S 1975 Anatomical perivertebral influences on the intervertebral foramen. In: Goldstein M (ed.) The research status of spinal manipulative therapy. US Department of Health, Education, and Welfare, Public Health Service, National Institutes of Health, National Institute of Neurological and Communicative Disorders and Stroke, Bethesda, Maryland. NINCDS Monograph No. 15, pp 129–140.

Teasell R W 1997 The denial of chronic pain. Pain Research Management 2: 89–91.

Travell J, Rinzler S H 1952 Myofascial genesis of pain. Postgraduate Medicine 11: 425–434.

Turner J A, LeResche L, Von Korff M, Ehrlich K 1998 Back pain in primary care. Patient characteristics, content of initial visit, and short-term outcomes. Spine 23: 463–469.

van Norel G J, Verhagen W I M 1996 Drop attacks and instability of the degenerate cervical spine. Journal of Bone and Joint Surgery 78B: 495–496.

van Oostenbrugge R J, Herpers M J, de Kruijk J R 1999 Spinal cord compression caused by unusual location and extension of ossified ligamenta flava in a caucasian male. Spine 24: 486–488.

Videman T, Leppavuori J, Kaprio J, Battie M C, Gibbons L E, Peltonen L, Koskenvue M 1998 Intragenic polymorphisms of the vitamin D receptor gene associated with intervertebral disc degeneration. Spine 23: 2477–2485.

Watts C, Dickhaus E 1986 Chemonucleolysis: A note of caution. Surgical Neurology 26: 236.

Weitz E M 1984 Paraplegia following chymopapain injection. Journal of Bone and Joint Surgery 66A: 1131.

White A A, Gordon S L 1982 Synopsis: workshop on idiopathic low back pain. Spine 7: 141–149.

White A A (III), Johnson R M, Panjabi M M, Southwick W O 1975 Biomechanical analysis of clinical stability in the cervical spine. Clinical Orthopaedics 109: 85–96.

Wiley J J, MacNab I, Wortzman G 1968 Lumbar discography and its clinical applications. Canadian Journal of Surgery 11: 280–289.

Wilkinson J L, 1986 Neuroanatomy of medical students. John Wright and Sons, Bristol, p 29.

Willen J H, Danielson B, Gaulitz A, Niklason T, Schonstrom N, Hansson T 1997 Dynamic effects on the lumbar spinal canal. Axially loaded CT-myelography and MRI in patients with sciatica and/or neurogenic claudication. Spine 22: 2968–2976.

Yochum T R, Barry M S 1996 Diagnostic imaging of the musculoskeletal system. In: Yochum TR, Rowe LJ (eds) Essentials of skeletal radiology, 2nd edn. Williams & Wilkins, Baltimore, pp 373–545.

Yonenobu K, Ebara S, Fujiwara K, et al 1987 Thoracic myelopathy secondary to ossification of the spinal ligament. Journal of Neurosurgery 66: 511–518.

Young A C 1967 Radiology and cervical spondylosis. In: Brain L, Wilkinson M (eds) Cervical spondylosis and other disorders of the cervical spine. William Heinemann, London, pp 133–196.

Lumbar spine cases

INTRODUCTION

Before presenting the low back pain cases it is important to consider the following summary of some possible causes of low back pain with or without radiculopathy (Table iii).

Table iii   Some possible causes of lumbar spine pain

Acute spinal pain
  Febrile disorders
  Injury

Chronic spinal pain

1. Traumatic, mechanical or degenerative
   Low back strain; fatigue, obesity; pregnancy causing
     altered biomechanics
   Injuries of bone, joint, intervertebral disc or ligaments
   Degenerative or traumatic changes of the spine
     (osteoarthrosis; spondylosis)
   Lumbar spine instability syndromes e.g. spondylolisthesis
   Scoliosis: primary and secondary
   Spinal or intervertebral canal stenosis
   Sacroiliac joint strain

2. Joint dysfunction
   Zygapophysial
   Intervertebral disc

3. Metabolic
   Osteoporosis
   Osteomalacia
   Hyper- and hypo-parathyroidism
   Ochronosis
   Fluorosis
   Hypophosphataemic rickets

4. Unknown causes
   Inflammatory arthropathies of the spine, such as
     ankylosing spondylitis and the spondylitis of Reiter's
     (Brodie's) disease, psoriasis, ulcerative colitis,
     Whipple's and Crohn's diseases
   Rarely polymyositis and polymyalgia rheumatica
   Paget's disease of bone
   Scheuermann's 'disease'

5. Infective conditions of bone, joint and theca of the spine
   Osteomyelitis
   Tuberculosis
   Melioidosis
   Undulant fever (abortus and melitensis)
   Typhoid and paratyphoid fever and other *Salmonella*
     infections
   Syphilis
   Yaws
   Very rarely Weil's disease (leptospirosis icterohaemorrhagica)
   Spinal pachymeningitis
   Chronic meningitis
   Subarachnoid or spinal abscess
   Herpes zoster
   Poliomyelitis
   Tetanus

continued

Table iii   Continued

6. Psychogenic
   Anxiety
   Depression
   Hysteria
   'Compensation neurosis'
   Malingering

7. Neoplastic – benign or malignant, primary or secondary
   Osteoid osteoma
   Eosinophilic granuloma
   Metastatic carcinomatosis
   Bronchial carcinoma
   Oesophageal carcinoma
   Sarcoma
   Myeloma
   Primary and secondary tumours of spinal canal and
     nerve roots: ependymoma; neurofibroma; glioma;
     angioma; meningioma; lipoma; rarely cordoma
   Reticuloses, e.g. Hodgkin's disease

8. Cardiac and vascular
   Subarachnoid or spinal haemorrhage
   Luetic or dissecting abdominal aorta aneurysm
   Enlarged aortic aneurysm
   Grossly enlarged left atrium in mitral valve disease

9. Gynaecological
   Tuberculous disease
   Rarely prolapse or retroversion of uterus
   Dysmenorrhoea
   Chronic salpingitis
   Pelvic abscess or chronic cervicitis
   Tumours

10. Gastrointestinal
    Pancreatitis
    Rarely appendicitis, or from new growth of intra-abdomi-
      nal viscus (colon, stomach, pancreas), or from retroperi-
      toneal strutures

11. Renal and genito-urinary
    Carcinoma of kidney
    Calculus
    Hydronephrosis
    Polycystic kidney
    Necrotizing papillitis
    Pyelitis and pyelonephritis
    Perinephric abscess
    Infection or new growth of prostate

12. Blood disorders
    Sickle-cell crises
    Acute haemolytic states

13. Drugs
    Corticosteroids
    Methysergide
    Compound analgesic tablets

14. Normality
    (Non-disease, i.e. 'mechanical' spinal pain)

Modified from Hart F D 1985 Back, pain in. In: Hart FD (ed.)
French's index of differential diagnosis 12th edn. Butterworth
& Co. Ltd, Oxford, pp 72–73.

PHYSICAL EXAMINATION

The physical examination should be orderly and systematic and should include the lumbar and pelvic examinations as indicated by the patient's presenting complaint(s) in Table iv.

Figure v represents the clinical features of the posterolateral lumbar intervertebral disc herniation and Figure vi the motor innervation of the lower limb; central disc herniation may cause spinal pain alone without radiculopathy (Postacchini & Gumina 1999) or lower limb involvement.

Table iv Some elements of the lumbar spine physical examination

Erect posture examination

Observe for
  Fluidity of movement
  Body build
  Skin markings – café-au-lait spots,
    lipomata & hairy patches often denote
    underlying neurologic or bone pathology
  Posture
  Deformities
  Pelvic obliquity
  Spine alignment

Sacroiliac joint
  Examine for joint motion or joint pain

Test spinal column motion, with caution, for
  Flexion
  Extension
  Side bending
  Rotation

Palpate for
  Iliac crest levels
  Anterior and posterior superior iliac spine levels
  Any break in contour of spinous processes
    (spondylolisthesis)
  Muscle spasm
  Myofascial trigger points
  Supraspinous and interspinous ligament tenderness
  Adjacent muscle tenderness
  Sciatic nerve tenderness
  Posterior aspect of coccyx
  Relative motion between adjacent vertebrae (by motion
    palpation) in an attempt to find restricted movement

Observe gait
  Walking on heels (tests foot and great toe dorsiflexion)
  Walking on toes (tests calf muscles)

Seated

Neurological tests
  Ankle jerk
  Knee jerk
  Plantar response (Babinski test*)
  Pinprick sensation of lower limbs
  Vibration sensation

Slump test
Slump test plus straight leg raising
Thigh/calf circumference measurement bilaterally

Supine

Straight leg raising
Flex thigh on pelvis then extend knee with foot dorsiflexed
  (sciatic nerve stretch)
Hoover test*
Kernig test (spinal cord stretch)*

Tests to increase intrathecal pressure
  Milgram test*
  Naffziger test*
  Valsalva manoeuvre*

Sacroiliac joint
  Compression test
  Pelvic rock test
  Gaenslen's sign*

Hip joint
  Fabere/Patrick test*
  Hip flexion, internal and external rotation

Palpate abdomen
Palpate for peripheral pulses and skin temperature
Palpate for flattening of lumbar lordosis during straight leg
  raising
Measure leg lengths (anterior superior iliac spine to medial
  malleolus) for a very *approximate* clinical impression of
  leg lengths
Test sensation and motor power
Listen for bruit (abdominal and inguinal)

Prone

Palpate
  Sciatic nerve between ischial tuberosity and greater trochanter
  Ischial bursa
  Cluneal nerves crossing the iliac crest for local tenderness

Palpate trochanteric bursa
Spine extension
  Femur extension test for hip extension

*See abbreviations and definitions chapter.
Adapted from Hoppenfeld 1976, Mackenzie 1985, Keim & Kirkaldy-Willis 1987.

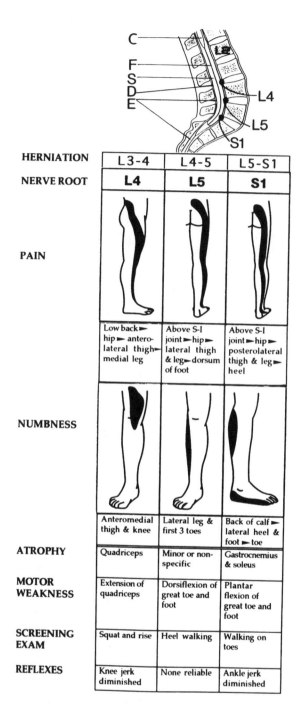

HERNIATION	L3-4	L4-5	L5-S1
NERVE ROOT	**L4**	**L5**	**S1**
PAIN			
	Low back ► hip ► antero-lateral thigh► medial leg	Above S-I joint ► hip ► lateral thigh & leg►dorsum of foot	Above S-I joint ► hip ► posterolateral thigh & leg ► heel
NUMBNESS			
	Anteromedial thigh & knee	Lateral leg & first 3 toes	Back of calf ► lateral heel & foot ► toe
ATROPHY	Quadriceps	Minor or non-specific	Gastrocnemius & soleus
MOTOR WEAKNESS	Extension of quadriceps	Dorsiflexion of great toe and foot	Plantar flexion of great toe and foot
SCREENING EXAM	Squat and rise	Heel walking	Walking on toes
REFLEXES	Knee jerk diminished	None reliable	Ankle jerk diminished

Figure v   Anatomy and clinical features of a posterolateral lumbar intervertebral disc herniation. C = conus medularis; D = dural tube; E = epidural space; F = filum terminale; S = subarachnoid space. (Modified from Wilkinson J L 1986 Neuroanatomy for medical students. John Wright and Sons, Bristol, p. 46; Keim & Kirkaldy-Willis (1987); Bigos S, Bowyer O, Braen G et al 1994 Acute low back problems in adults. Practice guideline, Quick Reference Guide Number 14. US Department of Health and Human Services, Public Health Service, Agency for Health Care Policy and Research, Rockville, MD, AHCPT Pub. No. 95-0643.)

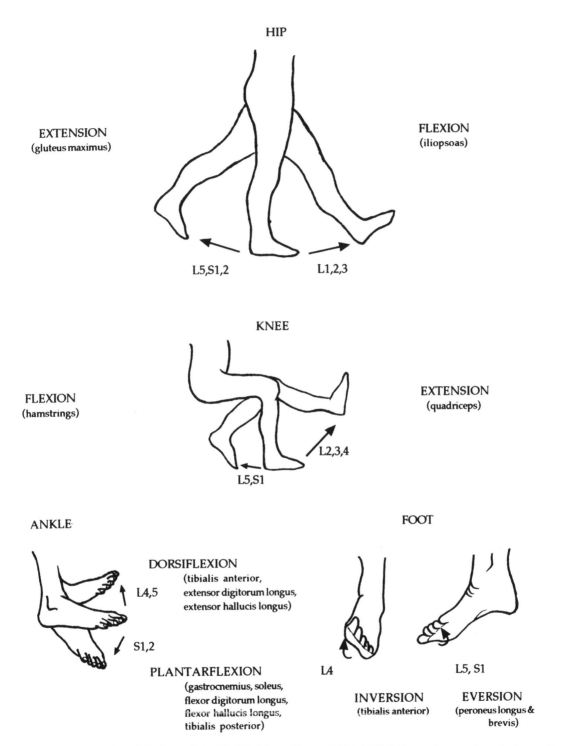

HIP

EXTENSION
(gluteus maximus)

FLEXION
(iliopsoas)

L5,S1,2   L1,2,3

KNEE

FLEXION
(hamstrings)

EXTENSION
(quadriceps)

L2,3,4

L5,S1

ANKLE

FOOT

DORSIFLEXION
(tibialis anterior,
extensor digitorum longus,
extensor hallucis longus)

L4,5

S1,2

PLANTARFLEXION
(gastrocnemius, soleus,
flexor digitorum longus,
flexor hallucis longus,
tibialis posterior)

L4

L5, S1

INVERSION
(tibialis anterior)

EVERSION
(peroneus longus &
brevis)

Figure vi Motor innervation of the lower limb. (Modified from: Hoppenfeld S 1977 Orthopaedic neurology. A diagnostic guide to neurologic levels. JB Lippincott, Philadelphia; Keim & Kirkaldy-Willis (1987); Moore KL 1992 Clinically Oriented Anatomy, 3rd edn. Williams & Wilkins, Baltimore.)

REFERENCES

Bigos S, Bowyer O, Braen G et al 1994 Acute low back problems in adults. Practice Guideline, Quick Reference Guide Number 14. US Department of Health and Human Services, Public Health Service, Agency for Health Care Policy and Research, Rockville, MD, AHCPT Pub. No. 95-0643.

Hart F D 1985 Back, pain in. In: Hart F D (ed) French's index of differential diagnosis. 12th edn. Butterworth & Co. Ltd, Oxford, pp 72–73.

Hoppenfeld S 1976 Physical examination of the spine and extremities. Appleton-Century-Crofts, New York.

Hoppenfeld S 1977 Orthopaedic neurology. A diagnostic guide to neurologic levels. J.B. Lippincott, Philadelphia.

Keim H A, Kirkaldy-Willis W H 1987 Low back pain. Clinical Symposia 39: 18.

Mackenzie I 1985 Spine, tenderness of. In: Hart FD (ed.) French's index of differential diagnosis, 12th edn. Butterworth & Co. Ltd, Oxford, p 788.

Moore K L 1992 Clinically Oriented Anatomy, 3rd edn. Williams and Wilkins, Baltimore.

Postacchini F, Gumina S 1999 Clinical features. In: Postacchini F (ed.) Lumbar disc herniation. Springer, New York, pp 207.

Wilkinson J L 1986 Neuroanatomy for medical students. John Wright and Sons, Bristol, p 46.

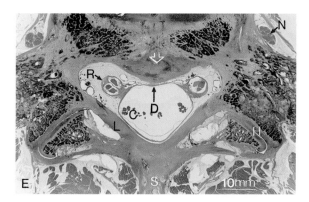

Figure 1.2 (E)

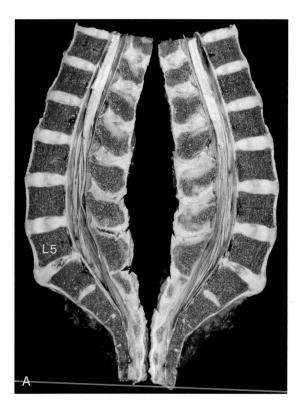

Figure 11.3 (A)

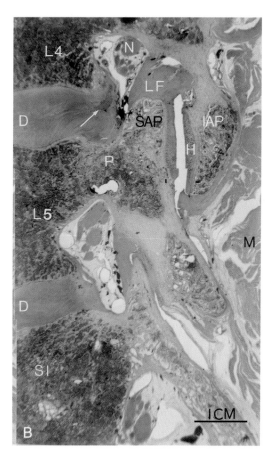

Figure 11.3 (B)

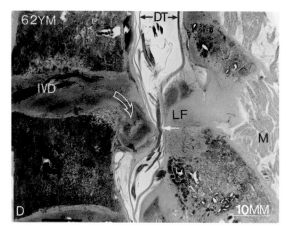

Figure 14.2 (D)

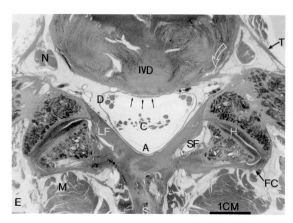

Figure 22.3

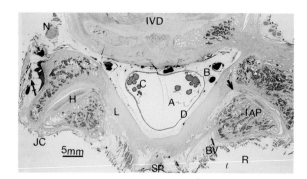

Figure 25.4

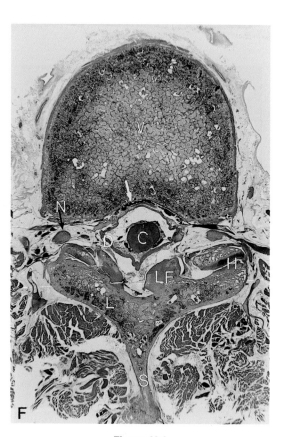

Figure 40.3

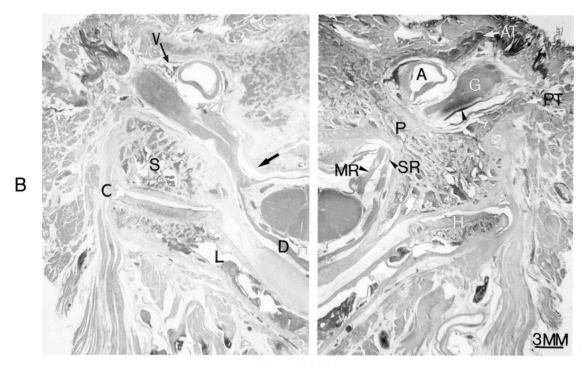

B

Figure 27.4 (B)

Case 1   Intervertebral disc protrusion

COMMENT
Lumbosacral disc thinning and retrolisthesis of
L5 on S1 is indicative of disc bulge or prolapse.

PROFILE

A 31-year-old man who worked in a manual
capacity who is a non-smoker and only drinks
alcohol socially.

PAST HISTORY

He had not experienced any unusual childhood
illnesses or unusual adult illnesses. He said he had
not had any significant falls and had never been
unconscious. He had no surgical history. The first
episode of low back pain that he ever experienced
occurred about 10 years ago and was 'minor'; it
lasted for approximately 7 days. That low back
pain resulted from helping his father to lift a 'not
too heavy' box from the back of a panel van. His
father was a masseur so gave him massage
treatment over 2–3 days; he became asymptomatic
within 7 days and went back to work without any
low back pain. He said he subsequently passed a
pre-employment medical examination before
starting to work as a carpenter.

PRESENTING COMPLAINT (Fig. 1.1)

He presented with constant low back pain that
radiates to the left or right upper buttock region.
At times, the pain radiates to the left buttock
then to the thigh and calf posteriorly and he
experiences a 'tingling' sensation in the left heel.
Sometimes, but less frequently, he experiences
pain radiating into the posterior aspect of the
right thigh as far as the knee. After driving the
car for approximately 1 hour the anterolateral
part of his left thigh develops an 'aching pain'.
There is no night pain. He awakens once or twice
each night due to low back pain when he
changes position. Coughing and sneezing do not
aggravate his low back or leg pain although these
actions did so when he injured his low back

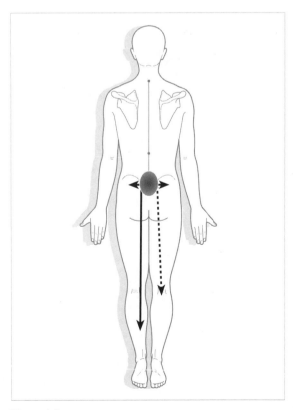

Figure 1.1

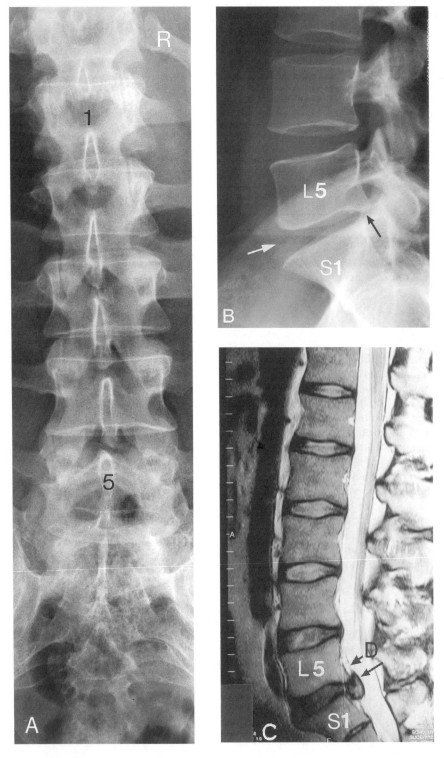

Figure 1.2 Caption is on next page.

10 months ago. Sometimes the pain radiates up the right side of the lumbar spine and he experiences an increase in low back pain on trying to walk up stairs. Arising from the seated position aggravates his low back pain; he finds it difficult to straighten his low back after bending forward.

Non-steroidal anti-inflammatory drug (NSAID) medication and physiotherapy have not helped and no imaging had been performed. He had seen an orthopaedic specialist whose opinion was: '(1) False rotation gave equal pain as true rotation. (2) There were inappropriate signs and symptoms. (3) The best form of treatment would be for this man to resume his normal activities in the work force'.

AETIOLOGY

Ten months ago he lifted heavy and awkward shaped boxes that caused a gradual onset of low back pain at that time and, by next morning, his low back was 'extremely painful'.

EXAMINATION

In the erect posture, there was no obvious pelvic obliquity from a clinical point of view, nor was there any obvious scoliosis. Percussion of the spine elicited some low back pain (L4–S1 level). Deep palpation of the paraspinal muscles elicited pain at the L5–S1 level. Testing the sacroiliac joints in the erect posture did not

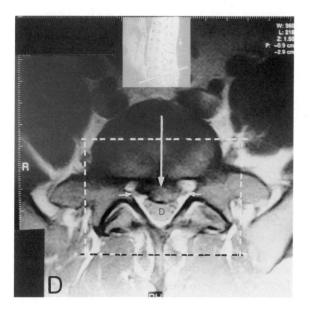

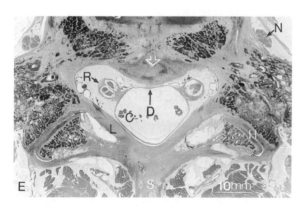

Figure 1.2 (A) Anteroposterior (A-P) pelvis and lumbar spine plain X-ray view (cropped and viewed from posterior to anterior). 1 = first lumbar vertebra, 5 = spinous process of fifth lumbar vertebra; R = right side of patient. (B) Lateral lumbosacral spine plain X-ray. Note the L5–S1 disc height thinning (white arrow) as compared to the L4–5 disc space height above. Also, note the retrolisthesis (black arrow) of L5 on S1. L5 = fifth lumbar vertebra. S1 = first sacral segment. (C) Lateral T2 weighted MRI scan showing the lumbosacral spine. S1 = first sacral segment. The posterior disc protrusion at the L5–S1 level is shown by the black arrow; it can be seen compressing the anterior part of the dural tube (D) (thecal sac). Note that the disc is becoming 'black' between L5 and S1 which indicates that it is undergoing dehydration (desiccation) as a result of injury. The L4–5 disc shows some early desiccation with essentially normal disc hydration at the levels above. (D) Axial T2-weighted MRI scan at the lumbosacral level. The arrow shows the degree of disc protrusion and the effect that it is having on the pain sensitive anterior part of the dural tube (D) and, to some extent, on the S1 nerve roots (small white arrows). R = right side of patient. The rectangle shows the approximate area shown in (E). (E) A 200-micron thick histological section from a cadaver with a similar, but less extensive, disc protrusion; this is to orientate the reader to the various anatomical structures. The histological section is represented approximately by the area within the rectangle on (D). R = right nerve roots budding off from the dural tube (D) containing small nerve roots from the cauda equina (C). H = hyaline articular cartilage on the zygapophysial joint facet surfaces. L = ligamentum flavum; N = spinal nerve; S = spinous process. Open arrow head = intervertebral disc protrusion. (Erhlich's haematoxeylin and light green counterstain.) See also colour plate section.

cause any sacroiliac joint pain but he did feel pain on the left of the L5 vertebra. Toe walking power (S1) was normal as was heel walking power (L5), although the latter caused some sciatica to extend into the left calf from the buttock.

The deep reflexes in the upper and lower extremities were normal. Pinprick sensation of the lower extremities was normal apart from hypoaesthesia along the lateral side (S1) of each foot and below the heels (S1). Vibration sensation at the ankles was normal.

In the seated and slumped forward position, there was low back pain, and the addition of left straight leg raising (SLR) caused an increase in low back and left leg pain posteriorly at a measured 45° elevation. Right SLR to 55° caused similar low back pain.

Lumbar spine active ranges of movement were as shown below:

1. Flexion – with cautious movement his out-stretched fingers were able to go two-thirds of the way down his shins; further movement was then limited by increasing low back pain. He had difficulty in straightening his spine due to an increase in low back pain.
2. Extension was limited by approximately 10% due to low back pain.
3. Left rotation was limited by approximately 10% due to pain on the left side of the lumbosacral joint.
4. Right rotation was limited by approximately 10% due to pain on the right side of the lumbosacral joint.
5. Left lateral bending – his fingers were able to reach approximately 2 cm below his knee before limitation due to low back pain.
6. Right lateral bending – his fingers reached to approximately 10 cm below the right knee before limitation due to low back pain.

Power in the lower limbs was normal, as was the case with the foot pulses. On palpation the foot temperature appeared equal bilaterally. The circumference of the calf, 14 cm below the patella, was 40 cm bilaterally. The Milgram active bilateral SLR caused low back pain at approximately 30° elevation of the legs from the examination table. Supine SLR was limited to a measured 60° (right) due to right leg pain posteriorly, and 65° (left) due to left thigh and calf pain posteriorly. Left SLR plus foot dorsiflexion caused an increase in low back pain and left sciatica; right SLR plus foot dorsiflexion did not cause any additional pain. The Lasegue sign for the left side caused low back and left leg pain and the right side caused slight right leg pain. Bilateral hip flexion caused a significant increase in low back pain at approximately 110° elevation of the thighs from the examination table.

There were no physical signs of malingering. For example, there was no positive Hoover's sign. In addition, false rotation of the pelvis did not elicit any pain. Although left straight leg raising with foot dorsiflexion was painful, straight leg raising with plantar flexion of the foot was reported as not aggravating his low back pain or left leg sciatica.

IMAGING REVIEW

An imaging review was not possible, as no imaging had been performed.

CLINICAL IMPRESSION

A central L5–S1 disc prolapse.

WHAT ACTION SHOULD BE TAKEN?

Erect posture lumbar spine and pelvis plain film radiographs were performed. The radiologist noted that 'there is narrowing of the L5–S1 disc space' (Fig. 1.2A). In addition, note that there is a retrolisthesis of L5 on S1 due to the disc narrowing which is secondary to disc prolapse at L5–S1. A lumbar spine MRI scan confirmed 'a central L5–S1 disc protrusion indenting the thecal sac anteriorly and abutting the proximal descending nerve roots. There is some narrowing of both L5 neural foraminae due to a combination of reduction in disc height and some bulging disc material extending into the inferior portion of both L5 neural foraminae'.

TREATMENT

Following the case history, examination, plain film and MRI studies (Fig. 1.2), the patient was told what was causing his low back pain syndrome. He was grateful that his problem had been diagnosed and that he had not been arbitrarily dismissed as a malingerer. He decided to take a conservative treatment approach now that he fully understood his condition and he decided to perform light work only and said he would manage on analgesics as required. He would only contemplate surgery if his condition became intolerable.

RESULTS

This man managed to cope reasonably well on light duties and occasional analgesics in spite of his disability and impairment.

Key point

Retrolisthesis at L5–S1 is indicative of L5–S1 intervertebral disc prolapse.

FURTHER READING

Giles L G F 2000 Mechanisms of neurovascular compression within the spinal and intervertebral canals. Journal of Manipulative and Physiological Therapeutics 23: 107–111.
Postacchini F, Cinotti G 1999 Spinal fusion and disc prosthesis at primary surgery. In: Postacchini F (ed.) Lumbar disc herniation. Springer-Verlag, New York, pp 521–538.

Case 2   Carcinoma of the pancreas

COMMENT
Always listen to the patient!

PROFILE

A 57-year-old married woman who smokes cigarettes but does not drink alcohol was referred by her medical practitioner for evaluation and treatment.

PAST HISTORY

There is nothing relevant in her past history.

PRESENTING COMPLAINT (Fig. 2.1)

Constant mild to severe low back pain of 1 year duration for which she had seen several general medical practitioners. When the low back pain is severe, it sometimes radiates upwards to the mid-thoracic spine and her legs 'feel weak'. She required two analgesic injections in the week prior to consultation as the low back pain was so severe. There is no night pain other than the constant low back pain.

Physiotherapy treatment provided limited help and a NSAID was of no help, but caused constipation. She then used another NSAID as required; this eased the pain but caused gastric upsets, therefore, she ceased that medication. She takes four to six Panadol tablets per day. She is post-menopausal and experiences some 'sweating' or 'cold spells' and, though there was some minor weight loss, a pelvic examination and pap smear test 9 months before this consultation were normal.

She had been referred to a psychologist because 'there are certainly many psychosocial issues exacerbating this lady's pain'. She said: 'I am told the low back pain is in my head – but it is not!'

AETIOLOGY

Unknown, but she periodically lifts approximately 35 kg weights at work.

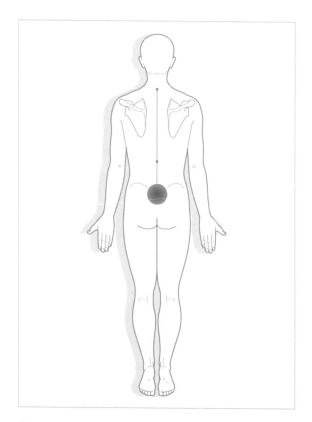

Figure 2.1

EXAMINATION

On examination, deep palpation of the lumbar paraspinal muscles indicated that she was tender over the entire lumbar spine. Active lumbar spine flexion, extension and rotation aggravated her low back pain. Supine SLR was to 90° bilaterally and painless, indicating no nerve root impingement. Muscle power was normal. The deep tendon reflexes at the knees and ankles were normal, as was the case with pinprick sensation of the lower limbs.

IMAGING REVIEW

Plain lumbosacral spine radiographs showed some thinning of the L3–4 disc space with some anterior lipping at the disc–vertebral body margins. The left and right oblique view films showed some osteoarthrotic changes of the L4–5 and L5–S1 zygapophysial joint facets. A lumbar spine CT scan performed from L3 to S1 levels did not show any spinal canal lesions. An ultrasound scan of the pelvis and abdomen showed three haemangiomas on the liver.

CLINICAL IMPRESSION

Referred pain from a visceral organ as she was neurologically intact and supine SLR was to 90° bilaterally and painless and the CT lumbar spine scan did not show any spinal lesions. In addition, the ultrasound scan had shown what appeared to be haemagiomas on the liver. The unexplained minor weight loss was of concern while the 'sweating' and 'cold spells' suggested sympathetic nervous system involvement.

WHAT ACTION SHOULD BE TAKEN?

A bone scan was ordered but the result was normal. Numerous laboratory tests were performed, as shown in Boxes 2.1 and 2.2.

In view of the slightly elevated C-reactive protein and ESR, a CT scan of the upper abdomen was performed with oral contrast and with and without intravenous contrast using a spiral technique. This showed a 5-cm pancreatic tail

carcinoma encasing adjacent arteries and veins (Fig. 2.2E).

TREATMENT

When the patient was told of her condition she sadly said 'so it is not in my head!'

Box 2.1 Chemical pathology

		Units	Reference range
Sodium	140	mmol/l	(135–145)
Potassium	3.7	mmol/l	(3.2–4.5)
Chloride	107	mmol/l	(100–110)
Bicarbonate	24	mmol/l	(22–33)
Anion gap	9	mmol/l	(8–17)
Urea	4.7	mmol/l	(3.0–8.0)
Creatinine	0.07	mmol/l	(0.05–0.10)
AST (Aspartate aminotransferase)	19	U/l	(<35)
Protein (total)	70	g/l	(62–83)
Albumin	43	g/l	(33–47)
Globulin	27	g/l	
ALP (alkaline phosphatase)	80	U/l	(40–120)
Gamma GT	22	U/l	(<50)
ALT (alanine aminotransferase)	8	U/l	(<40)
Bilirubin (total)	14	μmol/l	(<20)
C-reactive protein	**14**	mg/l	(<6)
Tumour marker (carcinoembryonic antigen)	3.7	μg/l	(<5)

Box 2.2 Haematology

		Units	Reference range
Haemoglobin	135	g/l	(115–160)
White cell count	6.9	×10⁹/l	(4.0–11.0)
Platelets	216	×10⁹/l	(140–400)
Haematocrit	0.41		(0.39–0.52)
Red cell count	4.63	×10¹²/l	(3.80–5.20)
MCV (mean corpuscular volume)	88.1	fl	(80.0–98.0)
Neutrophils	3.6	×10⁹/l	(2.0–8.0)
Lymphocytes	2.6	×10⁹/l	(1.0–4.0)
Monocytes	0.5	×10⁹/l	(0.1–0.8)
Eosinophils	0.1	×10⁹/l	(<0.2)
Basophils	0.0	×10⁹/l	(<0.2)
ESR (erythrocyte sedimentation rate)	**23**	mm/hr	(<15)

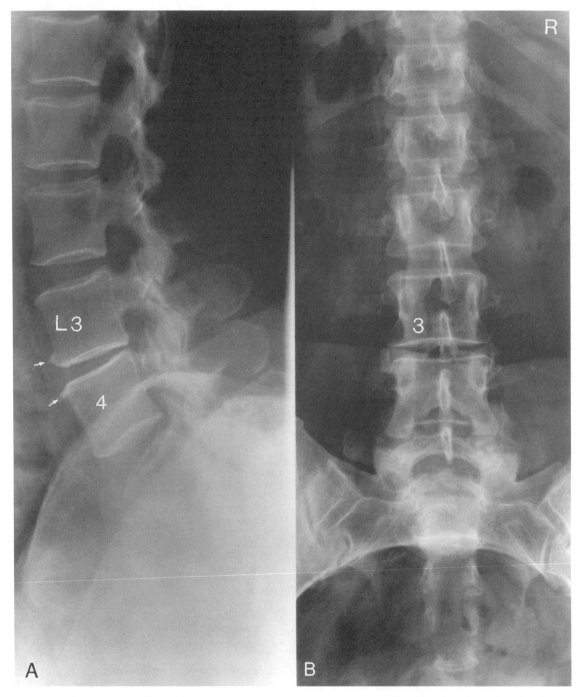

Figure 2.2 The plain X-ray films (A, B, C and D) were taken in the erect posture. The lateral lumbar spine view (A) shows disc thinning at the L3–4 level with anterior lipping (small white arrows) of the vertebral bodies adjacent to the intervertebral disc space. (C) and (D) represent the right and left oblique views and show zygapophysial joint facet early osteoarthrosis (black arrows) at the L5–S1 level with some imbrication (subluxation) of the opposing facet surfaces at the L3–4, L4–5 and L5–S1 levels. (R = right side of patient.)

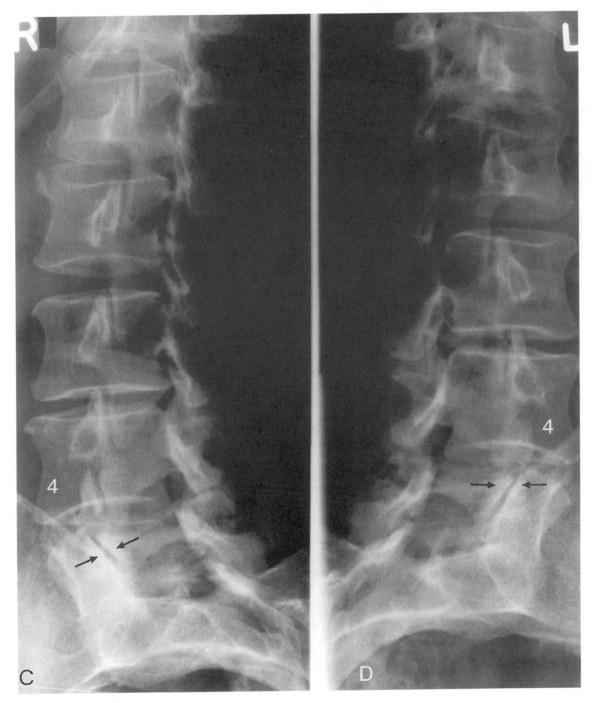

Figure 2.2   Continued.

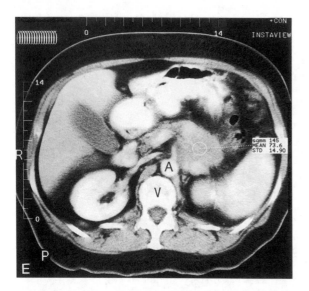

Figure 2.2   (E) An axial (horizontal) CT scan slice through the upper abdomen, with contrast, showing the pancreatic tumour (with a circle placed over part of it), the adjacent proximal aorta (A) and vertebral body (V). (R = right side of patient.)

The patient underwent surgical removal of the main tumour and she received good symptomatic benefit from coeliac plexus blocks. This, in combination with MS Contin and paracetamol, resulted in her pain being 'very slight', although she became constipated and required lactulose for this problem.

RESULT

It is interesting to note that the tumour marker, carcinoembryonic antigen did not reach the positive range (5.1) until approximately 3 months after the diagnosis was made; she passed away one month after this test became positive.

Key point(s)
1. The patient's low back pain was remote from the serious pathology. 2. The tumour maker test was normal until approximately 3 months after the diagnosis was made and did not reveal a serious tumour. 3. The combination of somewhat elevated CRP and ESR confirmed the presence of an inflammatory process but, of course, did not define the pathology involved. 4. Always take spinal pain patients seriously and never consider them to be malingerers unless you are sure of your facts.

FURTHER READING

Arslan A, Buanes T, Geitung J T 2001 Pancreatic carcinoma: MR, MR angiography and dynamic helical CT in the evaluation of vascular invasion. European Journal of Radiology 38: 151–159.

Kuzucu M K 2001 Imaging of pancreatic disease. European Journal of Radiology 38: 77.

Lankisch P G, DiMagno E P 1999 Pancreatic disease. State of the art and future aspects of research. Springer-Verlag, New York.

Lindblom A, Liljegren A 2000 Tumour markers in malignancies. British Medical Journal 320: 424–427.

Case 3   Seropositive inflammatory arthropathy

COMMENT
Always look at the imaging films and never rely only on the imaging report.

PROFILE

A 44-year-old man who kept fit by going to the gymnasium and running regularly.

PAST HISTORY

His history included psoriasis and he recalled that his maternal grandmother had rheumatoid arthritis and that his mother had some form of mild arthritis.

PRESENTING COMPLAINT (Fig. 3.1)

Low back pain of about 5 years duration that he said was worse in the cold weather and if he slept on a soft mattress. Sometimes he had severe low back pain, although he is usually free of pain. Occasionally, running caused slight low back pain but he preferred to keep fit, so kept on running. Lifting reasonably heavy items did not cause an increase in low back pain. There was no night pain. During the 2 weeks prior to his consultation the pain had been noticeable on a daily basis but a diagnosis had not been made.

AETIOLOGY

Unknown.

EXAMINATION

The physical examination showed that reflexes, tone, power, and sensation were normal. Lumbar spine ranges of movement appeared to be normal and there was no evidence of nerve root tension on SLR.

IMAGING REVIEW

An imaging review was not possible, as no imaging had been performed.

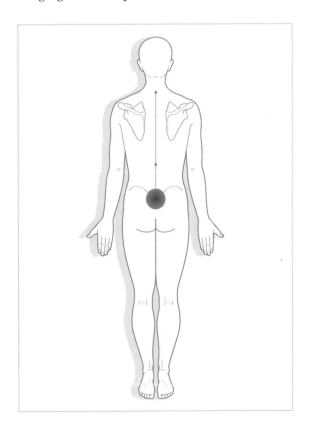

Figure 3.1

CLINICAL IMPRESSION

The history suggested a probable rheumatological condition.

WHAT ACTION SHOULD BE TAKEN?

Plain lumbar and pelvis X-ray films and appropriate laboratory tests. The plain film X-ray

examination performed (Fig. 3.2) was reported as showing 'degenerative marginal osteophytes at all lumbar levels, especially at L2–3. The sacroiliac joints appear normal. There is a minimal lumbar scoliosis'.

However, the thin bridging osteophytes, particularly at the anterior margins of the L2–3 intervertebral disc, with adjacent sclerotic changes anteriorly adjacent to the intervertebral

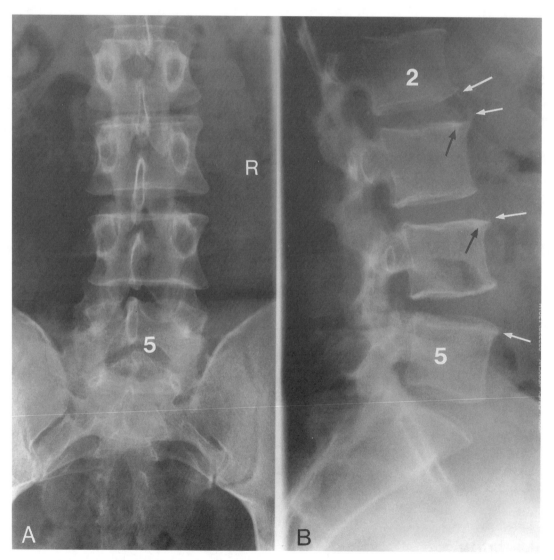

Figure 3.2 (A) Erect antero-posterior pelvis and lumbar spine plain X-ray image (cropped). Note the minimal lumbar scoliosis and the apparently normal sacroiliac joints. 5 = fifth lumbar vertebra; R = right side of patient. (B) Lateral lumbosacral plain X-ray image. Note the early thin bridging osteophytes, particularly at the anterior margins of the L2–3 intervertebral disc space (white arrows), with adjacent sclerotic changes in the intervertebral body endplates anteriorly (black arrows). 2 and 5 represent the second and fifth lumbar vertebrae, respectively.

disc space, suggested an arthritic process. Therefore, some haematology and serology laboratory tests were performed; the full blood count, ESR (3 mm/hr; range 2–15), and C-reactive protein (1 mg/l; range <6) were normal. Anti-nuclear serum antibodies were negative as was the HLA B27. However, the rheumatoid factor was 274 IU/ml (normal range <30). Therefore, a diagnosis of seropositive inflammatory arthropathy was made.

TREATMENT

The patient was given a NSAID to be used only as necessary; this proved to be very helpful and he was referred to a rheumatologist for further management.

RESULT

He made excellent progress, and he was able to keep up his gymnasium activities and running so as to keep fit.

Key point(s)

1. Always look at the imaging films.
2. Laboratory tests have their limitations, as shown in this case with respect to the ESR and the CRP as indicators of inflammation; these are not infallible markers of inflammation. However, based on a thorough history, clinical examination and imaging findings a clue as to which tests should be performed is possible.

FURTHER READING

Axford J S 1996 Rheumatic disease. In Axford J (ed.) Medicine. Blackwell Science, Oxford.
Weinstein J N, Rydevik B J, Sonntag V K H 1995 Essentials of the spine. Raven Press, New York.
Yochum T R, Rowe L J 1996 Essentials of skeletal radiology, 2nd edn. Williams & Wilkins, Baltimore.

Case 4   Sacroiliac joint dysfunction

COMMENT
Clinicians treating low back pain syndromes
should be appropriately trained in the diagnosis
and management of such conditions.

PROFILE

A 25-year-old married woman with three young
children was referred by her general medical
practitioner for evaluation and treatment.

PAST HISTORY

Her surgical history was that of an appendectomy
7 years ago and two caesarean sections; otherwise
she had been healthy.

PRESENTING COMPLAINT (Fig. 4.1)

Constant chronic low back pain that is central to
right sided, including the sacroiliac joint. This
pain radiates into the right buttock, the right leg
posteriorly and into the sole of the right foot.
The pain prevents her from playing with her
young children and undertaking normal home
duties because of constant aggravation of the
chronic low back pain syndrome. She said her
appetite is reduced and that she has inexplicably
lost 5 kg in weight during the last few weeks.
Domestic relations are becoming strained
because she feels her husband is 'sick and tired
of my pain' and he asks 'why can't doctors fix
it?'. At presentation she was tearful and anxious.
She moved slowly and stiffly.

Extensive neurological investigations had
apparently found no organic cause for the
'intolerable pain'. She was taking oxycontin
(20 mg, 1–2 per day) and endep (150 mg at night).
She had tried various NSAIDs, paracetamol,
diazepam, and pethidine injections without
relief.

She sleeps with a pillow between her knees in
an attempt to get some relief from the right-
sided low back pain. There is no night pain other
than her constant right-sided low back pain.

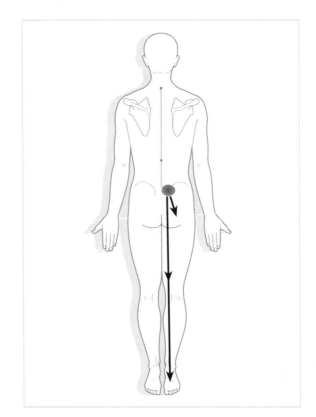

Figure 4.1

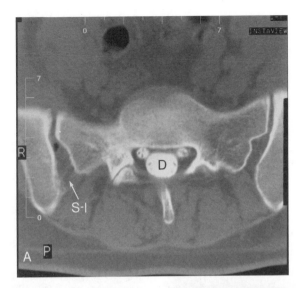

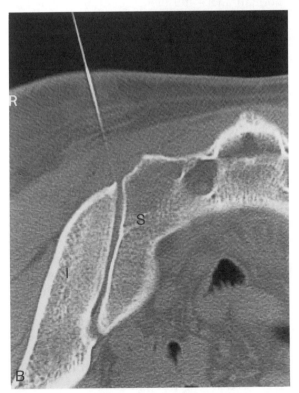

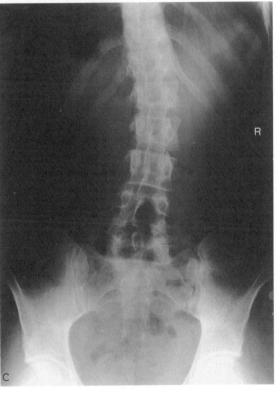

Figure 4.2   (A) A CT myelogram axial view through the lower region of the lumbosacral zyapophyseal joints and through the corresponding sacroiliac joint (SI) level which is above the synovial part of the sacroiliac joint. D = dural tube containing contrast material and some cauda equina nerve roots (grey dots) with adjacent nerve roots in the dural sleeve on the left and right sides, respectively. (B) A CT view of the right sacroiliac joint showing needle placement for injection of the joint. I = ilium; S = sacrum. (C) Erect posture anteroposterior plain X-ray view (viewed from behind) showing the sacroiliac joints and the mild idiopathic scoliosis of the lumbar spine. R = patient's right side.

Coughing and sneezing cause an increase in the low back pain.

She had been investigated with a CT myelogram (Fig. 4.2A) and a lumbar MRI study. A steroid and anaesthetic injection into the right sacroiliac joint had not provided any benefit (Fig. 4.2B).

She was dismayed at having been told that the pain was 'psychological' and her husband was distressed by her pain and incapacity.

AETIOLOGY

She fell 4 years ago onto her right buttock in particular and this caused her central to right-sided low back pain syndrome.

EXAMINATION

In the erect posture there was some clinical evidence of an idiopathic lumbar scoliosis, convex to the right side. Toe walking (S1) and heel walking (L5) power were normal. Erect posture straining of the left and right sacroiliac joints, respectively, caused a significant increase in right sacroiliac joint pain. Active lumbar spine ranges of movement were all limited due to significant pain on the right side of the lumbosacral joint and over the right sacroiliac joint. The deep reflexes at the knees and ankles were normal. Pinprick sensation of the lower extremities was normal, as was vibration sensation. Sitting in the slumped forward position aggravated the pain on the right of L5–S1 and over the right sacroiliac joint; the addition of right straight leg raising caused an aggravation of this pain. Supine SLR on the right was limited to approximately 25° elevation due to similar pain. The Valsalva manoeuvre caused a significant increase in her pain.

IMAGING REVIEW

Supine plain film radiographs showed a minor right convex thoracolumbar junction scoliosis. The CT lower lumbar myelogram and the lumbar spine MRI were normal.

CLINICAL IMPRESSION

Chronic right sacroiliac joint strain/subluxation in view of the history and normal neurology, in spite of the positive SLR on the right side.

WHAT ACTION SHOULD BE TAKEN?

An erect posture pelvis and lumbar spine radiograph (Fig. 4.2C) was taken to evaluate the degree of idiopathic scoliosis and to complement existing supine radiographs. Although the diagnosis of sacroiliac joint strain was made, because of the history of the right sacroiliac joint injection having not provided any relief and because her condition was so acute, it was considered prudent to perform a bone scan (reported as normal) and a full blood count as well as ESR and C-reactive protein tests; all the results were within normal limits.

TREATMENT

It was considered safe to manipulate the sacroiliac joint, although she found it intolerably painful to be positioned for the manipulation. In spite of her pain, the sacroiliac joint moved easily and an audible 'release' was heard. The patient found the manipulation to be very painful but said she felt better on getting off the manipulating table. She was advised to speak to her referring family doctor about stopping all narcotics but advised to continue with the NSAIDs until her re-assessment. She was told not to lift the young children or perform any housework or shopping before returning for a re-assessment 3 days later.

RESULTS

At the following visit 3 days later it was gratifying to see the cheerful 'grin' on her face and she stated that she was very much better. A follow-up manipulation resulted in a slight audible 'release' and she was advised to return if her symptoms persisted. Both she and her husband were delighted at the result. The patient's husband asked why several specialists to whom she had been referred had suggested her symptoms were in her head and stated that this had almost wrecked their marriage.

The patient did stop taking oxycontin and endep medication following the first sacroiliac joint manipulation.

This case is a good example of multidisciplinary co-operation leading to a satisfactory outcome for the patient.

The patient returned voluntarily 1 month later for a minor recurrence of right sacroiliac joint pain due to turning over in bed. Erect posture straining test for the sacroiliac joint caused pain over the right sacroiliac joint, so the joint was manipulated once more. She returned again approximately 2 months later with a further minor recurrence of symptoms in the right sacroiliac joint and one manipulation again provided relief. She was advised to return should symptoms recur, which she did on one occasion some 5 months later.

Key point(s)

1. Sacroiliac joint stress tests can localize pain to a particular sacroiliac joint.
2. No improvement in sacroiliac joint pain following a steroid and anaesthetic injection into the joint does not mean that the joint is not the site of pain.

FURTHER READING

Giles L G F, Crawford C M 1997 Sacroiliac joint. In: Giles LGF, Singer KP (eds) Clinical anatomy and management of low back pain. Butterworth-Heinemann, Oxford, pp 173–182.

Mior S A, Ro C S, Lawrence D 1999 The sacroiliac joint. In: Cox JM (ed.) Low back pain: mechanism, diagnosis and treatment, 6th edn. Williams & Wilkins, Baltimore, pp 209–234.

Walker J M 1992 The sacroiliac joint: a critical review. Physical Therapy 72: 903–916.

Yong-Hing K 1994 Sacro-iliac joint pain: etiology and conservative treatment. La Chirugia degli Organi di Movimento 79: 35–45.

Case 5   Reabsorption of intervertebral disc material

COMMENT
Prolapsed disc material may be reabsorbed with cautious conservative care.

PROFILE

A 49-year-old man who is a non-smoker and only drinks alcohol socially and who is involved in manual work was referred by his general medical practitioner for evaluation and treatment.

PAST HISTORY

The referring doctor's letter stated that the patient had experienced intermittent low back problems for approximately 10 years but that there was no other past medical history of note, which the patient confirmed.

PRESENTING COMPLAINT (Fig. 5.1)

Periodic low back pain that has occurred since he sneezed 10 years ago whilst bending forwards and lifting; this painful episode caused him to spend 8 days in bed. Two weeks ago he developed severe acute low back pain and, for the first time, right sciatica with parasthaesiae in the right foot and a 'cold' feeling in the right foot.

He was trying NSAID medication and Panadeine Forte without much success. He had undergone several physiotherapy traction sessions which gave some temporary relief.

AETIOLOGY

Nothing specific; the symptoms had begun during his work 2 weeks ago; he thought he may have twisted his back getting in and out of the car.

EXAMINATION

Because of the acute low back pain and right sciatica with paraesthesiae in the right foot, he sat on the chair on his left buttock with his right leg extended, in order to minimize the low back pain and sciatica. The right ankle jerk (S1) was

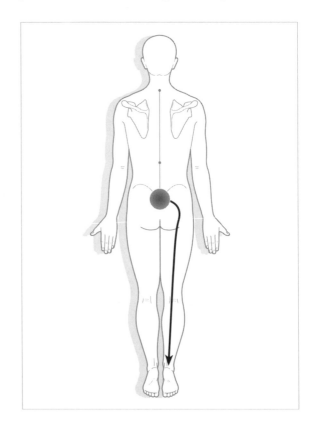

Figure 5.1

36

absent but other deep reflexes in the lower extremities were normal. Supine SLR was normal on the left but right SLR to 20° caused an increase in the low back pain and radiation into the right buttock. Active lumbar spine movements were considerably restricted due to low back pain and an increase in pain radiating into the right buttock.

IMAGING REVIEW

Plain lumbosacral spine and sacroiliac joint radiographs taken 6, 4 and 1 year previously were reviewed; these showed a complete left-sided lumbarization of S1 and a partial right-sided lumbarization. Minimal lipping changes were present at the anterior margins of most lumbar vertebral bodies, although the disc space heights were intact at the time of these investigations.

CLINICAL IMPRESSION

An acute right-sided disc protrusion at the L4–5 or L5–S1 level.

WHAT ACTION SHOULD BE TAKEN?

A CT scan was ordered of the lower lumbosacral spine (L3 to S1). The radiology report stated that, at the L4–5 disc level, there was a 'disc prolapse impinging upon the right L5 nerve root with effacement of the epidural fat. The differential diagnosis includes a right paracentral focal disc protrusion/oedema of the adjacent L5 or S1 nerve root, or a small neurofibroma'. A further possible differential diagnosis of epidural haematoma could be considered (as the clinical findings in spontaneous epidural haematoma are identical to those in acute disc herniation (Gundry & Heithoff 1993)).

TREATMENT

The patient was told that he had a disc prolapse at the L4–5 level that was pressing on the adjacent nerve root (Fig. 5.2A). He was advised to continue with his NSAID medication and, in order to resolve his acute low back pain and sciatica, that

it would be prudent to give him a few trial treatments using a chiropractic flexion–distraction technique modified from Cox (1999), i.e. 4×15 seconds of traction. He was told that the prolapse may become worse, requiring urgent surgical intervention. As he already was in so much pain, surgery was a likely possibility in any case. He signed a release form and treatment was begun immediately and a letter was written to his referring medical practitioner asking for the patient to be given 3–4 weeks off work. The patient was told to rest in bed before being seen 3 days later. He experienced some temporary soreness immediately after the flexion–distraction treatment but that had soon settled, so he decided to go to a wedding reception that evening where he sat for approximately 2 hours without undue pain. He then rested in bed. When he returned 3 days later he reported that he was 'much better' overall and that the pain had virtually gone from the right lower limb.

He was then seen again 2 days later for further flexion–distraction treatment and he said he was much better still. He had two further treatments and, because he was so much better, a CT scan was performed two weeks after the first CT scan through the L4–5 disc with a request to the radiographer to position the patient as closely as possible to the previous CT scan examination position. The disc prolapse was still evident but was perhaps a little smaller (Fig. 5.2B). Following a total of seven flexion–distraction treatments during a 2-week period he was so much better that he wanted to go back to work, in spite of still having a valid off-work certificate; his general medical practitioner was asked to give him a 'Return to Work' certificate for light duties for a 3-month period at which time he would be reviewed again before he returned to normal duties. As a differential diagnosis had included the conditions mentioned above, an MRI scan was performed approximately 3 months after the initial CT scan as he still had some minor residual low back pain and some intermittent paraesthesiae in the right leg (see Fig. 5.2C and D). This confirmed the L4–5 right-sided disc protrusion.

Approximately 8.5 months following the original MRI scan (Fig. 5.2C and D) a further MRI scan was performed (Fig. 5.2E). This showed no disc protrusion. Ten months after the initial CT scan was performed the patient was asked whether he would mind having a further CT scan performed (just through his L4–5 disc) to see what the spinal canal looked like now that he was virtually asymptomatic and was performing normal duties. He replied that he was interested to know and that he would be pleased to have this done, so a CT scan was performed (see Fig. 5.2F).

RESULT

The final MRI and CT scans (Fig. 5.2E and F), which again were taken in almost exactly the same position as the prior scan positions, showed that there was complete re-absorption of the disc protrusion.

The patient was asymptomatic for 1 year and 8 months until he fell onto his lower back and caused some pain in the upper lumbar spine but there was no recurrence of low back pain or right leg symptoms.

Note

Many papers have been written stating that prolapsed disc material has been re-absorbed. However, this can only be stated with certainty when initial and follow-up imaging is performed

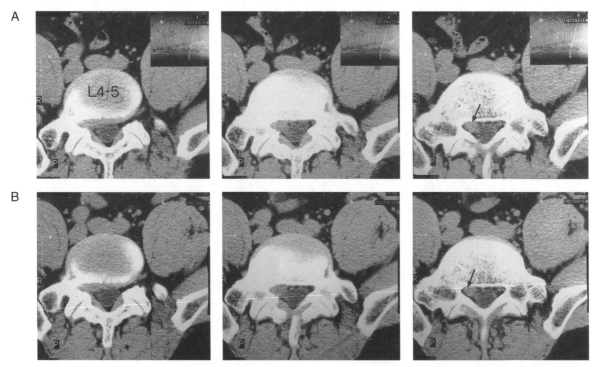

Figure 5.2 (A) Initial axial CT scan at the L4–5 disc level. Note that the radiology report stated: 'A fairly large right sided soft disc prolapse at L4–5 that is impinging upon the right L5 root as it buds off from the theca (arrow). No other significant feature is apparent'. (B) First follow-up axial CT scan at the L4–5 disc level 2 weeks after the initial CT scan. Note that the disc prolapse (arrow) remains essentially the same. (C) A parasagittal T1 weighted MRI scan (3 weeks after the CT scan in B). Note the L4–5 disc protrusion is still present. This parasagittal view shows the disc protrusion in another dimension and that it migrated inferiorly (arrow). (D) An axial T1 weighted MRI scan (3 weeks after the CT scan in B) showing the right lateral protrusion of the L4–5 disc (arrow) impinging upon the right L5 nerve root. (E) A sagittal T1 weighted MRI scan, taken approximately 8 months after the original MRI shown in (D), shows that the right-sided soft disc prolapse at L4–5 has been absorbed. (F) An axial CT scan at the L4–5 disc level taken 10 months after the initial CT scan in (A) to confirm that reabsorption, as compared with the original CT scan, was maintained. Note that the right-sided disc protrusion at L4–5 remains re-absorbed.

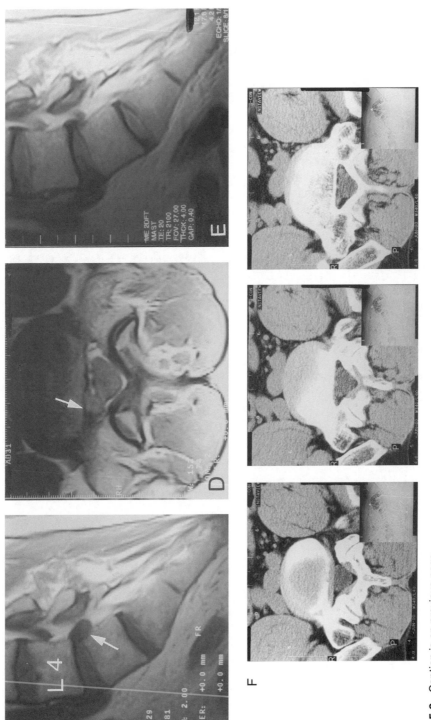

Figure 5.2 Caption is on previous page.

in a manner that produces follow-up imaging slices at the same anatomical level and in the same plane, or very close to the initial anatomical position and imaging plane. The bony and soft tissue structures in the CT and MRI slices show that this requirement was met in this case. Therefore, the absorption of prolapsed disc material in this case is a real phenomenon.

This case, and the writings of Dr James Cox (1999), raise the question of whether surgery should be undertaken without prior appropriate multidisciplinary conservative management having been tried to help patients with acute low back pain and sciatica.

Key point(s)

1. Prolapsed disc material may be reabsorbed with conservative treatment.
2. Surgery should not be considered as an initial option unless there are symptoms and signs of cauda equina syndrome.
3. Because the protrusion was right sided and impinged upon the right L5 nerve root the patient experienced typical low back pain and right sciatica.

REFERENCES

Cox J M 1999 Low back pain. Mechanism, diagnosis and treatment, 6th edn. Williams & Wilkins, Baltimore.
Gundry C R, Heithoff K B 1993 Epidural hematoma of the lumbar spine: 18 surgically confirmed cases. Radiology 187: 427–431.

FURTHER READING

Cox J M 1999 Low back pain. Mechanism, diagnosis and treatment, 6th edn. Williams & Wilkins, Baltimore.
Editor 1999 Major sciatica treatment proves ineffective in landmark randomized trial. The BackLetter 14: 25.
Editor 1999 Disturbing level of disagreement over the surgical treatment for spinal stenosis. The BackLetter 14: 13–14.
Editor 1999 Is it safe to treat massive disc herniations nonoperatively? The BackLetter 14: 51–52.
Herron L D, Pheasant H C 1980 Prone knee-flexion provocative testing for lumbar disc protrusion. Spine 5: 65–67.
Ito T, Takano Y, Yuasa N 2001 Types of lumbar herniated disc and clinical course. Spine 26: 648–651.
Saal J S 1990 The role of inflammation in lumbar pain. Physical Medicine and Rehabilitation: State of the Art Reviews 4: 191.
Saal J A, Saal J S, 1989 Nonoperative treatment of herniated lumbar intervertebral disc with radiculopathy. An outcome study. Spine 14: 431–437.
Saal J A, Saal J S, Herzog R J 1990 The natural history of lumbar intervertebral disc extrusions treated nonoperatively. Spine 15: 683–686.

Case 6   Ewing's sarcoma

COMMENT

Prompt and accurate diagnosis, initially using plain X-ray films, is imperative, bearing in mind serious pathological conditions that may mimic 'benign' low back pain. To 'wait for 6 weeks before X-raying' can be a dangerous practice.

PROFILE

A 45-year-old non-smoker who only drinks alcohol socially.

PAST HISTORY

There was no history of trauma and he said he was very fit.

PRESENTING COMPLAINT (Fig. 6.1)

He presented with left buttock/hip pain and some thigh pain that has been present for 3–4 weeks. There is no involvement of other joints. Active lumbar spine flexion causes an increase in his pain. The bowel and bladder function normally and there is no weight loss. There are no neurological symptoms and the pain does not radiate to the groin. There is no night pain.

AETIOLOGY

Unknown.

EXAMINATION

On examination he had a slight left-sided antalgic gait. He was able to touch his toes but with an increase in low back pain. The paraspinal muscles were not tender on deep palpation. Left hip joint ranges of movement were as follows – flexion to 50° with pain, abduction to 5° with pain, adduction to 20° without pain and internal rotation was limited by 50%.

He was tender to deep muscle palpation over the greater trochanter and the gluteus medius muscle. Neurologically, he was intact. The abdomen was not tender and had no masses on palpation. There was a left leg length deficiency of approximately 0.5 cm on clinical estimation.

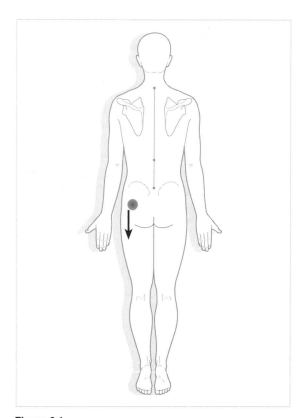

Figure 6.1

IMAGING

There was no previous imaging.

CLINICAL IMPRESSION

Suspicion of two possible conditions:

1. As there was absolutely no history of trauma and the pain was essentially localized to the left buttock/hip area with pain on deep palpation, a deep-seated bone pathology was suspected.
2. Possible L4–5 or L5–S1 disc changes as suggested by his slight left-sided antalgic gait.

WHAT ACTION SHOULD BE TAKEN?

- Pelvis and lumbar spine radiographs; these showed a lytic lesion in the left ilium (Fig. 6.2A).
- A pelvis CT scan; this showed 'considerable osseous erosion and a large extra-osseous mass as is typical of Ewing's sarcoma'.
- Plain chest X-ray films and CT chest films; these were found to be normal.
- A bone scan; this indicated that there was no evidence of metastatic disease.
- Biopsy; the patient was referred for a biopsy of the lytic lesion in the left iliac wing and a diagnosis of Ewing's sarcoma was made. Therefore, bone marrow aspirate and trephine was performed on the opposite iliac crest but this showed no evidence of infiltration with Ewing's sarcoma.

TREATMENT

The patient was referred to a medical oncologist where he was given on-going courses of chemotherapy to maximal tumour response. A repeat CT scan of the affected area was performed at 6-weekly intervals following courses of chemotherapy until maximum tumour response was attained. He required eight courses of chemotherapy administered at 3-weekly intervals and this treatment was well tolerated. He then underwent surgery approximately

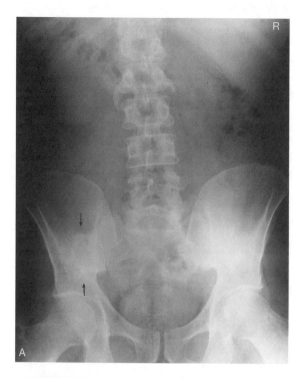

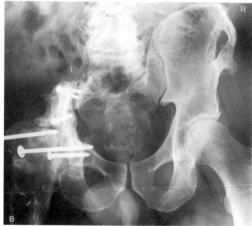

Figure 6.2 (A) Pelvis and lumbar spine anteroposterior view X-ray showing a lytic lesion in the left ilium (Ewing's sarcoma) (arrows). R = right side of patient. (B) Anteroposterior pelvis view showing previous resection of the ilium and arthrodeses of the left hip. Degenerative changes are noted at the lumbosacral level. No focal bony erosive change is demonstrated.

6 months following diagnosis, radiotherapy and then adjuvant chemotherapy.

Four months following resection of the original tumour he underwent bone graft surgery to the area of original treatment. This was followed by chemotherapy for a further 6 months (making a total of 70 weeks of chemotherapy).

RESULTS

The patient had a very positive outlook on life and is now 11 years post surgery and, although he has experienced bouts of considerable low back pain since the time of the operation, he manages to walk reasonably well, in spite of developing pseudoarthroses at the left hip joint.

Key point(s)

1. Be wary of patients who present with pain and absolutely no history of trauma.
2. Bogduk's 1999 'Modified criteria for the use of plain films in low back pain' that are based on the paper by Deyo and Diehl (1986) are shown to be questionable by this case.

REFERENCES

Bogduk N 1999 Evidence-based clinical guidelines for the management of acute low back pain. National Medical Research Council, Canberra, Australia, November 1999.
Deyo R A, Diehl A K 1986 Lumbar spine films in primary care: current use and effects of selective ordering criteria. Journal of General Internal Medicine 1: 20–25.

FURTHER READING

Christner J G 2000 Index of suspicion. Case 2. Diagnosis: Ewing's sarcoma. Pediatric Reviews (United States) 21: 281, 283.
Parsons V 1980 A colour atlas of bone disease. Wolfe Medical Publications, Holland.
Porsch M, Kornhuber B, Hovy L 1999 Functional results after partial pelvic resection in Ewing's sarcoma of the ilium. Archives of Orthopaedic and Trauma Surgery (Germany) 119: 199–204.
Sucato D J, Rougraff B, McGrath B E, et al 2000. Ewing's sarcoma of the pelvis. Long-term survival and functional outcome. Clinical Orthopaedics (United States) 373: 193–201.

Case 7 Abdominal aorta aneurysm

COMMENT

This is another example to show how important it is to look at the imaging films and not to rely only upon a radiological report.

PROFILE

A 76-year-old man of average build.

PAST HISTORY

He underwent surgery for the removal of a cyst on the right knee 8 years ago. He has been on medication for hypertension for 2 years.

PRESENTING COMPLAINT (Fig. 7.1)

Chronic low back pain intermittently since a work-related injury 42 years ago. The chronic low back pain does not trouble him unduely, although he has noted 'sharp stabs of pain in the low back' during the last month or two. There is no night pain.

AETIOLOGY

He slipped and fell, landing on his right buttock 42 years ago.

EXAMINATION

The examination was unremarkable apart from minor low back pain on right rotation of the lumbar spine. Supine SLR was to 90° on the left and right sides without any increase in low back pain. The deep reflexes in the lower extremities were normal as was the case with muscle tone, power, pinprick sensation, and vibration sensation.

IMAGING REVIEW

No recent imaging was available.

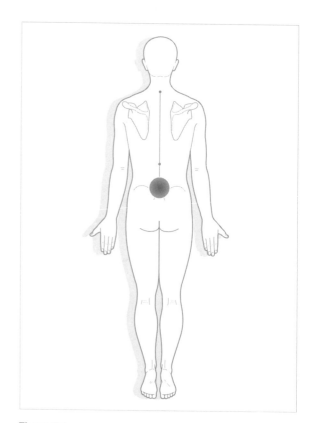

Figure 7.1

44

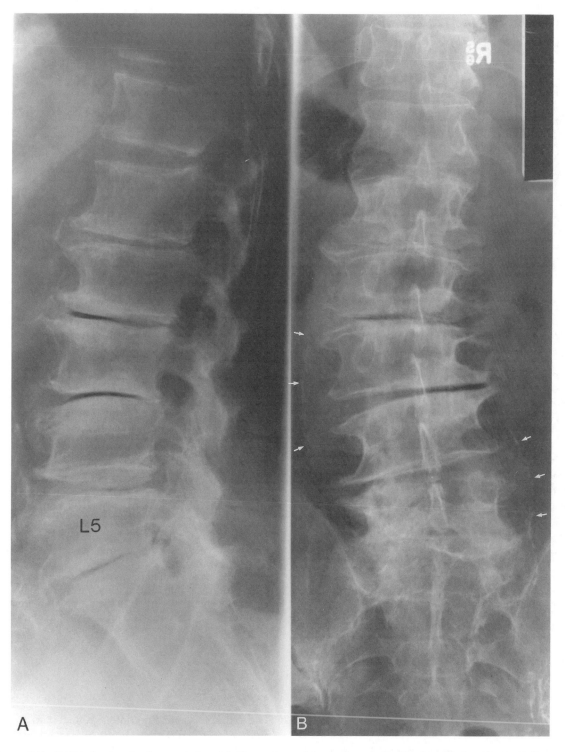

Figure 7.2   (A,B) Lateral and anteroposterior plain X-ray views of the lumbosacral spine showing the advanced discogenic spondylosis with partial calcification in the abdominal aorta aneurysm (small arrows). L5 = fifth lumbar vertebra.

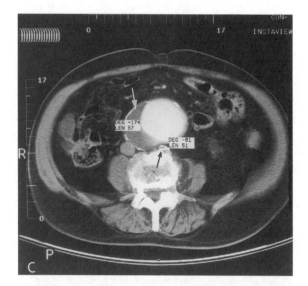

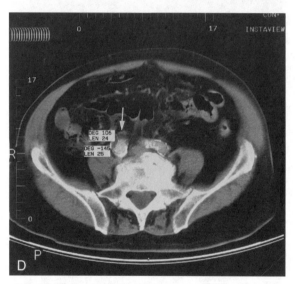

Figure 7.2 (C) Axial CT scan with contrast showing the large abdominal aortic aneurysm (8×6 cm) with the right lateral eccentric thrombus (white arrow). Note how the lumbar spondylosis (small black arrow) is indenting the aortic aneurysm posteriorly which could make the wall of the aneurysm vulnerable to bleeding. (D) Axial CT scan showing that the aneurysm involves the origin of the right common iliac artery which has a maximal diameter of 2.4×2.5 cm (arrow).

CLINICAL IMPRESSION

Although he was neurologically intact and he had a 42-year history of chronic intermittent low back pain, it was necessary to be sure of the pathology causing his low back pain so as to exclude pathology other than lumbar spine 'wear and tear'.

WHAT ACTION SHOULD BE TAKEN?

Laboratory tests were performed as a precaution in view of his age, with the following results: Serum prostate specific antigen was 3.5 ng/ml (range = 0.0–13.1). A full blood count was normal as was the ESR at 4 mm/1 hr (range 2–20).

Lumbar spine plain film radiographs were ordered in the erect posture (Fig. 7.2A and B) and the radiology report stated:

Advanced degenerative change is noted throughout the lumbar spine with disc narrowing and gas in the disc space at all five lumbar discs. There is an associated lumbar scoliosis convex to the left and centred at L3 with a mild rotational component. There is severe degenerative change in the zygapophysial joints at all levels, particularly from L3 to S1.

A vitally important finding was missed on the plain X-ray report. Note the large aneurysm in the abdominal aorta at the L3 to S1 level (small arrows). Therefore a CT abdomen scan was ordered using the technique of post contrast axial scans performed from the diaphragms to the symphysis. This confirmed the extent of the large abdominal aortic aneurysm:

There is an ectatic fusiform abdominal aortic aneurysm with a maximal diameter of 8×6 cm. It has right lateral eccentric thrombus. It arises well below the origins of the renal arteries. There is diffuse calcification and atheroma within the abdominal aorta. The aneurysm involves the origin of the right common iliac artery that has a maximal diameter of 2.4×2.5 cm. Both kidneys perfuse normally. (Fig. 7.2C and D).

TREATMENT

The patient was immediately referred to a vascular surgeon and underwent successful surgery to repair the aneurysm. This gave him great relief from most of his low back pain.

RESULT

Some months following surgery the patient required intermittent relief for minor residual low back pain symptoms for which he was given needle acupuncture treatment that resulted in great relief. Occasionally, he returns for a course of 6–10 needle acupuncture treatments to relieve his chronic intermittent low back pain.

Key point(s)
1. Be wary of patients presenting with a long history of intermittent low back pain who may subsequently have developed life-threatening pathology that apparently mimics the 'longstanding low back pain'. 2. Always look at the imaging films and not only the report.

FURTHER READING

Kramer P W 1980 Back and leg pain secondary to abdominal aortic aneurysm. Neurosurgery 7: 626–628.
Orsnes T, Fallentin E M, Gebuhr P H 1993 Back pain in abdominal aortic aneurysm. Ugeskrift for Laeger 155: 2412–2413.
Tollefsen I, Jorgensen I K, Woie L, Fossdal J E 2001 Aortic dissection: natural course of disease? Report of two cases representing the extremes of the condition. European Journal of Radiology 40: 68–72.
Vernon L F, Peacock J R, Esposito A P 1986 Abdominal aortic aneurysms presenting as low back pain: a report of two cases. Journal of Manipulative Physiological Therapy 9: 47–50.

Case 8   Small aortic aneurysm

COMMENT
When necessary, 3-D CT reconstruction can be useful for looking at the relationship between adjacent anatomical structures in greater detail.

PROFILE

A 64-year-old man who smokes approximately 40 cigarettes daily and drinks six beers a day.

PAST HISTORY

Nothing contributory. There is a family history of ischaemic heart disease.

PRESENTING COMPLAINT (Fig. 8.1)

Constant low back pain, varying in intensity from a mild ache to severe pain, with considerable sciatic radiation into the right hip, groin and down the back of the right leg during the last 6 months. Coughing and sneezing makes the pain worse. He can get some relief from the low back pain syndrome by lying on his right side. NSAIDs have not been helpful so he was referred by his general medical practitioner for an opinion and treatment; his prostate-specific antigen (PSA) level was normal.

AETIOLOGY

There was no obvious cause for the low back pain syndrome that becomes worse as the day progresses.

EXAMINATION

Lumbar spine movements were of full range and painless, except for extension of the lumbar spine which caused some lumbosacral pain. External rotation of the right hip caused slight pain in the right groin. Supine SLR was of a good range for his age and painless. Neurologically he was intact. Muscle tone and power, as well as pinprick sensation and

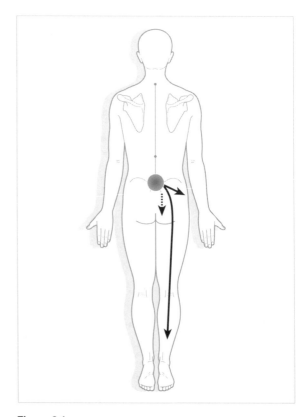

Figure 8.1

reflexes, were normal. His peripheral pulses were all intact. A small aortic aneurysm was palpable on abdominal examination.

IMAGING REVIEW

A previous lower lumbar CT scan suggested minor L4–5 spinal canal stenosis.

CLINICAL IMPRESSION

A degree of abdominal aortic aneurysm and probable L4–S1 degenerative stenosis changes.

WHAT ACTION SHOULD BE TAKEN?

Plain film radiographs were taken of the pelvis and lumbar spine in the erect posture and these showed minor osteoarthrosis in the lower lumbosacral zygapophysial joints with minor lipping of the vertebral bodies anteriorly; in addition, patchy atheromatous plaques were noted in the abdominal aorta (Fig. 8.2A).

Therefore, he was sent for an ultrasound examination of the abdominal aorta that showed:

Evidence of calcification with atheroma within the abdominal aorta. The antero-posterior diameter of the abdominal aorta just distal to the superior mesenteric artery is 2.2 cm. The renal origins are identified and the abdominal aorta at this level measures 2.2 × 1.8 cm. Below the renal arteries there is a focal aneurysmal dilatation of the abdominal aorta with an anteroposterior diameter of 2.6 cm and a transverse diameter of 3 cm. There is calcification of the iliac arteries with no evidence of aneurysmal dilatation.

A CT abdomen and pelvis was then performed to further evaluate the aneurysm using a technique of pre-contrast scans followed by contrast-enhanced dynamic helical scans of the abdominal aorta and iliac arteries with 3-D reconstruction of the abdominal aorta. The findings were:

Extensive calcification of the abdominal aorta and iliac arteries. There is no evidence of intraluminal thrombus (Fig. 8.2B). The CT confirms the presence of focal aneurysmal dilation below the renal arteries

(Fig. 8.2C). The maximum transverse diameter is 3.2 cm. There is no evidence of aneurysmal extension into the iliac arteries, normal spleen and both kidneys with no mass in the pancreas and no retroperitoneal lymphadenopathy.

The reconstruction view (Fig. 8.2D) clearly shows the spatial relationship between the kidneys, various blood vessels and the aneurysmal dilatation below the renal arteries.

A CT lumbar spine was ordered to examine the spinal canal prior to consideration of treatment options. This showed that:

At the L4–5 disc level, there is significant canal stenosis due to a combination of a very diffuse disc bulge, hypertrophy of the ligamenta flava and hypertrophic degenerative change in the zygapophysial joints. At the L5–S1 disc level there is also a prominent generalized disc bulge and hypertrophy of the ligamenta flava causing a minor degree of relative canal stenosis. There is advanced degenerative change in the zygapophysial joints occurring bilaterally.

The conclusion was: 'Canal stenosis and hypertrophic degenerative change in the zygapophysial joints leads to foraminal stenosis, which is most marked at the L5–S1 level but the most significant overall finding is the canal stenosis at the L4–5 level'.

TREATMENT

In view of the low back pain with considerable right sciatica he was advised to stop smoking, lose weight and stop lifting heavy containers during his work. He was given a trial of needle acupuncture while waiting to see a vascular surgeon for an opinion but this treatment was not helpful. As he had intact peripheral pulses and only a small aortic aneurysm that was palpable on abdominal examination, it was decided by the vascular surgeon that no surgery was necessary at this time. However, should the aneurysm eventually reach 5 cm in size (as found on follow-up ultrasound or CT scans), elective repair would be indicated.

The patient elected to stop working as he was of approximately retirement age and he agreed to 6-monthly follow-up abdominal ultrasound

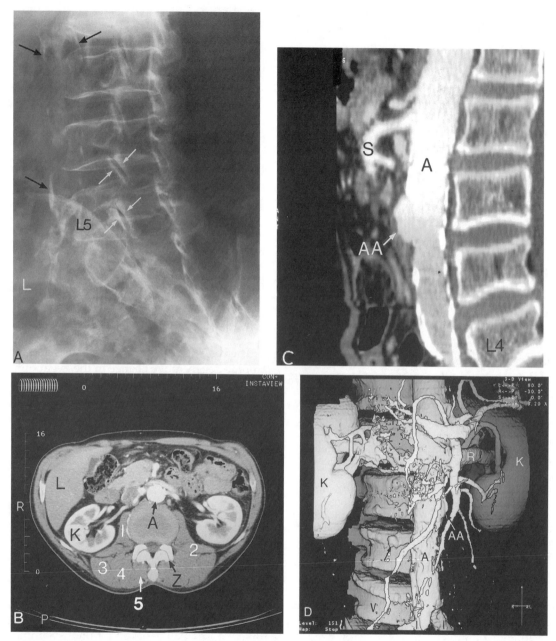

Figure 8.2 (A) Plain lumbar spine oblique X-ray view. L = left side of the patient. Note the osteoarthrotic changes in the zygapophysial joints as indicated by subchondral sclerosis (white arrows). The patchy atheromatous plaques in the abdominal aorta are indicated with black arrows. L5 = fifth lumbar vertebra. (B) Axial CT scan showing the aorta (A), right kidney (K) and blood vessels leaving it, and the liver (L). Z = left zygapophysial (facet) joint; 1= psoas major muscle; 2 = quadratus lumborum muscle; 3 = iliocostalis lumborum muscle; 4 = longissimus thoracis muscle; 5 = multifidus muscle. (C) 3-D reconstruction CT scan showing the infra-renal small abdominal aortic aneurysm (AA), abdominal aorta (A) and superior mesenteric artery (S). L4 = fourth lumbar vertebral body. (D) 3-D CT reconstruction view showing the kidneys (K), renal artery (R), abdominal aorta (A), small aneurysm of the abdominal aorta (AA) and common iliac arteries (I). V = vertebral body of the fourth lumbar vertebra. Black arrows indicate osteoarthrotic lipping along the superior margin of the L3 vertebral body; lipping can also be seen at some of the other vertebral body levels adjacent to the intervertebral disc spaces.

scans to determine whether the aneurysm progressed.

RESULTS

On review 6 months after he stopped working, he said his pain had improved considerably since ceasing work, although he required occasional antidepressant medication and analgesics to help to control his chronic low back pain syndrome symptoms. A follow-up ultrasound scan showed no progression of the small aortic aneurysm at that time.

Key point(s)

1. A small palpable aortic aneurysm should be investigated by ultrasound and further studies as indicated.
2. Further sophisticated imaging such as 3-D CT reconstruction may be useful to augment an ultrasound examination.

FURTHER READING

See Case 7.

Case 9 L4 discectomy

COMMENT
Spinal surgery has its limitations even when all
conservative treatments have failed.

PROFILE

A somewhat overweight 34-year-old male of solid
build who performed manual work and smokes
approximately 20 cigarettes a day but does not
drink alcohol.

PAST HISTORY

No past history of any significance.

PRESENTING COMPLAINT (Fig. 9.1)

Unbearable low back pain that radiates posteriorly to the left leg as far as the ankle; he
describes the low back pain as a 'sharp pain in
the low back'. The pain may awaken him in the
early hours of the morning but is not a deep-
seated 'night' pain.

He had tried NSAIDs and analgesics from his
general medical practitioner. He had also seen
an anaesthetist for an epidural block. A
discogram had been performed for the two
lower discs but this procedure had, unfortunately, caused an increase in his left-sided
sciatica. He was taking 120 mg MS Contin daily
and he was on antidepressants because of his
chronic low back pain syndrome. He found
that physiotherapy treatment, manipulation and
acupuncture did not help; traction had caused a
'burning' sensation at the lower lumbar spine
level at 30 kg of traction.

He was concerned that he could not completely empty his urinary bladder, but bowel

function was normal. Coughing did not exacer-
bate his symptoms but sneezing did, as did
bearing down; the latter caused a significant
increase in low back pain. His general medical
practitioner referred him for a further opinion.

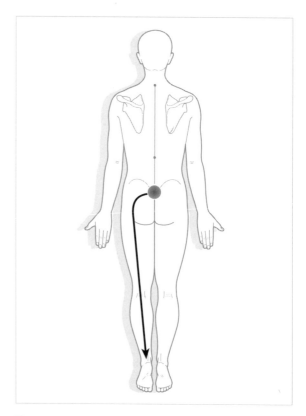

Figure 9.1

AETIOLOGY

Four months before consultation he had lifted a 40-kg tin of paint and while doing so, he slipped and twisted his low back, causing an immediate 'sharp pain in the low back'. He continued to work on light duties for approximately 6–8 weeks with low back pain, then there was no longer any light work to be performed so he was dismissed.

EXAMINATION

He did not have a temperature and felt well apart from his presenting complaint. Lumbar spine active ranges of movement were as follows:

1. Flexion limited by 80% due to pain at the L4–5 level.
2. Extension limited by 90% due to pain at the L4–5 level.
3. Left and right lateral bending limited by 50% due to L4–5 pain.
4. Left and right rotation with the pelvis fixed were painless.

Toe walking power (S1) was normal but he felt there was an increase in his low back pain. Heel walking power (L5) was normal but caused an increase in his low back pain. The ankle and knee jerks were normal. Bilateral hip flexion caused a significant increase in low back pain. The foot pulses were normal. Pinprick sensation over the lower extremities was normal apart from an area of hypoaesthesia of approximately 2 cm in diameter on the anterolateral aspect of his left thigh. There was hypoaesthesia in the left little toe (S1 dermatome) and in the big toe (L5 dermatome). Supine SLR was limited by low back pain to a measured 15° on the left and to 20° on the right. Hoover's sign was normal, i.e. there was no attempt to malinger. The circumference of the thighs, 15 cm above the knee, was equal and within normal limits, as was the circumference of the calves. The Naffziger test caused an increase in low back pain. The Milgram test (actively lifting both straight legs together) caused an increase in low back pain.

In the supine position, cervical spine flexion caused an increase in low back pain.

IMAGING REVIEW

Plain film radiographs were within normal limits and a myelogram (Fig. 9.2A), followed by a CT, had shown, at the L4–5 level, 'mild waisting of the thecal sac with a broad-based anterior impression on the thecal sac due to generalized anular bulging, without significantly compromising the spinal canal or exiting L4 nerve roots'. A recent bone scan showed a normal examination.

CLINICAL IMPRESSION

A left posterolateral L4–5 intervertebral disc bulge/protrusion.

WHAT ACTION SHOULD BE TAKEN?

In view of existing imaging and his clinical presentation, an MRI was performed of his lumbar spine to further evaluate his lower lumbar discs. The MRI showed that 'the left L4–5 intervertebral foramen appeared narrowed by disc material' (Fig. 9.2B). As he was depressed by his chronic low back pain syndrome and his invalidity, he was referred for a surgical opinion that led to a discogram being performed at L3–4–L5–S1 (Fig. 9.2C). This showed posterior leakage of contrast and reproduced his symptoms. A CT scan following the discogram showed a full thickness tear of the posterior disc fibres with leakage of contrast material (Fig. 9.2D).

TREATMENT

He was advised to lose weight and to have a trial of acupuncture treatment but he did not make much progress in either attempt. Therefore, in view of the CT, discogram and MRI results, the patient elected to have a discectomy at the L4–5 disc level, in spite of advice regarding the unpredicability of spinal surgery, as he found his symptoms unbearable.

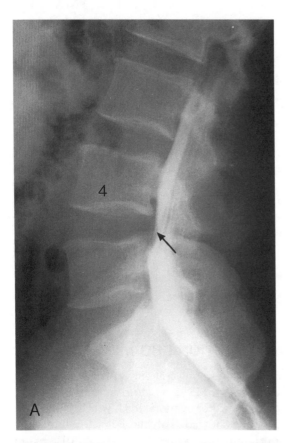

A

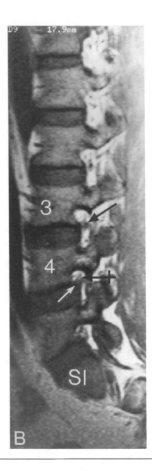

B

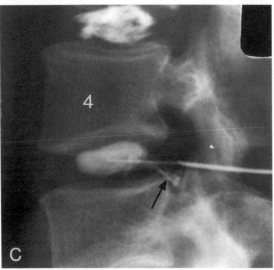

C

Figure 9.2 (A) Lateral lumbar spine myelogram contrast view showing some indentation of the thecal sac at the L4–5 level (arrow). (B) Sagittal MRI T1 weighted image of the lumbar spine showing a normal intervertebral foramen at the L3–4 level with normal neural structures in the foramen (black arrow). Note the encroachment of disc material into the left L4–5 foramen (white arrow) with some pressure upon the nerve root at this level (tailed black arrow). Note how the disc material extends into the lower part of the intervertebral foramen narrowing its anteroposterior dimension considerably when compared with the L3–4 foramen. The nerve root at the L5–S1 disc level is normal, and lies within a normal intervertebral foramen. S1 = first sacral segment. (C) Lateral lumbar spine view of the discogram procedure at the L3–4 and L4–5 disc levels; at the L4–5 level, leakage of contrast material posteriorly is noted (arrow). (D) Axial CT post-discogram views of the contrast in the L4–5 disc. This shows some internal disc disruption (white arrow) with posterior leakage of contrast material (tailed arrow) with a full thickness tear of the posterior disc fibres and repro-duction of his pain.

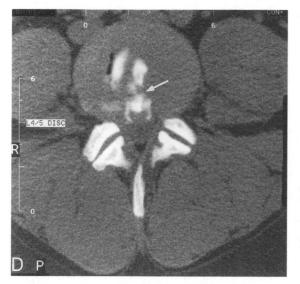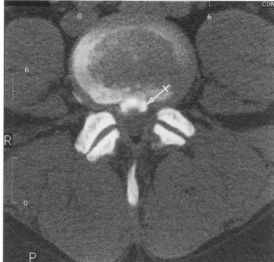

Figure 9.2 Caption is on previous page.

RESULTS

Following surgery he had 'good and bad days' and, although he walked for 2.5 km daily, he experienced severe pins and needles in the soles of both feet which he felt were 'cold' since surgery. Unfortunately, in the long term, surgery was not successful and he has been left with a chronic mixed mechanical and neuropathic low back pain that occasionally radiates to both legs despite the L4–5 discectomy.

Key point(s)

1. The results of spinal surgery are unpredictable, even when the patient sees a good surgeon.
2. The long-term results of standard lumbar discectomy are not very satisfying (Loupasis et al 1999), supporting the notion that disc surgery involves a high rate of failure (Postacchini 2001).

REFERENCES

Loupasis G A, Stamos K, Katonis P G, Sapkas G, Korres D S, Hartofilakidis G 1999 Seven- to 20-year outcome of lumbar discectomy. Spine 24: 2313–2317.
Postacchini F 2001 Lumbar disc herniation. A new equilibrium is needed between nonoperative and operative treatment. Spine 26: 601.

FURTHER READING

Keim H A, Kirkaldy-Willis W H 1987 Clinical symposia. Low back pain, Vol 39. Ciba-Geigy, Jersey.
Postacchini F 1998 Lumbar disc herniation. Springer-Verlag, New York.
Weinstein J N, Rydevik B L, Sonntag V K H 1995 Essentials of the spine. Raven Press, New York.

Case 10   Disc protrusion

COMMENT
It is unwise not to promptly order at least erect posture pelvis and lumbar spine anteroposterior and lateral lumbosacral X-ray films for low back pain with radiculopathy; oblique views should also be considered. An appropriate and prompt diagnosis should be a clinician's goal – not a 'wait and see approach'.

PROFILE

A 33-year-old man of muscular build who is somewhat overweight.

PAST HISTORY

At approximately 18 years of age he developed some neck and upper thoracic spine pain due to lifting at work, and following X-rays it was concluded that he had aggravated an old neck injury. He had always been involved in sport such as touch football and indoor cricket up until injuring his low back 5 years ago.

PRESENTING COMPLAINT (Fig. 10.1)

He presented with low back pain and pointed to the lumbosacral level, particularly the right side. In addition his low back pain can radiate to the left buttock, the posterior aspect of his left thigh and calf, then as far as his ankle. The left leg radicular pain began approximately 4.5 years ago, i.e. approximately 6 months after injuring his low back.

On the day of the accident, he went to his general medical practitioner who thought a 'muscle had been pulled'; the patient was told to take 2 days off from work and to use anti-inflammatory medication, then to return for a review. The pain 'subsided a lot' as a result of taking NSAIDs, Panadeine Forte and Mersyndol.

He went back to work where there was some light lifting to be done but within a few minutes, the low back pain became 'intense'. Therefore,

his general medical practitioner referred him to a physiotherapist for 2 weeks of treatment. He was given 20 minutes of traction daily which 'worked well' coupled with the anti-inflammatory medication. He believes he was off work for approximately 2 weeks. He returned to light

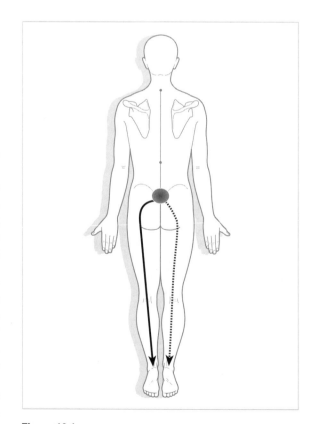

Figure 10.1

duty work but had to terminate his employment approximately 2.5 years after the accident as there were no longer any light duty positions for him.

AETIOLOGY

He was shovelling sand and clay to cover an electrical cable when the bank of the trench collapsed. He was unable to prevent himself from falling across the trench; as he fell backwards across the trench his low back hit the opposite side of the trench. The trench was approximately 105 cm deep and 60 cm wide and he fell into it. He kept working for 2–3 hours, thinking that he had just 'strained' his low back. He sat and had lunch for approximately 20–30 minutes and, on getting up, he felt considerable low back pain.

EXAMINATION

In the erect posture his pelvis appeared to be approximately level without clinical evidence of pelvic obliquity. Percussion of the spine was painless and deep palpation of the paravertebral muscles did not elicit any pain. Lumbar spine active ranges of movement were as follows:

1. Flexion – limited by approximately 10% due to lumbosacral pain extending into the left leg posteriorly. He bent forward cautiously and slowly until the left leg pain (sciatica) occurred.
2. Extension – limited by approximately 10% due to low back pain.
3. Left lateral bending – full range but caused pain on the right side of L5.
4. Right lateral bending – full range and painless.
5. Left and right rotation – normal range and painless.

The deep reflexes in the legs were normal, as was the plantar response. Pinprick sensation of the legs and feet was normal. Left SLR in the seated and slumped forward position (slump test) caused left sciatic pain. No pain was felt on raising the right leg. Supine straight leg raising was limited to a measured 75° on the left due to pain in the left buttock and thigh posteriorly. Right SLR was unremarkable. Active SLR of both his legs, while lying in the supine position (Milgram test), caused considerable low back pain with some radiation into the lower abdomen. Bilateral hip flexion was of full range and painless but he felt low back pain on actively lowering his legs. In the supine position, flexion of the cervical spine did not cause any low back pain. Coughing caused low back pain. The pulses in his feet were normal and the temperature was equal in both the left and right feet. Power in the big toes, feet and legs was normal.

IMAGING REVIEW

No X-ray films or any other imaging films had been taken until approximately 4 years and 3 months following the injury when he was referred to an orthopaedic surgeon for continuing low back pain and left sciatica management; he was then sent for a supine lumbar spine plain film X-ray examination including anteroposterior, lateral and oblique views and told to continue with NSAIDs. The radiology report on these films read: 'there is some narrowing of the L4–5 and L5–S1 disc spaces; the remaining disc spaces appear normal. The facet joints and posterior elements appear normal.'

CLINICAL IMPRESSION

Central to left-sided disc protrusion at the L5–S1 level (or at the L4–5 level).

WHAT ACTION SHOULD BE TAKEN?

An erect posture pelvis and lumbar spine and a lateral lumbosacral spine X-ray view were performed (Fig. 10.2A and B). The former figure showed that the lumbar spine was antalgic above the L4 level with a 'lumbar curvature convex to the left'. As a diagnosis of L5–S1 disc protrusion was considered highly likely

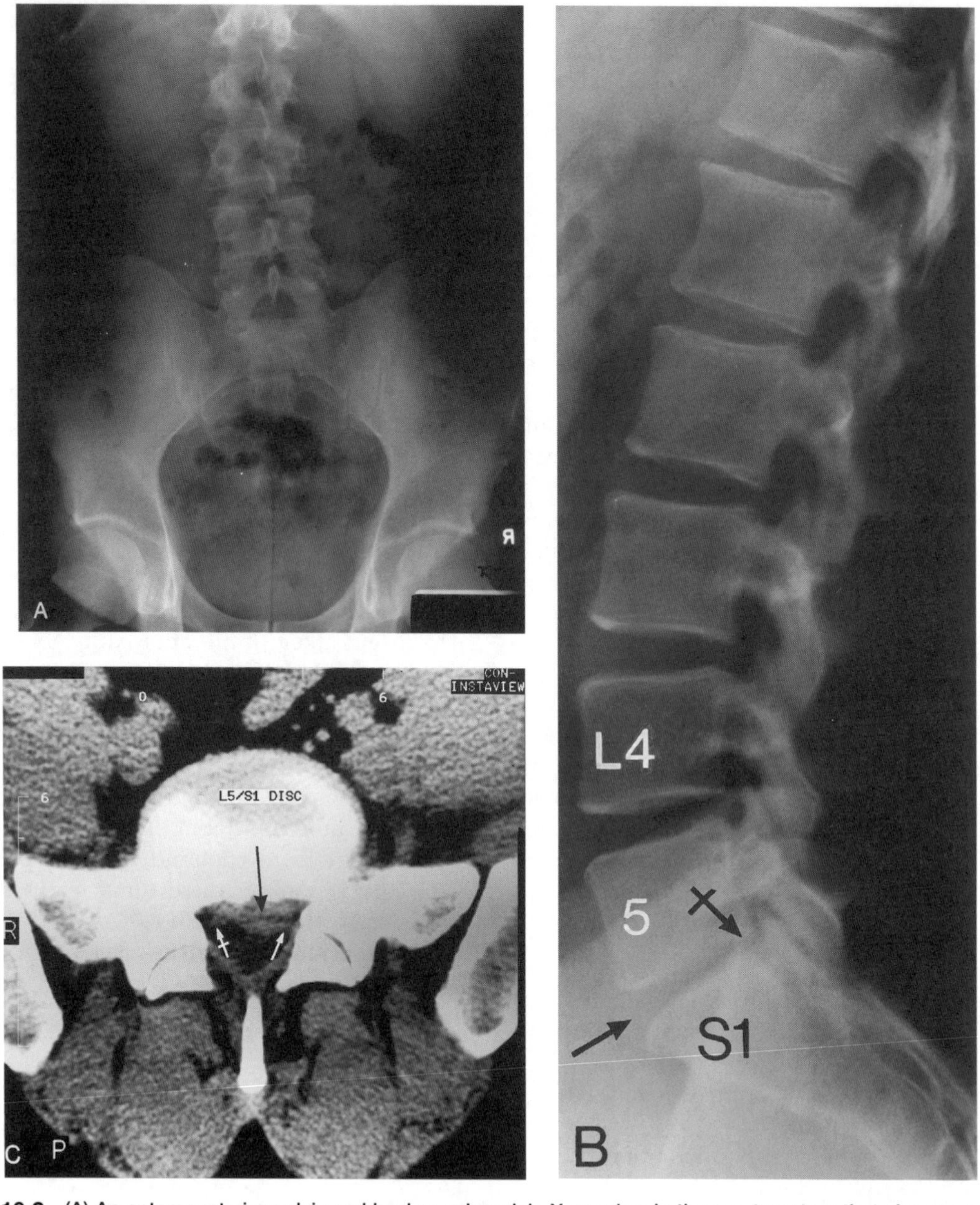

Figure 10.2 (A) An anteroposterior pelvis and lumbar spine plain X-ray view in the erect posture that shows some degree of antalgic scoliosis (lumbar curvature convex to the left). (B) A lateral lumbar spine plain X-ray view showing the fourth (L4) lumbar vertebra and the disc thinning at L5–S1 (black arrow), with retrolisthesis of L5 on S1 (tailed arrow). (C) An axial CT scan at the L5–S1 level showing the large left paracentral disc protrusion (black arrow) compressing the left S1 nerve root (small white arrow). The small white-tailed arrow shows the right S1 nerve root which appears not to be compromised.

because of his history and symptoms, and the disc thinning with retrolisthesis of L5 on S1 noted on the lateral view (Fig. 10.2B), a CT scan was performed of the lower lumbar spine (L3–S1); this showed, at the L5–S1 level, 'a large left paracentral disc protrusion compressing the S1 nerve root' (Fig. 10.2C).

TREATMENT

The patient was very relieved to find that he had a genuine pathological condition causing his low back pain and left sciatica, having tried for approximately 4 years and 8 months to obtain a diagnosis. He decided to take a conservative approach to his problem by losing weight, exercising (i.e. going for long walks) and cutting down his anti-inflammatory medication. He said he did not want to consider a surgical approach and would let me know whether the proposed conservative approach did not help him. He was given exercises to perform to strengthen the abdominal, buttock and lumbar muscles (see Figs 10.3 and 10.4), as well as an exercise to mobilize the lower lumbar nerve roots (see Fig. 10.5) and he decided to find a light duty occupation in which he was virtually self-employed so that he could accommodate his low back and left leg pain.

RESULTS

To date, some 9 years post injury, he has managed to avoid surgery for his intervertebral disc prolapse by losing weight, going for long walks and performing exercises to strengthen the muscles mentioned above. The main reason for his cooperation was that a definitive diagnosis had been made and his condition clearly explained to him.

Key point

When buttock and leg symptoms occur on the left and right sides in varying degrees, expect a central intervertebral disc protrusion. If the symptoms are predominantly left sided, the disc protrusion will most likely be central to left sided, as in this case.

FURTHER READING

See Case 9.

APPENDIX: BASIC LOW BACK EXERCISES

(Modified from: Burton C, Nida G 1977 *Be good to your back*. The Sister Kenny Institute Low Back Clinic. Rehabilitation Publication No. 738, Minneapolis, MN, with permission.)

If no adverse reaction

Day 1:   5 repetitions of each exercise.
Day 2:   10 repetitions of each exercise.
Day 3 onwards: 20 repetitions of each exercise, then build up to 50–100 repetitions.

1. Begin in a relaxed position, lying on your back with knees bent and feet flat on the floor (Fig. 10.3).
2. Tighten the buttocks closely together.
3. Still holding the buttocks together, tighten and pull in the stomach.
4. Your low back should roll flat against the floor.
5. Hold for a slow count of 5, then relax.
6. Do *not* push with your feet.

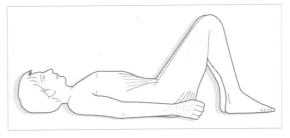

Figure 10.3

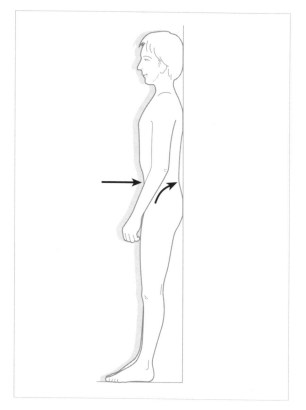

Figure 10.4

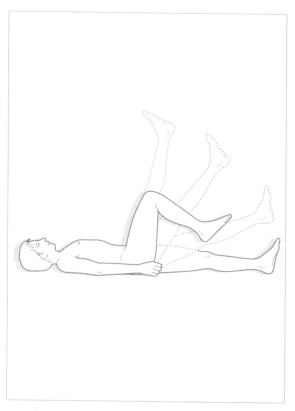

Figure 10.5

1. Stand with your back touching a wall (Fig. 10.4).
2. Move your feet about 20–30 cm away from the wall, resting your back against the wall.
3. Squeeze your buttocks together and hold.
4. Now pull in your abdomen. The space between your back and the wall should have gone.
5. Holding your low back flat against the wall, gradually move your feet closer to the wall.
6. When you can stand straight with no curve, try walking around the room with your back in the same position, returning to the wall to double check your ability to maintain proper posture.

This exercise (Fig. 10.5) stretches and strengthens muscles of the back, abdomen, and legs and improves range of motion; it also promotes movement of nerve roots within the lower intervertebral foraminae.

1. Begin in a relaxed position, lying on your back with one knee bent.
2. Slowly raise the bent leg, straightening the leg as it moves upward and keeping the low back flat.
3. Raise the leg as far as possible without causing discomfort.
4. Slowly lower this leg, keeping the low back flat as the leg approaches the floor.
5. Relax a few seconds.
6. Repeat the motions, as outlined above, using the other leg.

Be good to your back!

The human body has a remarkable ability to adapt to almost any form of activity if that activity is begun slowly and increased gradually over a period of time. Recommended activities include:

1. Walking – on a daily basis, gradually increasing distance day-by-day.
2. Hiking – once walking is well established.
3. Swimming – it is with swimming that the paravertebral muscles can be gently exercised since the gravity-induced weight of the body is modified by the presence of water. Swimming is the closest that a low back pain patient can come to exercising in a gravity-free environment. Once again, frequent swimming, using gentle motion and progressively increasing effort and time is most desirable.

Case 11   Internal disc disruption

COMMENT
When a MRI study appears to be normal, in spite of a patient having a history and physical findings suggesting a disc problem, it is important to have a clinical suspicion of internal disc disruption.

PROFILE
A 20-year-old young man with muscular athletic build who is a non-smoker and non-drinker.

PAST HISTORY
He had always been very fit.

PRESENTING COMPLAINT (Fig. 11.1)
Constant moderate to severe low back pain centrally at the L4 to S1 level with some pain radiating to the left thigh posterolaterally and down the back of the left leg with paraesthesiae in the left foot. Coughing aggravates the low back pain and sneezing aggravates the paraesthesiae in the left foot. Walking causes an increase in low back and left thigh pain as do long standing and sitting. The pain is sometimes felt as a 'sharp throbbing low back pain'.

The degree of pain causes him difficulties when trying to sleep as he feels that there are 'severe muscle spasms' in the left leg.

Nerve conduction studies had been performed and reported as being normal. He was particularly upset as the clinicians whom he had consulted (medical practitioners, chiropractor and physiotherapist) thought he was malingering and, in fact, one comment recorded stated '? supratentorial component'.

He tried NSAIDs, needle acupuncture, chiropractic manipulation and physiotherapy treatment without success and was currently depressed by his genuine symptoms that have been trivialized.

AETIOLOGY
While lifting a heavy weight with three work colleagues, 6 months before consultation, he felt a central 'moderate' low back pain. He thought he had 'pulled a muscle' in the low back,

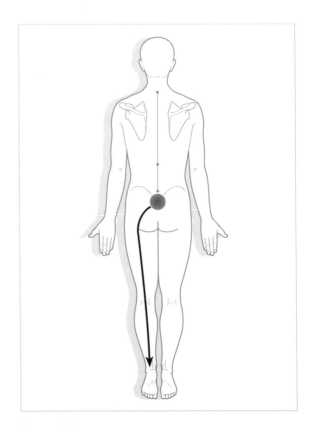

Figure 11.1

so performed some exercises that he normally performed to keep fit; these caused a marked increase in the low back pain and radiation down the lateral aspect of his left thigh and down the back of the left leg, with paraesthesiae in the left foot. He was hospitalized and treated with bed rest, analgesia, muscle relaxants and physiotherapy but with little, if any, improvement.

EXAMINATION

Percussion of the spine elicited L4–S1 pain, as did deep palpation of the paraspinal muscles in the same region. Lumbar spine active ranges of movement were as follows:

1. Flexion – limited by approximately 60% due to L4–S1 pain with a 'flat back' on forward bending.
2. Extension – limited by approximately 15% due to L4–S1 pain.
3. Left rotation – limited by approximately 10% due to L4–S1 pain.
4. Right rotation – painless and of full range.

Sitting slumped forward caused an increase in low back pain. Seated straight leg raising was limited due to low back pain to a measured 30° (left) and 45° (right). Supine SLR was limited due to low back pain to a measured 30° (left) and 45° (right). Pinprick sensation was diminished in the lateral aspect of the left calf (L5) and foot (S1). The foot pulses were normal and the temperature of the feet and legs appeared equal and normal bilaterally on palpation. Axial loading on the shoulders caused an increase in low back pain, whereas gentle axial loading of the skull did not cause any low back pain. Power in the big toes, feet and legs was normal. Sacroiliac joint stress tests were normal. Active bilateral SLR was very limited due to L5–S1 pain.

CLINICAL IMPRESSION

L5–S1 intervertebral disc bulge/protrusion at the lumbosacral disc level; definitely not psychosomatic!

IMAGING REVIEW

A review of his plain film radiographs (Fig. 11.2A and B) showed normal imaging, as did the oblique views.

WHAT ACTION SHOULD BE TAKEN?

An MRI of the lumbosacral spine. This was essentially normal, apart from some T10–11 and T12–L1 Schmorl's nodes (Fig. 11.2C and D). The axial view at L5–S1 shown in Fig. 11.2E shows that there is no disc protrusion and the nerve roots, spinal ganglion and spinal nerves are normal. Because this young man was going to lose his employment as he was considered a malingerer, steps were taken to try to prove that he had internal disc disruption or an anular tear.

Erect posture left (Fig. 11.2F) and right (Fig. 11.2G) lateral bending radiographs were taken. It can be seen that the disc spaces above the L5 vertebra wedge from being narrow on the concave side to wide on the convex side on lateral bending. However, there is apparently no movement between the transverse processes of L5 and the sacral ala on comparing the left and right sides for both left and right lateral bending. Because further evidence was required to confirm that he did have internal disc disruption and a probable tear of the anular fibres, it was necessary to perform a discogram, a procedure which, according to Clifford (1986), Shapiro (1986) and Wiley et al (1968), is a barbaric and a non-efficacious procedure that can have significant complications (Yochum and Rowe, 1996). However, a discogram had to be ordered to override the suggestions that he was a malingerer and the lateral view of the L5–S1 disc is shown in Fig. 11.2H. This figure clearly shows tracking of the contrast medium posteriorly. A CT scan of the L5–S1 disc containing contrast material (following the discogram) clearly shows a full thickness left posterolateral tear in the anular fibres with some internal disc disruption (Fig. 11.2I).

Referral to an orthopaedic surgeon for a second opinion confirmed that 'the posterior anular tear would cause his low back pain syndrome'.

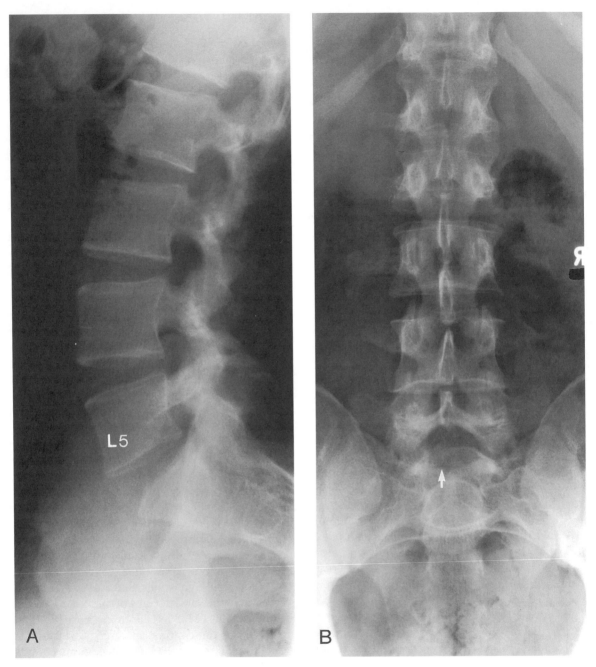

Figure 11.2 Caption is on next page.

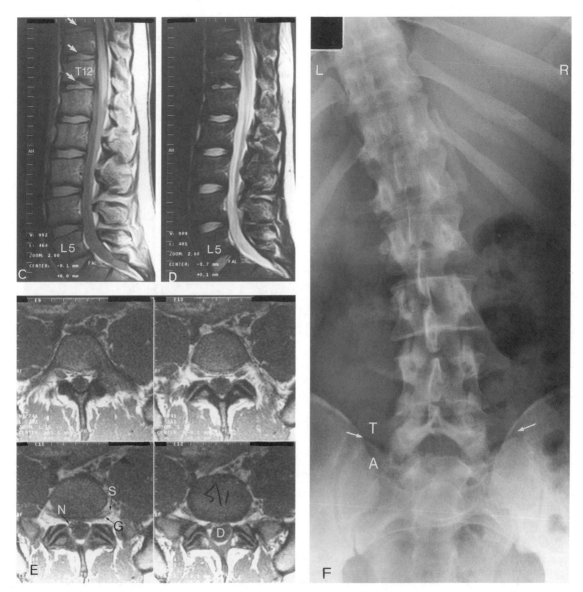

Figure 11.2 (A) A normal plain X-ray lateral view of the lumbosacral spine. L5 = fifth lumbar vertebra. (B) A normal plain X-ray anteroposterior view of the lumbosacral spine apart from a very minor spina bifida occulta at the S1 level (arrow). (C) MRI sagittal T1-weighted image of the lumbosacral spine. Note the Schmorl's nodes (vertebral body end plate fractures due to vertical rupture of nucleus pulposus material) at the T10, T11 and T12 levels (white arrows). (D) MRI sagittal T2-weighted image of the lumbosacral spine. (E) Normal MRI axial images of the L5–S1 level. Note the nerve root (N), spinal ganglion (G) and spinal nerve (S). D = Dural tube; RF = right side of patient. (F) Erect posture left lateral bending anteroposterior radiograph of the lumbosacral spine. Note that the disc spaces above the L5 vertebra wedge from being narrow on the left to wide on the right. However, there is apparently no movement between the transverse processes (T) of L5 and the sacral ala (A) (white arrows).

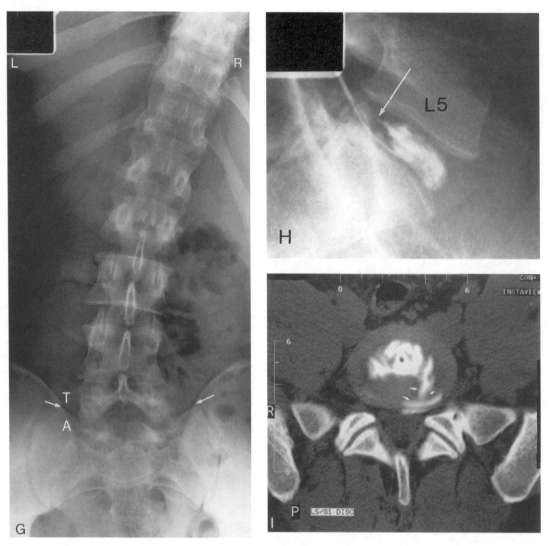

Figure 11.2 (G) Erect posture right lateral bending anteroposterior radiograph of the lumbosacral spine. Note that the disc spaces above the L5 vertebra wedge from being narrow on the right to wide on the left. However, there is apparently no movement between the transverse processes (T) of L5 and the sacral ala (A) (white arrows). (H) Lateral view discogram of the L5–S1 disc which shows tracking of the contrast medium posteriorly (arrow). (I) A CT scan of the L5–S1 disc containing contrast material following the discogram which clearly shows a full thickness left posterolateral tear in the anular fibres (arrows) with some internal disc disruption centrally.

TREATMENT

The patient was told exactly what was causing his symptoms. He was greatly relieved to finally have a diagnosis made and to be told that he had an organic cause for his pain that clearly was not in his head. He agreed to have an epidural block injection and this gave some relief and he was advised to only perform light duties and to keep fit and ensure that his muscles remained strong and supportive for his low back. Apart from walking and swimming, he was advised to perform the same exercise programme as those exercises advised for Case Number 10.

RESULTS

The patient continues to experience minor inter-mittent low back pain with some pain and paraesthesiae extending into his left lower limb, some four years after his injury. He is reluctant to have any invasive procedure and only per-forms light duties.

Note

It is important to visualize what internal disc disruption looks like at the gross anatomical level (Fig. 11.3A) and what it can look like in the early histopathological stage (Fig. 11.3B).

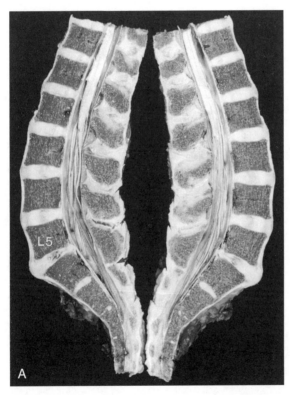

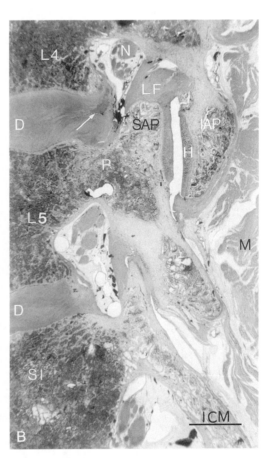

Figure 11.3 (A) Anatomical specimen of a sagittally sectioned spine. Note the approximation (black arrow) of the elongated fifth lumbar spinous process and the adjacent sacral spinous tubercle, in spite of the normal lumbar lordosis in this 70-year-old female. The L5 intervertebral disc shows degenerative changes which include (i) anterior 'bulging' of the disc, and (ii) posterior herniation of the disrupted nucleus pulposus which has elevated the posterior longitudinal ligament above and below this disc level. (Reproduced with permission from Giles LGF. Miscellaneous pathological and developmental (anomalous) conditions. In: Giles L G F, Singer K P (eds) 1997 *Clinical anatomy and management of low back pain*. Butterworth-Heinemann, Oxford, pp 196–216.) (B) A 200-micron thick histopathology sagittal section showing a tear within the L4–5 intervertebral disc with retrograde movement of nuclear material in this disc (arrow). In this post-mortem material the L5–S1 intervertebral disc is essentially normal and does not show movement of nuclear material within it. However, a few small blood vessels (dark dots) are seen within the posterior fibres of the disc. D = intervertebral disc; H = hyaline articular cartilage on the inferior articular process of L4; IAP = inferior articular process of the L4 vertebra; L4 = part of the fourth lumbar vertebral body; L5 = part of the fifth lumbar vertebral body; LF = ligamentum flavum; M = muscles; N = neural structures within the nerve root sheath located in the pear-shaped intervertebral foramen; P = pedicle of the L5 vertebra; SAP = superior articular process of the L5 vertebra; S1 = part of the first sacral segment. (Erhlich's haematoxylin and light green counterstain). See also colour plate section.

It should be noted that *internal disc disruption and anular tears are not part of the normal ageing process*. Discs can be perfectly normal even in the 70-year age group as shown by the specimen in Fig. 11.3A where the discs are normal except for at the L5–S1 level where there is internal disc disruption with anterior and posterior bulging of disc material. Clearly this is a phenomenon related to injury and it is not related to the ageing process, as only one disc in the 70-year-old spine showed internal disc disruption and those above are perfectly normal with a normal nucleus pulposus and anulus fibrosus.

Key point(s)

1. A 'normal' MRI study does not mean the disc is normal – there may be internal disc disruption and/or an anular tear allowing disc material to inflame the adjacent neural structures.
2. Osti and Fraser (1992) in their study of lumbar discs showed that 'discography is more accurate than MRI for the detection of anular pathology'. Furthermore, the study by Schellhas et al (1996) on cervical spine discs showed that 'significant cervical disc anular tears often escape magnetic resonance imaging detection'.

REFERENCES

Clifford J R 1986 Lumbar discography. An outdated procedure (letter). Journal of Neurosurgery 64: 686.

Osti O L, Fraser R D 1992 MRI and discography of annular tears and intervertebral disc degeneration. Journal of Bone and Joint Surgery 74-B (3): 431–435.

Schellhas K P, Smith M D, Gundry C R, Pollei S R 1996 Cervical discogenic pain. Prospective correlation of magnetic resonance imaging and discography in asymptomatic subjects and pain sufferers. Spine 21: 300–312.

Shapiro R 1986 Current status of lumbar discography (letter). Radiology 159: 815.

Yochum T R, Rowe L J 1996 Essentials of skeletal radiology, 2nd edn. Williams & Wilkins, Baltimore, p 555.

Wiley J J, MacNab I, Wortzman G 1986 Lumbar discography and its clinical applications. Canadian Journal of Surgery 11: 280–289.

FURTHER READING

Cooke P J, Lutz G E 2000 Internal disc disruption and axial back pain in the athlete. Physical Medicine and Rehabilitation Clinics of North America 11: 837–865.

Crock H V 1970 A reappraisal of intervertebral disc lesions. Medical Journal of Australia 1: 983–989.

Sachs B L 1989 Discography as a diagnostic modality for use in low back pain. In: Guyer RD (ed.) Spine, lumbar disc disease, Vol 3 (1). Hanley and Belfus, Philadelphia, pp 49–55.

Shalen P R 1989 Radiological techniques for diagnosis of lumbar disc degeneration. In: Guyer RD (ed.) Spine, lumbar disc disease, Vol 3 (1). Hanley and Belfus, Philadelphia, pp 27–48.

Case 12 Lumbosacral metastasis

COMMENT
There are three important lessons to be learned from this case viz: (i) beware of spinal night pain, (ii) always carefully examine imaging films and never just read the report, and (iii) remember that laboratory tests can be normal in spite of pathological processes.

PROFILE

A 40-year-old woman of average build who is a non-smoker and a non-drinker.

PAST HISTORY

She had always been very fit.

PRESENTING COMPLAINT (Fig. 12.1)

Constant chronic central low back pain with a 'burning and aching' quality following a fall approximately 1 year prior to consultation. She had seen a chiropractor for low back manipulation and her general medical practitioner for NSAIDs but without any relief of pain. The pain is of variable intensity and she was beginning to develop pain in the right buttock and hip joint region extending to the lateral aspect of the thigh. On awakening in the morning, her back pain was minimal, but as the day progressed her pain increased, even though she did not perform heavy work as an office worker.

The low back pain is aggravated by any sudden movements or twisting and with sneezing and coughing. The low back pain increases with menstruation. She takes two analgesics on going to bed in order not to be awakened by low back pain during the night. She had had a cortisone injection into the right hip joint for bursitis but without any relief.

AETIOLOGY

This was considered to be due to having fallen approximately 1 year prior to consultation, and the significance of night pain previously had been overlooked.

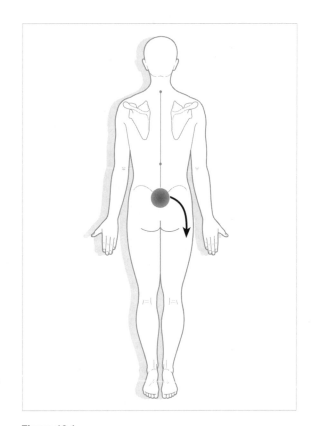

Figure 12.1

69

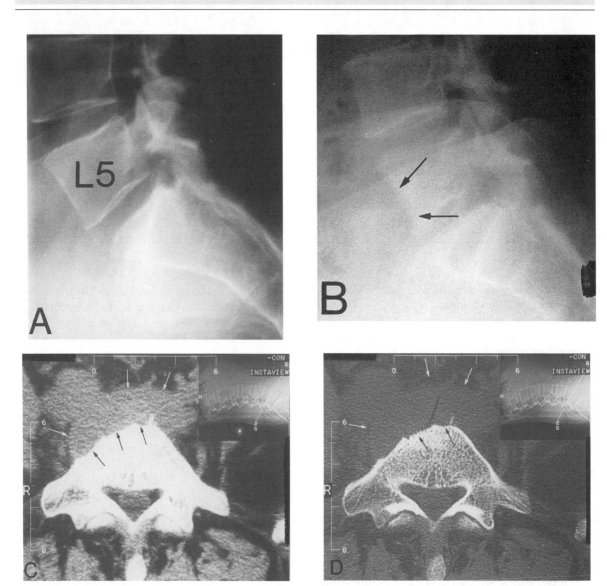

Figure 12.2 (A) A plain X-ray lateral view of the L4–S2 level. Note the 'minimal narrowing of the L5–S1 intervertebral disc'. (B) A plain X-ray lateral view of the lumbosacral spine region taken 12 months after the X-ray shown in (A). Note the minor concave appearance of the anterior aspect of the L5 vertebral body (arrows). (C) A CT axial soft tissue view through the upper one-third of the L5 vertebral body. Note the pre-vertebral soft tissue density, with similar density to muscle tissue, anterior to the vertebral body margin (white arrows) and the bony erosion along the anterior cortical margin of the L5 body (black arrows). R = right side of patient. (D) A CT axial bone window view showing the features mentioned in (C). R = right side of patient. (E) Bone scan coronal views showing increased uptake in the L5 vertebral body (arrow). (F) Bone scan horizontal view through the L5 body showing the increased uptake in the L5 vertebral body (arrows) and what appears to be a hotspot in the T11 body, although this is at the very edge of the SPECT scanning and therefore could be due to possible 'edge effect' (short black arrows). (G) A sagittal T2-weighted MRI scan of the lumbosacral spine showing 'significant soft tissue mass in the subligamentous location' anterior to the L5 vertebral body (white arrows) with some post-contrast enhancement within the L5 vertebral body consistent with inflammatory response related to this erosive process (black arrows). Note the Schmorl's node in the upper endplate of the T11 vertebra. (H) A MRI axial T1-weighted view, through the upper one-third of the L5 vertebral body, showing the subligamentous soft tissue mass (white arrows) with erosion of the anterior aspect of the right half of the vertebral body (black arrows). R = right side of patient.

E
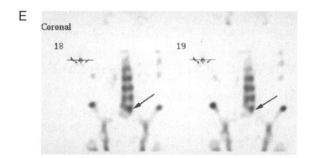

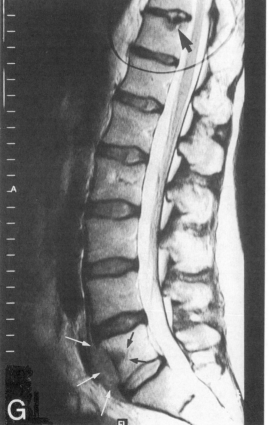

F
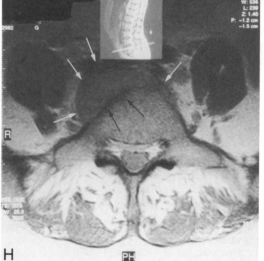

Figure 12.2 Caption is on previous page.

EXAMINATION

The deep reflexes in the lower extremities were normal as was muscle power. Pinprick sensation and vibration sensation were normal. There was no evidence of leg length inequality. Sitting in the slumped forward position did not aggravate the low back pain; the addition of SLR did not cause any increase in low back pain. Active supine SLR was of full range and painless. Hip joint tests were normal apart from slight discomfort on performing the right Fabere Patrick test.

Lumbar spine active ranges of movement were as follows:

1. Flexion was full and painless.
2. Extension was limited by approximately 10% due to slight low back 'discomfort'.
3. Right lateral bending was limited by approximately 10% but painless, while left lateral bending caused some low back 'discomfort' with approximately 10% limitation of movement.

The abdomen appeared to be normal.

CLINICAL IMPRESSION

Lumbosacral significant pathology in view of the *night pain* and because the deep reflexes, SLR, vibration sensation and pinprick sensation were normal.

IMAGING REVIEW

Pelvis and lumbar spine radiographs performed 12 months prior to consultation were reported as normal apart from 'minimal narrowing of the L5–S1 intervertebral disc'. However, upon review, the oblique view indicated some minor concavity of the right anterolateral part of the L5 body, even though the lateral view (Fig. 12.2A) and other views appeared to be normal.

WHAT ACTION SHOULD BE TAKEN?

In view of the night pain that required two Neurofen tablets upon going to bed, in order to minimize the pain, the following laboratory (Boxes 12.1 and 12.2) and imaging tests were performed.

Repeat plain radiographic anteroposterior and lateral views were taken of the lumbosacral spine; the report stated 'no significant bony abnormality shown'. However, this was clearly incorrect, as there was a minor concave appearance of the anterior aspect of the L5 vertebral body (see Fig. 12.2B). Therefore, a CT scan and a bone scan were ordered.

Box 12.1 Chemical pathology			
Specimen type		**Units**	**Reference range**
ALP (alkaline phosphatase)	69	U/l	(30–115)
C-reactive protein	5.8	mg/l	(0–10)

Box 12.2 Haematology			
		Units	**Reference range**
Haemoglobin	120	g/l	(115–165)
White cell count	7.6	$\times 10^9$/l	(3.5–12.0)
Platelets	329	$\times 10^9$/l	(150–400)
Haematocrit	0.37		(0.35–0.47)
Red cell count	4.3	$\times 10^{12}$/l	(3.9–5.6)
MCV (mean corpuscular volume)	86	fl	(81–97)
MCH (mean corpuscular haemoglobin)	28	pg	(27–34)
MCHC (mean corpuscular haemoglobin concentration)	322	g/l	(310–360)
Neutrophils	4.16	$\times 10^9$/l	(2.5–8.0)
Lymphocytes	2.83	$\times 10^9$/l	(1.2–4.0)
Monocytes	0.54	$\times 10^9$/l	(0.0–0.8)
Eosinophils	0.07	$\times 10^9$/l	(0.0–0.6)
Basophils	0.01	$\times 10^9$/l	(0.0–0.3)
ESR (erythrocyte sedimentation rate)	18	mm/hr	(2–20)

Ovarian tumour markers were very slightly increased

The CT soft tissue axial scan at L5–S1 (Fig. 12.2C) and the bone window scan (Fig. 12.2D) both showed some loss of the right anterolateral margin of the L5 body with an adjacent soft tissue mass.

The bone scan views (Fig. 12.2E and F) showed 'very minimally increased uptake in the superior aspect of the anterior part of the L5 vertebral body, suggesting a minor degree of non-specific osteoblastic activity in the anterior aspect of the L5 body'. A focus of increased uptake was also seen in the region of the T10 vertebral body. Therefore, a lumbar MRI study was ordered. The MRI (Fig. 12.2G and H) showed:

Pre-vertebral subligamentous mass eroding the anterior aspect of the L5 vertebral body with maintenance of the adjacent disc spaces, suggesting that an inflammatory process is less likely than a neoplastic process with metastatic deposit or subligamentous lymphoma; consideration should be given to a granulomatous type infection. An acute Schmorl's node is demonstrated involving the upper endplate of T11 (Fig. 12.2G) accounting for the hot spot seen on the bone scan.

Upon consultation with the radiologist about the T11 'Schmorl's node', he felt confident that this is a Schmorl's node and not a secondary deposit.

In view of these findings, a CT-guided fine needle aspiration was performed for microscopic cytology examination and Ziehl–Neelsen's stain for acid fast bacilli. This showed 'inflammatory cells and inflammatory debris. Some apoptotic cells with epithelial appearance very suspicious of neoplasia rather than infective or just purely inflammatory condition. No acid fast bacilli seen; no growth and cultures. Follow-up suggested'.

A chest X-ray study and a CT thorax were ordered to look for possible metastases; these showed 'clear lungs and a normal heart and mediastinum with no significant axillary, mediastinal or hilar adenopathy; superior aspect of liver and spleen unremarkable'. A CT abdomen and pelvis found 'the liver, spleen, pancreas and gall bladder to be normal' and confirmed the 'ill-defined soft tissue anterior to the L5 body'.

The patient was advised to have a gynaecological examination by a gynaecologist and a hysteroscopy showed no abnormality.

She was referred to an orthopaedic surgeon for review and she was sent for a nuclear medicine whole body scan using cells labelled with technetium and single proton emission computerized tomography (SPECT) that 'suggested infiltration of the L5 body is more likely than inflammatory pathology; the liver is enlarged'.

A follow-up needle aspiration biopsy found tumour cells of undifferentiated epithelial origin, so a diagnosis was made of a secondary tumour from an unknown primary location.

TREATMENT

The patient was referred to an oncologist for ongoing management.

Key point(s)
1. Beware of night pain!
2. Always carefully examine imaging in spite of a 'normal' report.
3. Routine laboratory tests can be normal in spite of serious pathology.

FURTHER READING

Ellis H 1996 Back, pain in. In: Bouchier IAD, Ellis H, Fleming PR (eds) French's index of differential diagnosis, 13th edn. Butterworth-Heinemann, Oxford. pp 44–53.

Frymoyer J F 1997 The adult spine: principles and practice, 2nd edn. Lippincott, Raven, Philadelphia.

Moll R 1998 Cytokeratins as markers of differentiation in the diagnosis of epithelial tumors. Subcellular Biochemistry 31: 205–262.

Yochum T R, Rowe L J 1996 Essentials of skeletal radiology, 2nd edn. Williams & Wilkins, Baltimore.

Case 13   Grade 1 spondylolisthesis

COMMENT
Spinal surgery can be helpful in carefully selected cases.

PROFILE

A 44-year-old slim man with reasonably good muscle tone who smokes approximately 50 cigarettes per week and drinks beer.

PAST HISTORY

He said he had fallen through a ceiling 3 years ago but did not injure his low back although he had previously experienced intermittent low back pain.

PRESENTING COMPLAINT (Fig. 13.1)

Severe low back pain that radiates to the right buttock and intermittently to the ankle since lifting heavy boxes at work 1 month ago.

Walking up steps aggravated the low back pain, as did coughing. On awakening in the morning he experienced low back pain. Heat was of no help. Cold aggravated the low back pain so he wore a low back support belt during the winter months to keep his lower back warm.

He had been treated with rest, NSAIDs and analgesics which had given him some relief and this was followed by physiotherapy treatment. He returned to work approximately 2 weeks later but found that his back was too painful for working so he stopped.

AETIOLOGY

Sudden onset of severe low back pain which came on while lifting heavy boxes.

EXAMINATION

On deep palpation of the paraspinal muscles, there was tenderness throughout the lumbo-sacral spine and in the right buttock centrally. Power in the lower extremities was normal and SLR was to 90° bilaterally before he experienced

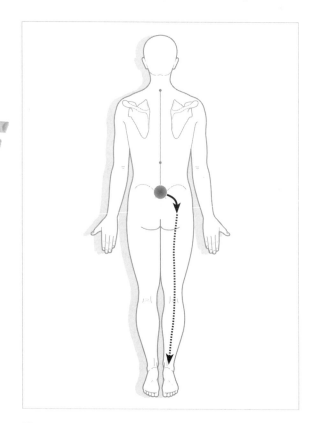

Figure 13.1

low back pain on right SLR. The right knee and ankle deep tendon reflexes were reduced to 1 plus (2 plus being normal).

IMAGING REVIEW

A plain film radiograph showed a Grade 1 spondylolisthesis of L5 on S1 with bilateral pars defects (Fig. 13.2A). A bony spicule projecting into the L5–S1 intervertebral foramen was present on the right side. The L5–S1 intervertebral disc was very thin and there were anterior osteophytes adjacent to it on the L5 and S1 bodies.

CLINICAL IMPRESSION

Grade 1 spondylolisthesis of L5 on S1 with right L5 nerve root entrapment and probable L5–S1 disc bulge/protrusion.

WHAT ACTION SHOULD BE TAKEN?

A CT scan was ordered and this showed a large central and right-sided disc herniation.

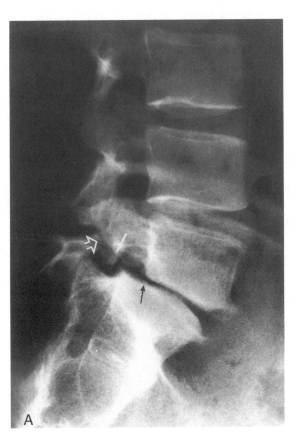
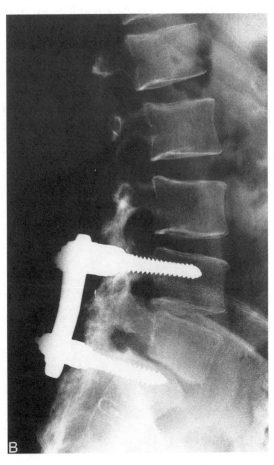

Figure 13.2 (A) A lateral view X-ray of the lumbosacral region showing the grade 1 spondylolisthesis of L5 on S1 with advanced thinning of the intervertebral disc at this level and osteophytic lipping at the anterior margins of the L5 and S1 bodies. The open arrow shows the fractured pars interarticulares. The white arrow indicates the bone spicule projecting into the right L5–S1 intervertebral foramen. The black arrow shows the degree of spondylolisthesis, i.e. the L5 body has moved approximately one quarter of the distance along the sacral body, hence the grade 1 classification according to Meyerding's (1932) classification (Giles & Singer 1997, Yochum & Rowe 1996). (B) A post-surgical lateral view of the lumbosacral region showing the pedicle screw fixation from L4 to S1 and the patent L5–S1 intervertebral foramen following removal of the bony spicule.

The patient was referred to an orthopaedic surgeon for an opinion regarding possible stabilization of the spondylolisthesis and removal of the bony spicule projecting into the right L5–S1 intervertebral foramen and a discectomy.

TREATMENT

A posterolateral spinal fusion was performed from L4 to the sacrum (Fig. 13.2B) with decompression of the nerve roots on the right side, and removal of the central and right-sided disc herniation. The post fusion result shown in Fig. 13.2B shows the pedicle screw fixation from L4 to S1 with a patent intervertebral foramen following removal of the bony spicule.

RESULTS

He reported that he had no more leg pain and also had excellent relief of back pain.

Following surgery, this man periodically suffered from low back pain and responded well to needle acupuncture treatment on a symptomatic basis.

Key point

In carefully selected cases, spinal surgery can be successful.

REFERENCES

Giles L G F 1997 Miscellaneous pathological and developmental (anomalous) conditions. In: Giles LGF, Singer KP (eds) Clinical anatomy and management of low back pain, Vol. 1. Butterworth-Heinemann, Oxford, pp 196–216.
Meyerding H W 1932 Spondylolisthesis. Surgery, Gynecology & Obstetics 54: 471–477.
Yochum T R, Rowe L J 1996 Essentials of skeletal radiology, 2nd edn. Williams & Wilkins, Baltimore, pp 237–372.

FURTHER READING

Postacchini F 1999 Lumbar disc herniation. Springer-Verlag, New York.
Weinstein J N, Rydevik B L, Sonntag V K H 1995 Essentials of the spine. Raven Press, New York.

Case 14 Cauda equina syndrome

COMMENT
Cauda equina syndrome is a condition that
demands prompt surgical intervention.

PROFILE

A 48-year-old male of solid build who normally
performs light duties. He does not smoke and only
drinks alcohol occasionally.

PAST HISTORY

He had previously experienced minor intermittent
low back pain, without radiation, for approximately
6 years for which he had periodically undergone
successful chiropractic manipulation and
physiotherapy, heat and exercises. There was no
other past medical history of significance.

PRESENTING COMPLAINT (Fig. 14.1)

He presented with central low back pain of
approximately 6 weeks duration that radiated
to the left buttock , left calf and ankle. His symptoms were worse in the morning but, on getting
up and moving around, they lessened somewhat. The symptoms had become acute 2 days
before, when he had sneezed.

AETIOLOGY

The original cause was due to bending forwards
to pick up a relatively light object.

EXAMINATION

In the erect posture, there was no pelvic obliquity and straining the sacroiliac joints did not
cause any sacroiliac joint pain but caused some
pain at the lumbosacral area. Active lumbar
spine ranges of movement were as follows:

1. Flexion – very limited due to an increase in
   low back pain.
2. Extension – full range and painless.

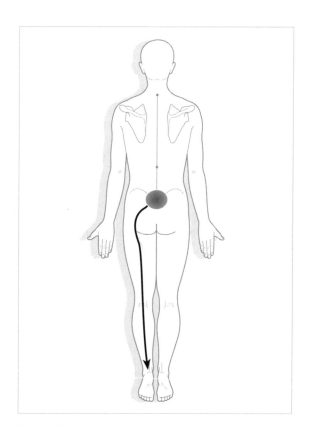

Figure 14.1

3. Left and right lateral bending – both movements caused an increase in pain on the left of the L5–S1 level.
4. Right rotation caused a significant increase in low back pain but left rotation caused only a slight 'pulling' sensation on the left of the lumbosacral level.

The deep reflexes in the lower extremities were normal as was the plantar response. Pinprick sensation elicited hypoaesthesia on the lateral aspect of the left calf (L5). Sitting slumped forward caused an increase in low back pain; addition of left SLR to a measured 15° caused a significant increase in low back pain that radiated to the left thigh posteriorly. Supine SLR was limited to 20° (left) and 75° (right) due to low back pain. Bilateral hip flexion caused slight low back pain. Vibration sensation at the ankles was normal.

IMAGING REVIEW

No previous imaging was available.

CLINICAL IMPRESSION

L4 or L5 disc protrusion.

WHAT ACTION SHOULD BE TAKEN?

He was referred for plain film radiographs and the report stated 'no obvious significant disc space narrowing'. However, he was referred for a CT scan of the L3, L4 and L5 discs and was given a NSAID. The CT scan showed a central to left-sided soft disc prolapse at L4–5 impinging upon the anterior part of the thecal sac.

TREATMENT

He underwent a trial of acupuncture treatment and was advised to walk but not to lift anything or twist his spine. He was also advised to sit down to dry his feet after showering and to rest periodically if the symptoms became aggravated.

RESULTS

Ten days later he noticed a significant improvement. However, prolonged sitting aggravated the left sciatica. On returning to work his symptoms were aggravated and he experienced a recurrence of sciatica extending to the left ankle. Flexion distraction chiropractic treatment (3×20 second distraction) was tried and this provided some relief. The combination of anti-inflammatory medication, acupuncture and flexion distraction treatment enabled him to perform some normal activities such as being able to personally remove his socks. Lumbar spine ranges of movement began to increase and he said he was sleeping well. Approximately 2 months after treatment was commenced he was carrying some items when he suddenly twisted his back and caused a severe exacerbation of low back pain with left buttock pain, sciatica and paraesthesiae in the left foot; he also had left leg cramps, so he returned for a further consultation. Examination showed that he now walked with difficulty, had a loss of pinprick sensation in the S1 dermatome of the left foot and a decrease in pinprick sensation in the anal region as well as a decrease of anal sphincter tone.

He was immediately referred for an emergency surgical opinion with a diagnosis of cauda equina syndrome because this condition demands prompt surgical intervention (Henriques et al 2001).

An MRI investigation (Fig. 14.2) was not performed until 7 hours after presentation with cauda equina syndrome and this showed 'L4–5 canal stenosis due to a broad-based disc protrusion, more prominent on the left, causing a moderately severe canal and lateral recess stenosis at the level of the disc with a developmentally small canal'.

He then noted that he could not move the toes on his left foot, although he could move the entire foot, and he felt numbness from the low back to his toes. He was catheterized as he now had urinary incontinence.

Approximately 23 hours following the diagnosis of cauda equina syndrome he underwent a laminectomy for the removal of a single large

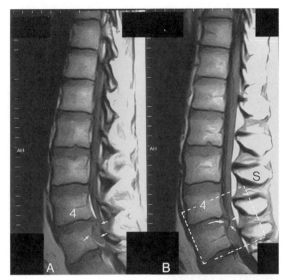

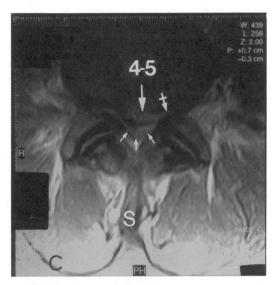

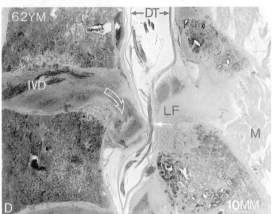

Figure 14.2 (A) Sagittal MRI T1-weighted image showing inferior extension of the large L4–5 disc protrusion (arrows) causing moderately severe canal stenosis. (B) Sagittal MRI T1-weighted image showing the large disc protrusion at the L4–5 level (arrow) that compresses the cauda equina posteriorly (small white arrows). S = spinous process. The rectangle shows the orientation for the histopathology section described in (D). (C) Axial MRI T1-weighted image showing the large L4–5 level broad based central to left-sided disc protrusion (large white arrow) producing moderately severe spinal canal and left lateral recess stenosis (tailed arrow). The small arrows show the considerable compression of the dural tube containing the cauda equina nerve roots. S = spinous process; R = right side of patient. A large central to lateral left-sided disc protrusion can be represented as shown in the postmortem histological preparation (D). (D) A 200-micron thick histopathology para-sagittal section from a 62-year-old male cadaveric spine. The large open arrow shows pro-truded disc material compressing the dural tube (DT) and a nerve root (small white arrow) between the protrusion and the ligamentum flavum (LF) posteriorly. As the section is 200 microns thick (1/5th of a millimetre thick) only one nerve root is seen being compressed. However, in a broad based disc protrusion a number of nerve roots would be com-pressed, thus causing the cauda equina syndrome. IVD = intervertebral disc. M = muscles. (Erhlich's haematoxylin and light green counterstain.) For orientation purposes, this para-sagittal plane histological section can be approximately equated to the rectangle in (B). See also colour plate section.

sequestration of nucleus pulposus at the L4–5 level.

Unfortunately, he had a very difficult few months with weakness of the left foot and having to use self-catheterization; he was left with impaired left lower limb power and sen-sory changes. Although bowel and bladder func-tion are now normal some months post surgery,

(a)

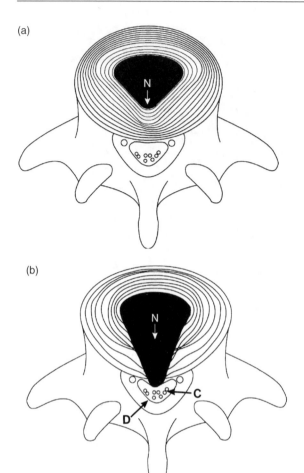

(b)

Figure 14.3 (a) The nucleus pulposus (N) is bulging into the approximately 90 layers of anular fibres located at the posterior of the disc. (b) The nucleus pulposus (N) has now ruptured through the anular fibres and is pressing upon the dural tube/thecal sac (D) containing the cauda equina (C) nerve roots which become compressed.

he has been left with left lower limb weakness, atrophy of some muscles and some neurological dysfunction.

Key point(s)

1. A patient with cauda equina syndrome requires very urgent surgical intervention to decompress the cauda equina otherwise serious complications will occur.
2. Figure 14.3(a) schematically represents how the nucleus pulposus may initially cause posterior bulging of the intervertebral disc then proceed to nuclear prolapse (Fig. 14.3(b)).

REFERENCE

Henriques T, Olerud C, Petren-Mallmin M, Ahi T 2001 Cauda equina syndrome as a postoperative complication in five patients operated for lumbar disc herniation. Spine 26: 293–297.

FURTHER READING

Ahn U M, Ahn N U, Buchowski J M, Garrett E S, Sieber A N, Kostuik J P 2000 Cauda equina syndrome secondary to lumbar disc herniation: a meta-analysis of surgical outcomes. Spine 25: 1515–1522.
Pattern J 1996 Neurological differential diagnosis, 2nd edn. Springer-Verlag, New York.
Postacchini F 1999 Lumbar disc herniation. Springer-Verlag, New York.
Shapiro S 2000 Medical realities of cauda equina syndrome secondary to lumbar disc herniation. Spine 25: 348–351.

Case 15 Lumbar vertebral body compression fracture

COMMENT
Some patients appear to have a higher threshold for pain than do other patients, so be wary of treating without a detailed history, physical examination and appropriate imaging.

PROFILE

A tall (approximately 195 cm; 6 feet 5 inches) 54-year-old fit man who works in the building industry.

PAST HISTORY

Episodes of low back pain when lifting heavy objects or on bending down to tie his shoe laces

PRESENTING COMPLAINT (Fig. 15.1)

Constant thoracolumbar junction pain that radiates bilaterally to his low back and which began 5 days after a motor vehicle accident 18 months ago. He awakens with increased pain in the morning and has to get up early as he cannot lie in bed due to this pain.

Coughing does not normally cause an increase in pain but taking a deep breath may aggravate the thoracolumbar pain which then radiates around his chest.

Lifting concrete building blocks, weighing approximately 20 kg each, causes a significant increase in his thoracolumbar pains. Before his motor vehicle injury, he used to lay 300 to 500 building blocks each day but this activity has been significantly curtailed as a result of the injury.

NSAIDs caused 'stomach pains' so had to be stopped.

AETIOLOGY

A motor vehicle accident, in which he was a passenger in a car that caught the edge of the bitumen strip causing it to skid severely before the car hit a bank; it became airborne before landing heavily on its wheels. The patient hit his head on the roof of the car in spite of wearing a seat belt.

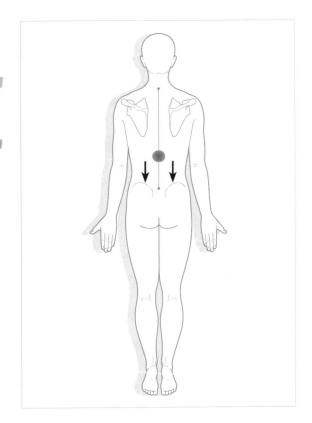

Figure 15.1

EXAMINATION

The knee jerks were asymmetrical in their response (++ on the left and + on the right). The ankle jerks were normal as were the pulses in both feet. Pinprick sensation of the thighs and calves was normal. Vibration sensation of the lower extremities was normal. The circumference of the thighs, 15 cm above the knee, was 47 cm (left) and 48 cm (right). The circumference of the calves, 13 cm below the knee, was 39 cm (left) and 38 cm (right). Power in the legs was normal. Left SLR caused slight lumbosacral pain at approximately 90° elevation. Bilateral hip flexion caused slight lumbosacral pain at approximately 120° elevation of the thighs from the examination table. The Naffziger test (compression of the jugular veins accompanied by coughing) caused some pain in the mid-thoracic spine. Percussion of the spine elicited pain from the thoracolumbar junction to the low back.

Active ranges of lumbar spine movement were as follows:

1. Flexion – the patient was able to touch the floor with his finger tips without any spinal pain.
2. Extension – limited by approximately 40% due to thoracolumbar pain.

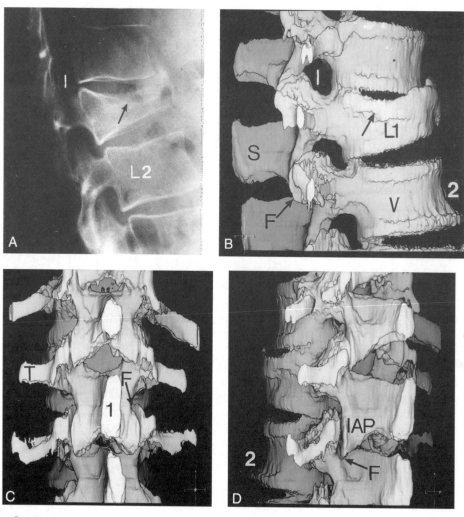

Figure 15.2 Caption is on next page.

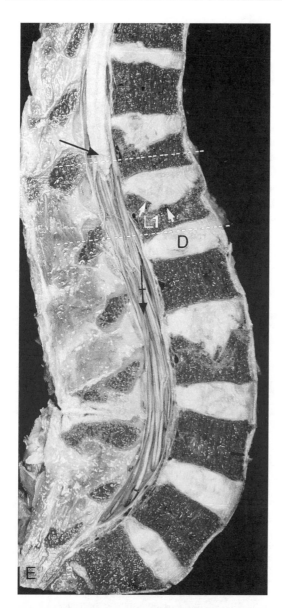

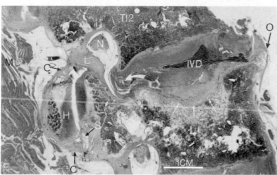

Figure 15.2 (A) A lateral thoracolumbar spine plain X-ray view showing a compression fracture of the superior endplate of the body of the L1 vertebra (arrow), consistent with a recent or relatively recent fracture. I = intervertebral foramen at the T12–L1 level; L2 = second lumbar vertebra. (B) A CT lateral 3-dimensional reconstruction view. This reconstruction view better shows the T12–L1 disc space with the compression of the superior endplate of the L1 vertebral body (arrow). There is some extension of the L1 vertebra on the L2 vertebra with subluxation/imbrication of the opposing facet surfaces (F) at L1–2. This subluxation is seen to be occurring bilaterally in the reconstruction (C) and is also clearly demonstrated in the oblique projection (D). I = intervertebral foramen; S = spinous process; V = vertebral body. Note how the intervertebral foramen at the L1–2 level (B) is distorted, when compared to the level above, because of the L1–2 subluxation of the facet surfaces due to the L1 vertebra tipping backwards ('extension') on the vertebra below. (C) CT postero-anterior 3-dimensional reconstruction view. T= transverse process; 1 = spinous process of the first lumbar vertebra; F = facet surface and subluxation. (D) CT oblique 3-dimensional reconstruction view. Note how the inferior articular process of the L1 vertebra (IAP) approximates the pars interarticularis area of the L2 vertebra below (2). F = facet surface and subluxation. (E) A gross anatomical postmortem specimen cut in the sagittal plane from a 78-year-old male showing several vertebral body fractures of the superior endplates at T12, L1 and L3 where disc material can be seen extending into the fractured vertebral body. D = intervertebral disc; L1 = first lumbar vertebra and the white arrows show how the disc material extends inferiorly. Large black arrow indicates the lower part of the spinal cord (conus medularis) from which the cauda equina (nerve roots) extend. The nerve roots are highly vascular and the tailed arrow shows a blood vessel on one of the nerve roots. The rectangle within the broken lines represents the area from which the histological section shown in (F) was obtained. (F) A 200-micron thick histopathology section cut in the sagittal plane through the L1 vertebral body compression fracture shown in (E). This shows an osteophyte (O) beginning to develop anteriorly. There is disruption of the intervertebral disc material (IVD) that extends inferiorly to the fractured vertebral body endplate (white arrows). There is some posterolateral bulging of disc material showing encroachment into the adjacent intervertebral foramen (curved white arrow). In this specimen, the intervertebral disc is bulging posteriorly (curved white arrow) into the lower part of the intervertebral foramen but it is still contained within the anular fibres. In addition, the subluxation of the opposing facet surfaces with their hyaline articular cartilage (H) is shown and this can result in tractioning of the joint capsule (C) and pinching of the synovial fold (S). H = hyaline articular cartilage on the inferior articular process of the T12 vertebral body; L = ligamentum flavum; L1 = first lumbar vertebra; M = muscle; N = neural structures within the intervertebral foramen. (Erhlich's haematoxylin and light green counterstain.)

3. Left and right rotation – slightly limited due to thoracolumbar 'stiffness'.

IMAGING REVIEW

No imaging was available.

CLINICAL IMPRESSION

Thoracolumbar injury to bone and or soft tissues.

WHAT ACTION SHOULD BE TAKEN?

Plain film thoracolumbar spine X-ray films were ordered (Fig. 15.2A) and showed a fracture of the L1 vertebral body. As more detail was deemed necessary to better visualize the L1 fracture, CT films were ordered, including a 3-D reconstruction (Fig. 15.2C and D). The CT scan report stated:

Some degeneration of the T12–L1 disc with gas seen in this disc space but there is no disc protrusion. There is no significant compromise of the spinal canal. The L1–2 disc is unremarkable and there is no disc protrusion at this level and no canal stenosis. The anterior wedge fracture of the L1 vertebral body is associated with only a very minimal bowing of the posterior vertebral body margin.

TREATMENT

He was advised to (i) change his employment so that he no longer has to lift heavy building blocks, (ii) perform only light duties, (iii) perform back muscle strengthening exercises (prone thoracic extension exercises), and (iv) to trial a course of needle acupuncture treatment to help with pain control as non-steroidal anti-inflammatory drugs caused gastric pain.

RESULTS

The above advice resulted in a satisfactory outcome for pain management.

Note

R. Maigne (1974, 1978) and J.-Y. Maigne (2000) pointed out that the cutaneous dorsal rami (cluneal nerve) of the T10–L1 or L2 root pass to the left and right iliac crests, explaining why pain may be felt in the low back area due to an injury at the thoracolumbar junction. The cluneal nerves pass over the iliac crest approximately 8 cm from the posterior iliac spine (Kostuik 1997).

In order to more clearly understand what may happen to the spine when a vertebral body compression fracture is sustained, a gross anatomical specimen is shown in the sagittal plane (Fig. 15.2E). This figure shows several vertebral fractures at the superior endplates of T12, L1 and L3; disc material can be seen extending into the fractured vertebral bodies. In this example there is no burst fracture with retropulsion of bone into the spinal canal. A histological section showing an endplate fracture in shown in Fig. 15.2F.

Key point(s)

1. Some patients with serious spinal injuries may have a high pain threshold that appears to trivialize a considerable injury.
2. When a vertebral body compression fracture is present it is important to determine whether only an endplate has fractured, as in this case, or whether there is an associated burst fracture component with bony material encroaching upon the spinal canal (see Case 45).

REFERENCES

Kostuik J P 1997 Failures after spinal fusion. In: Frymoyer JW (ed.) The adult spine. Principles and practice, 2nd edn. Lippincott-Raven, Philadelphia, pp 2277–2326.
Maigne J-Y 2000 Cervicothoracic and thoracolumbar spinal pain syndromes. In: Giles LGF, Singer KP (eds) Clinical anatomy and management of thoracic spine pain. Butterworth-Heinemann, Oxford, pp 157–170.
Maigne R 1974 Origine dorso-lombaire de certaines lombalgies basses. Role des articulations interapophysaires et des branches posterieures des nerfs rachidiens. Revue du Rhumatisme 41: 781–789.
Maigne R, Le Corre F, Judet H 1978 Lombalgies basses d'origine dorso-lombaire: traitement chirugical par excision des capsules articulaires posterieures. Nouvelle Presse Medicale 7: 565–568.

FURTHER READING

Frymoyer J W 1997 The adult spine. Principles and practice, 2nd edn. Lippincott-Raven, Philadelphia.

Case 16   Lumbosacral disc protrusion

COMMENT
Never label a patient as a malingerer unless you are absolutely certain of your facts.

PROFILE

A 25-year-old, tall, overweight woman who does not smoke and hardly ever drinks alcohol.

PAST HISTORY

Her past history was unremarkable.

PRESENTING COMPLAINT (Fig. 16.1)

She presented, upon referral from her general medical practitioner, with considerable low back pain and right greater than left leg pain. The leg pains extend down the posterolateral aspects of each leg to the heels. Apparently, it felt as though there was a 'permanent band of pain' across her low back as far as her hips, worse on the right side.

She had undergone an epidural block injection that caused numbness on the lateral aspect of her right thigh, just above the knee joint, and she had become unwell due to a severe post-epidural infection that required two antibiotics, via a drip, to resolve the infection. Approximately 1 month before consultation, she had been admitted to hospital for 2 weeks due to an acute recurrence of her low back and leg pains; Pethidine had been administered 4-hourly at one period because of her severe low back pain syndrome.

She had difficulty in getting to sleep because of the low back pain, so was taking two 5 mg Valium tablets before going to bed. This resulted in her having to take laxatives even though she was eating fruit and wholemeal bread. Coughing and sneezing caused an increase in low back pain. She stood with her right knee slightly flexed due to pain radiating to the right heel from her low back.

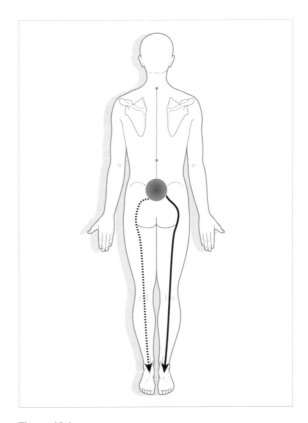

Figure 16.1

She had tried acupuncture but without long-lasting relief.

She now wore a rigid back support that does not allow her to bend or lift as her general medical practitioner thought this might help and, in fact, it does if she wears it at all times. The only time she takes it off is when she goes to bed and when she showers. A transcutaneous electrical nerve stimulator (TENS) and physiotherapy were of no help. Bladder and bowel functions were normal apart from constipation brought about by taking Valium. She tries not to use medication as she does not feel well on it and, when she recently took an analgesic, she developed an allergic reaction and the skin began to peel on the palms of her hands.

She had seen a number of neurosurgeons and orthopaedic surgeons, none of whom considered that surgery was a good option and she had, in fact, been labelled as a malingerer by the orthopaedic and neurosurgeons that she had consulted; this greatly distressed her and her family.

AETIOLOGY

The patient had first felt low back pain when working in a cramped space in which she had to bend and twist her spine. She said that, because she is tall, bending and twisting in the cramped space had placed a lot of strain on her low back. The work place was cramped because two people worked at the same time in a confined space. Apparently the pain began early during the course of her employment and it rapidly increased during several months of repetitive bending and twisting.

EXAMINATION

She stood up cautiously from the chair and removed the rigid back support. When she lay down on the examination table she was equally guarded about her movements and found it too painful to allow her right leg to lie flat on the table, so she kept it slightly flexed at the knee. SLR was limited by low back pain to 25° elevation (right) and to 30° (left). The slump test caused considerably increased low back pain at the lumbosacral area; the addition of SLR was greatly limited bilaterally due to increased low back pain. She could not perform active bilateral SLR as this caused a great deal of low back pain. Forward bending of the cervical spine, in the supine position, caused an increase in low back pain. Bilateral hip flexion was painful as soon as movement was felt at the lumbosacral region. The posterior tibial and dorsalis pedis pulses were normal. The left knee jerk (L2,3,4) was difficult to elicit, with only a slight response. The right knee jerk was normal, as was the case with the ankle jerks (S1,2) bilaterally. Pinprick sensation of the legs was normal, apart from an area of decreased sensation on the lateral aspect of the right thigh (L2,3) just above the knee joint, and her left fifth toe (S1). Vibration sensation at her ankles was normal. Her spine was very tender to palpation in the L4–S1 region.

Active lumbar spine ranges of movement were as follows:

1. Flexion – limited by 80% due to low back pain and her fingers could not reach to her knees.
2. Extension – limited by approximately 85% due to considerable low back pain.
3. Left and right rotation – limited by approximately 85% due to considerable low back pain.

There was no loss of power in her legs. The circumference of the calves, 11 cm below the knee cap, was 39.5 cm (left) and 40 cm (right); the thigh circumference was equal on both sides. Axial compression of the spine, due to pressing down on her shoulders, reproduced the low back pain.

IMAGING REVIEW

An MRI scan showed a moderately large central disc protrusion at the L5–S1 level that may be confined by the posterior longitudinal ligament which is displaced posteriorly (Fig. 16.2). The moderately severe degree of compression on the anterior aspect of the thecal sac is clearly visible. A much smaller posterior disc bulge at the L4–5

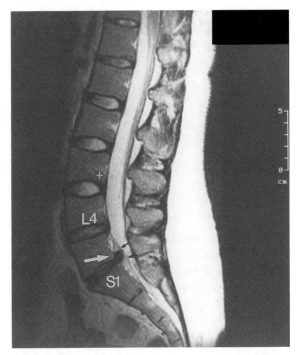

Figure 16.2 An MRI T2-weighted sagittal lumbar spine scan showing the moderately large central disc protrusion at the L5–S1 level (white arrow) that may be confined by the posterior longitudinal ligament which is displaced posteriorly. The moderately severe degree of compression on the anterior aspect of the dural tube/thecal sac is clearly visible (black arrows). Note that the L5–S1 intervertebral disc shows more advanced desiccation than does the L4–5 disc.

level was noted. The L5–S1 disc showed considerable desiccation as compared to the mildly desiccated L4–5 disc.

CLINICAL IMPRESSION

L5–S1 central disc protrusion.

WHAT ACTION SHOULD BE TAKEN?

She was sent to another surgeon who said surgery would not solve her problem. Over a period of approximately 10 months she developed a 2-cm loss of right thigh circumference, so she was sent interstate for a neurosurgical opinion.

TREATMENT

The surgeon to whom she was referred realized the significance of the L5–S1 posterior intervertebral disc protrusion and the associated clinical signs and symptoms and performed an L5–S1 discectomy.

RESULTS

The patient told me that the low back surgery was very helpful and that her pain had decreased dramatically. She occasionally felt slight pain in the right leg in the sciatic distribution and sometimes one foot felt 'colder' than the other. However, she stated that she is coping very well psychologically. In addition, she had considerably decreased her medication and had returned to work in a new light duties position. She still had some 'weakness' of her right leg intermittently, so she goes for frequent walks to exercise her low back and to strengthen her legs.

Key point(s)

1. Over the last 30 years it has been my experience that patients only very rarely malinger.
2. A careful history, physical examination and appropriate imaging will differentiate between genuine patients and malingerers.
3. When the history, physical examination and appropriate imaging correlate well with the patient's symptoms, it is negligent to label a patient as a malingerer.
4. Because a patient has a work-related injury it should not be automatically assumed that the patient is a malingerer.

FURTHER READING

Main C J, Waddell G 1989 Behavioural responses to examination. A reappraisal of the interpretation of 'nonorganic signs'. Spine 23: 2367–2371.
Margoshes B G, Webster B 2000 Why do occupational injuries have different health outcomes? In: Mayer TG, Gatchel RJ, Polatin PB (eds) Occupational musculoskeletal disorders, Lippincott Williams & Wilkins, Philadelphia, pp 47–61.

Case 17   Adolescent tethered cord syndrome

COMMENT
Always listen carefully to the patient, even when a complex and apparently bizarre symptom pattern is being described.

PROFILE

A 15-year-old schoolgirl who plays hockey and gets good grades for her school subjects.

PAST HISTORY

Her past history is non-contributory and she has no history of accidents or any serious infections. There is no history of bowel or bladder incontinence. Her general medical practitioner apparently did 'blood tests' approximately 2 months ago and said that there was nothing abnormal. An ultrasound scan performed of her abdomen in view of her unusual symptoms was normal. Her general medical practitioner considered that she had growing pains.

PRESENTING COMPLAINT (Fig. 17.1)

Chronic (approximately 3 years) increasing thoracolumbar junction pain that spreads down to the lower lumbar spine especially on the right side. She also experiences pain extending bilaterally into the buttocks and posterior to the hip joints, with some intermittent bilateral pain 'around the lower rib cage' laterally and anteriorly. The thoracolumbar pain begins in the morning and becomes progressively worse during the afternoon until it becomes 'really bad' by approximately 7.30 pm. Bearing down causes an increase in pain between the shoulder blades and at the thoracolumbar region with some increase in low back pain. Coughing aggravates the thoracolumbar junction pain. She feels generally 'tired' because of the pain which makes her feel 'weary'. She has taken Nurofen and Panadol without any relief. She is able to play hockey and this does not aggravate her symptoms while she is playing.

She thinks there is a night pain component (approximately 2.00 am) but is not certain.

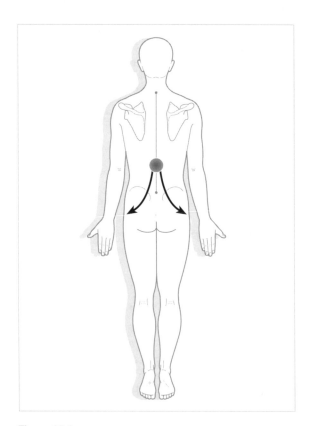

Figure 17.1

A secondary, and far less painful complaint, is some cervico-shoulder pain bilaterally, especially on the left side. There is no associated radiation and there are no arm symptoms. The minor neck pain has been present for approximately 6 months.

AETIOLOGY

Unknown. Gradual onset of progressive symptoms during the last 3 years.

EXAMINATION

In the erect posture there was no clinical evidence of pelvic obliquity or scoliosis. There was an increased lumbar lordosis. On the right side of the T10 region there was a faint skin blemish measuring 4.5×1.8 cm that does not blanch on pressure. She also had unusual horizontal striae across the thoracolumbar region. Toe and heel walking power were normal. The deep reflexes in the upper and lower extremities were normal. The plantar response was normal and pinprick sensation over the legs and the posterior part of the torso was normal. As she stated that she did not have any difficulty with sphincter control, pinprick sensation was not performed in the perianal area. Vibration sensation at the ankles was normal.

When seated in the slumped forward position, this aggravated the thoracolumbar pain; the addition of SLR caused a significant increase in this pain. Supine SLR caused low back pain at approximately 50° elevation of the left and right legs, respectively. Bilateral hip flexion aggravated her low back pain. Bilateral hip flexion with the addition of cervical spine flexion caused an increase in the thoracolumbar junction pain. Milgram's bilateral active SLR caused some low back pain but nothing significant. The Naffziger jugular compression test caused some increase in thoracolumbar junction pain. Hip joint mobility tests were normal. There was no paravertebral muscle spasm. Deep palpation of the paraspinal muscles between T10 and L5 elicited local tenderness. Pressure on the lumbosacral area with the patient prone caused some vague lumbar discomfort.

Active ranges of lumbar spine movement were as follows:

1. Flexion caused an increase in thoracolumbar pain when her fingers reached halfway down the tibia.
2. Extension caused an increase in pain at approximately the L3–4 level.
3. Left and right lateral bending caused some pain to extend from L2 to L5.
4. Left and right rotation caused pain in the approximately L2 to L4 region.

She had noted the following changes:

- She can walk less distance due to feeling 'tired', but walking does not cause numbness in the legs.
- Flexing the spine aggravates the thoracolumbar pain and extension causes some mid-lumbar spine pain.
- The thoracolumbar pain extends to the lumbosacral area, the sacrum and then to both inguinal areas and hips, with some knee pain.
- She cannot lie on her back at night due to lumbar spine pain, so she lies on her left side in a fetal position.
- Two of the three 'B' postures (Yamada et al 1996), i.e. sitting in the Budda pose and Bending slightly over the sink aggravated the lumbar spine pain; holding a small Baby or dog did not aggravate the lumbar spine pain.
- Sitting in a slouched position caused an increase in lumbar spine pain.
- Being driven in a car over an uneven surface, or for a long distance, caused an increase in thoracolumbar pain.
- After standing for 30 minutes, for example while cooking, the thoracolumbar pain becomes aggravated and, after an hour, extends into the hips.
- She had an exaggerated lumbar lordosis.
- There was no osseous or soft tissue anomaly involving the feet but she had an S1 spina bifida occulta.
- There was no obvious muscle weakness in the lower extremities, although she appeared to have minor instability of the ankle joints with slight inversion of the right ankle.

IMAGING REVIEW

Plain X-ray films taken 10 months previously were reported as normal. However, spina bifida occulta at the first sacral level was noted (Fig. 17.2A). The lateral lumbosacral view (Fig. 17.2B) did not show any abnormality.

CLINICAL IMPRESSION

1. A high suspicion of a functional tethered cord syndrome in view of the history, unusual symptoms and signs and the spina bifida occulta at S1.
2. A differential diagnosis of a neurofibroma at the T10 level in view of the faint skin blemish on the right side of the spine at this level.
3. Possible mechanical thoracolumbar joint pain.

Tests for nerve root tension did not provide a typical response for a space-occupying lesion, so such a lesion was considered unlikely.

WHAT ACTION SHOULD BE TAKEN?

Because of the clinical suspicion of a functional tethered cord syndrome an MR lumbar spine and sacrum was ordered. This was reported as follows: 'The vertebral bodies and disc spaces appear intact with no desiccation or narrowing. No focal disc herniation. The exit foramina and spinal canal appear normal in size. No paraspinal soft tissue abnormality. The conus is normal in position'. Because the filum appeared to approximate the posterior spinal structures within the spinal cord, the radiologist was asked to re-examine the imaging to check for a tethered cord but again reported that there was no evidence of tethered cord. Laboratory tests were ordered and the results are shown in Boxes 17.1 and 17.2.

As the results were essentially normal, apart from a very slight increased ESR and alanine transaminase, an opinion was sought from a specialist physician who was asked to consider this case in view of the spinal symptoms, the striae across the lumbar region and the skin blemish on the right side of the thoracolumbar region. The specialist physician performed the following laboratory tests and repeated several of the previous tests which were found to be normal (Boxes 17.3 and 17.4).

In addition, a bone scan was performed to look for any osseous lesion such as an osteoid osteoma. However, the bone scan was reported as normal with only mild increased uptake in the anterior ends of the ribs, the femoral growth plates and the sacroiliac joints, with

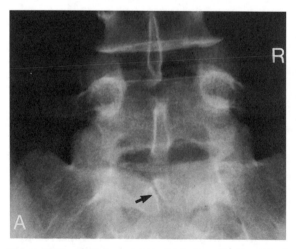
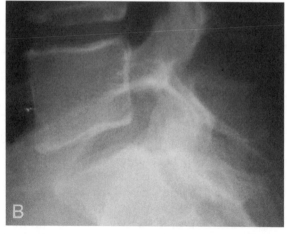

Figure 17.2 (A) Anteroposterior plain X-ray image of the lumbosacral region. Note the spina bifida occulta at the S1 level (black arrow). R = right side of patient. (B) This lateral lumbosacral plain X-ray image did not show any abnormality.

Box 17.1 Chemical pathology

		Units	Reference range
Status	Fasting		
Sodium	139	mmol/l	(135–145)
Potassium	**4.6**	mmol/l	(3.2–4.5)
Chloride	106	mmol/l	(100–110)
Bicarbonate	28	mmol/l	(22–33)
Anion gap	5	mmol/l	(4–13)
Osmolality (calculated)	277	mmol/kg	(270–290)
Glucose	5.5	mmol/l	(4–13)
Urea	3.7	mmol/l	(3.0–8.0)
Creatinine	0.06	mmol/l	(0.05–0.10)
Urea/creatinine	62		(40–100)
Protein (total)	75	g/l	(62–83)
Albumin	46	g/l	(33–47)
Globulin	29	g/l	(25–45)
Bilirubin (total)	8	μmol/l	(<20)
Alkaline phosphatase	63	U/l	(40–250)
Gamma-glutamyl transferase	13	U/l	(<50)
Alanine transaminase	**46**	U/l	(<40)
Aspartate transaminase	27	U/l	(<35)

Box 17.2 Haematology

		Units	Reference range
Haemoglobin	135	g/l	(120–160)
White cell count	6.1	×10⁹/l	(4.0–11.0)
Platelets	336	×10⁹/l	(140–400)
Haematocrit	0.39		(0.39–0.46)
Red cell count	4.52	×10¹²/l	(4.10–5.10)
MCV (mean corpuscular volume)	87	fl	(78–100)
Neutrophils	3.13	×10⁹/l	(2.0–8.0)
Lymphocytes	2.28	×10⁹/l	(2.0–8.0)
Monocytes	0.53	×10⁹/l	(0.10–1.00)
Eosinophils	0.15	×10⁹/l	(<0.60)
Basophils	0.01	×10⁹/l	(<0.20)
ESR (erythrocyte sedimentation rate)	**12**	mm/hr	(<10)
Rheum. factor (neph)	<20	IU/ml	(<20)

Box 17.3 Serum-specific protein chemistry

		Units	Reference range
Immunoglobulin G (total IgG)	9.87	g/l	(5.76–15.36)
Immunoglobulin A (total IgA)	**0.80**	g/l	(1.24–4.16)
Immunoglobulin M (total IgM)	1.34	g/l	(0.48–3.10)

Box 17.4 Serum autoantibodies

		Units	Reference range
Anti-nuclear antibody titre	Negative <1:40		
Anti-DNA (Farr assay)	<3	IU/ml	(<5)
Anti-ENA (ELISA)	Negative		
HIA B27	Peripheral blood negative		

ELISA, enzyme-linked immunosorbent assay

over the sacroiliac joints and in the region of the left hip joint, because her problem had developed over quite a time and appeared to be getting worse, and because her father suffers from psoriasis with a lot of aches and pains. The skin lesion on the right side of the spine was considered to be a plaque of morphea (a localized form of scleroderma); the striae were considered to be related to morphea having left characteristic scars. She was referred to a dermatologist regarding the skin changes and he concurred with the diagnosis of morphea.

TREATMENT

Three lumbar spine manipulations were performed to determine whether there was a mechanical component to her thoracolumbar pain but this was of no help. Naprosyn (750 mg) at night was prescribed to see if she would get pain relief through the night, with 500 mg Naprosyn in the morning. This provided some slight temporary relief, suggesting that she may have a rheumatological component.

these changes being related to growth plate activity in view of the patient's age. The specialist physician suggested that the patient very likely had a spondyloarthritis as there was approximately 4-cm restriction in the lumbar spine range of flexion, tenderness

However, the relief was short lived so the Naprosyn dose was increased to 2000 mg daily. Approximately 3 weeks later, she was started on Salazopyrin (1000 mg morning and night) but her symptoms gradually worsened.

A new lumbar spine MRI in the supine and prone positions was performed at a different facility with a specific request for careful examination for a 'functional tethered cord'. However, the report stated: *'There are no features of tethered cord or other dysraphic disorder'*. The full report follows:

The conus medullaris terminates normally at T12/L1 disc. The conus is normal in configuration and signal intensity with no focal lesion demonstrated. Cauda equina are normal. In the prone position the nerve roots are seen to separate freely with no evidence of arachnoiditis. There is no thickening of the filum terminale and there is no evidence of filum lipoma. There is no spinal stenosis. The intervertebral discs appear normal throughout. Marrow signal intensity of the vertebral elements is normal. No epidural or intradural mass lesion is identified. The paravertebral soft tissues appear normal.

A T2-weighted sagittal MRI view of the lumbosacral spine is shown in Fig. 17.3.

The patient determinedly kept going to school but, on returning home, would immediately lie down on the couch; she began to miss days at school and became depressed about her increasing thoracolumbar spine and buttock/hip joint pains and spent a lot of time in bed, lying prone in an attempt to lessen the lumbar spine pain.

Because of the persisting clinical impression of tethered cord syndrome, the patient was advised to obtain second opinions from another specialist physician, a neurologist and a neurosurgeon. The specialist physician could not provide a diagnosis for her symptoms and, because of clashing appointments, the patient did not see the neurologist but saw the neurosurgeon. The neurosurgeon suggested a further lumbar MRI and concluded that she did not have a tethered cord syndrome and strongly recommended against any surgical intervention but did state that he was not experienced enough to comment on the presence of tethered cord in the absence of MRI abnormality.

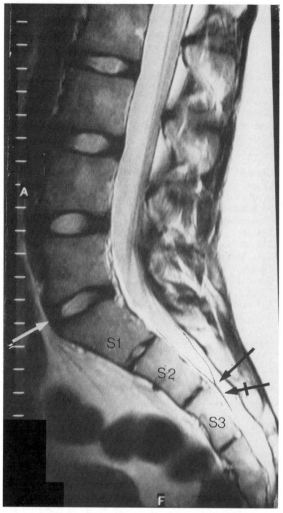

Figure 17.3 A sagittal T2-weighted lumbosacral MRI scan showing the thecal sac extending to the lower S2/upper S3 level (black arrow) with a suggestion of thickening of the filum at this level (tailed arrow). The L5–S1 intervertebral disc level is indicated by the white arrow.

The patient's MRI films were then sent to an authority on tethered cord who discussed the images with a radiologist and the conclusion was that, although there was no fat density found in the filum tip, the filum was displaced posteriorly to touch the posterior arachnoid membrane and the thecal sac extended to the lower S2 level (considered to be lower than usual) with a suggestion of thickening of the filum at this level. The patient was, therefore, advised to see another neurosurgeon, following a second bone scan that had been ordered by the specialist physician in view of the increasing symptoms, and which was, once again, reported as being within normal limits for her age. Meanwhile the patient stopped all medication to see if her symptoms would increase but they did not, so the specialist physician agreed that she did not have a rheumatological condition.

The second neurosurgeon decided that the symptoms could relate to a functional tethered cord syndrome and, because the patient was now beginning to get 'numbness in the legs and feet', he agreed to section the filum. An L5 laminectomy was performed to release the tethered spinal cord. At surgery, the filum was identified approaching the dorsal dura, and when the filum was divided, it spontaneously retracted cephalad.

RESULTS

The patient began to cautiously mobilize the next day, went home 4 days later and the staples were removed 6 days following surgery. She rapidly became asymptomatic and has made a complete physical and psychological recovery. Her mother says it is a pleasure to have her 'old' happy daughter back again.

Note

For a detailed understanding of tethered cord syndrome with its various presentations see the textbook edited by Yamada (1996).

Key point

In cases of unexplained lumbar, buttock and leg symptoms, clinical awareness of adult tethered cord syndrome due to cord dysfunction is important.

REFERENCE

Yamada S, Iacono R P, Douglas C C, Lonser R R, Shook J E 1996 Tethered cord syndrome in adults. In: Yamada S (ed.) Tethered cord syndrome. The American Association of Neurological Surgeons, Chicago, IL, pp 149–165.

FURTHER READING

Cartwright C 2000 Primary tethered cord syndrome: diagnosis and treatment of an insidious defect. Journal of Neuroscience Nursing 32: 210–215.
Marchiori D M, Firth R 1996 Tethered cord syndrome. Journal of Manipulative and Physiological Therapy 19: 265–267.
Oakes W J 1996 The borderlands of the primary tethered cord syndrome. Clinical Neurosurgery 43: 188–202.
Witkamp T D, Vandertop W P, Beek F J A, et al 2001 Medullary cone movement in subjects with a normal spinal cord and in patients with a tethered spinal cord. Radiology 220: 208–212.
Yamada S (ed.) 1996 Tethered cord syndrome. The American Association of Neurological Surgeons, Chicago, IL.
Yamada S, Lonser R R 2000 Adult tethered cord syndrome. Journal of Spinal Disorders 13: 319–323.

Case 18　Adult tethered cord syndrome

COMMENT
Patients with unexplained urinary incontinence should be fully investigated, including a MRI study of the lumbosacral spine when indicated.

PROFILE

A 49-year-old woman who does not smoke and only drinks alcohol socially.

PAST HISTORY

Urinary difficulties for many years which have gradually become worse over the last 2 years. She has undergone surgery for a bladder neck suspension procedure but without a change in incontinence.

PRESENTING COMPLAINT (Fig. 18.1)

A 13-year history of low back pain. The pain radiates bilaterally to the buttocks with leg pain extending particularly to the right thigh and right calf medially, with some aching in the right calf laterally, on prolonged standing. There is minor numbness intermittently in both feet with prolonged sitting. There is no groin pain but occasional genitorectal pain, especially premenstrually. She reported urinary urgency and occasionally was incontinent of urine, with very occasional faecal incontinence.

She has tried various abdominal muscle strengthening exercises, traction, gym work-outs, walking programmes, massage, acupuncture and anti-inflammatory medication. She currently uses Paracetamol and occasional Panadeine Forte.

AETIOLOGY

Pregnancy was thought to have been the precipitating factor.

EXAMINATION

She has a normal gait, an increased lumbosacral lordosis with a dimple centrally over the lumbosacral region and dropped arches with pronation of both feet. The left knee jerk was depressed (one plus instead of two plus) and

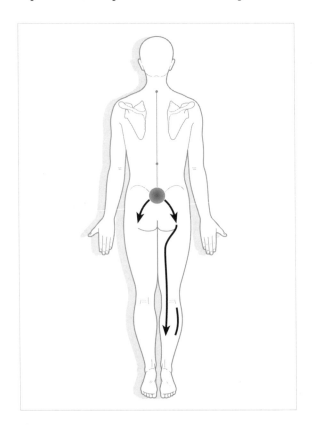

Figure 18.1

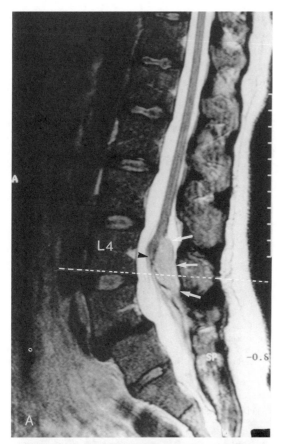

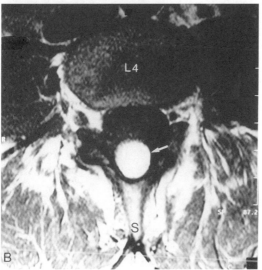

sensation was slightly impaired to light touch and pinprick on the dorsum of both feet in the L5–S1 dermatomes.

She could sit in the Budda position (cross-legged) but felt leg discomfort. Bending slightly at the waist increased the low back 'discomfort'. When carrying a light weight (2–3 kg) she had to hold it close to her abdomen, otherwise she experienced low back discomfort.

Urological examination, in spite of bladder neck suspension surgery, found the urodynamics basically showed evidence of detrusor instability and genuine stress incontinence with low urethral pressures; bladder compliance was quite good with a capacity of about 400 ml. An ultrasound scan showed a post-void urinary residual of 105 ml.

IMAGING REVIEW

Plain X-ray films showed a spina bifida occulta of L5 and lumbarization of the right transverse process of the transitional presacral segment; bilateral pars interarticularis defects at L5 were associated with a Grade 1 spondylolisthesis of L5 on the transitional segment below. Lumbar spine stress views showed no movement of the spondylolisthesis.

CLINICAL IMPRESSION

Adult tethered cord syndrome.

WHAT ACTION SHOULD BE TAKEN?

In view of the unexplained incontinence and spinal anomalies, a clinical suspicion of tethered cord syndrome lead to a lumbar MRI study, even though neurological findings were normal apart from only subtle abnormalities noted above.

The lumbar MRI showed a fatty mass (lipoma) in the posterior part of the spinal canal from L3 to the lumbarization level, with the conus unusually low at L4 level (Fig. 18.2A and B).

Figure 18.2 (A) Sagittal T2-weighted MRI scan showing the lipoma (white arrows) in the posterior part of the canal and the conus medullaris at the L4 level (arrowhead). The broken line shows the level at which the axial view was taken for (B). (B) Axial T2-weighted MRI scan through the area shown by the white broken line in (A). The arrow shows the lipoma. S = spinous process; L4 = 4th vertebral body endplate; R = right side of patient.

TREATMENT

Untethering of the spinal cord in order to prevent further neurological deterioration in the future was considered. However, an attempt to remove the lipoma was considered to be too risky in this particular case.

A conservative approach was taken: (1) a continued exercise programme to strengthen the lumbar, buttock and abdominal areas; (2) hormone replacement therapy by her general medical practitioner to help with the incontinence; (3) the patient was advised not to abuse her lumbosacral spine; she was told not to participate in any activities that could injure her low back and the tethered cord, as injury may well lead to a surgical emergency which would require an attempt to untether the cord.

RESULTS

The above conservative approach led to a considerable improvement in the symptoms, so surgery was not performed.

Note

Clinical awareness of the association between tethered cord syndrome and bladder dysfunction is essential. Bladder dysfunction is associated with tethered cord syndrome in 40–72% of adult cases (Yamada & Lonser 2000) and is the exclusive complaint in 4% (French 1990) and may represent the earliest sign of tethered cord syndrome (Hadley & Holevas 1996).

> **Key point**
>
> Bladder dysfunction is associated with tethered cord syndrome in 40–72% of adult cases and may represent the earliest sign of tethered cord syndrome.

REFERENCES

French B N 1990 Midline fusion defects and defects of formation. In: Youngmans JR (ed.) Neurological surgery. WB Saunders, Philadelphia, pp 1183–1185.
Hadley R, Holevas R E 1996 Lower urinary tract dysfunction in tethered cord syndrome. In: Yamada S (ed.) Tethered cord syndrome. The American Association of Neurological Surgeons, Chicago, pp 79–88.
Yamada S, Lonser R R 2000 Adult tethered cord syndrome. Journal of Spinal Disorders 13: 319–323.

FURTHER READING

See Case 17.

Giles L G F, Yamada S 2001 An unusual cause of incontinence. Australian Family Physician 30: 767–769.

Case 19 Lumbar neuroma

COMMENT

Beware of chronic recurring symptoms that mimic spinal mechanical dysfunction but may actually have a pathological basis.

PROFILE

A 57-year-old male who performed manual work.

PAST HISTORY

He fell from a height of approximately 8 m at the age of 26 years and this caused low back pain with left sacroiliac joint pain. He recovered with anti-inflammatory medication then aggravated his low back pain 12 years later while lifting heavy objects; again he recovered after using NSAIDs.

PRESENTING COMPLAINT (Fig. 19.1)

Severe pain in the left buttock with some low back pain that radiated to the lateral aspect of the left lower leg and medial aspect of the left foot. On this occasion anti-inflammatory and analgesic medication did not help his pain so he was referred by his general medical practitioner for a second opinion.

AETIOLOGY

One week before consultation he twisted his low back and caused the above presenting symptoms.

EXAMINATION

On examination there was loss of pinprick sensation on the lateral aspect of the left calf (L5) and the medial aspect of the left foot (S1). Supine SLR was limited by low back pain at 45° elevation (left) and by hamstring tightness at 90°

(right). The left knee jerk (L4) was absent. All lumbar spine movements were painful. Coughing and bearing down did not aggravate his symptoms. Hip joint movements were of normal range and painless.

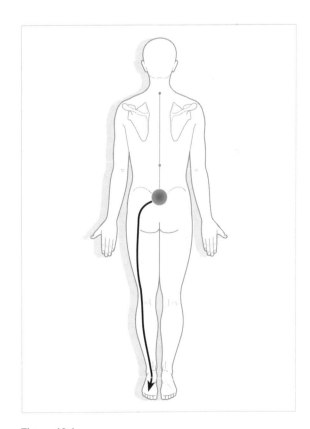

Figure 19.1

IMAGING REVIEW

Recent lumbar spine and pelvis radiographs were reported as showing only 'minor degenerative changes' (Fig. 19.2A and B).

CLINICAL IMPRESSION

A possible left-sided L4–5 or L5–S1 intervertebral disc prolapse.

WHAT ACTION SHOULD BE TAKEN?

As the plain radiographs did not correlate with the degree of low back and leg symptoms chemical pathology tests and haematology tests were performed as a precaution (Boxes 19.1 and 19.2) as well as a lumbar (L3–S1 levels) CT scan.

The chemical pathology and haematology results were considered to be essentially normal and not related to his low back pain.

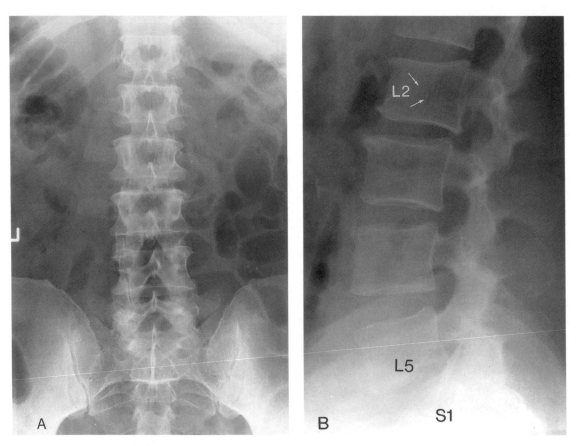

Figure 19.2 (A) Anteroposterior plane X-ray view of the lumbosacral spine showing minor lipping of most vertebral bodies and tropism of some zygapophysial joints. L = left side of patient. (B) Lateral plane X-ray view of the lumbar spine showing some thinning of the L2–3 intervertebral disc with lipping anteriorly on the adjacent bony margins and some retrolisthesis of L2 on L3 vertebra. Note the vertical 'corduroy' trabecular pattern in the L2 body (arrows) indicating a haemangioma. L5 = fifth vertebral body; S1 = first sacral segment. (C) A CT lumbar spine view at the L4–5 disc level showing a possible left far lateral L4–5 disc protrusion or a tumour of neural origin (arrow). P = posterior side of patient; R = right side of patient. (D) Sagittal T1-weighted MRI scan of the lumbosacral spine showing the haemangioma (arrow) involving the L2 vertebral body with some posterior bulging of the L2–3 intervertebral disc. (E) Axial T1-weighted pre-contrast MRI scan at the L4–5 disc area. The arrow shows apparent continuity between disc material and the far lateral 'lesion'. (F) Axial T1-weighted post-contrast MRI scan at the L4–5 disc area. The arrow clearly shows there is no continuity between the tumour (T) and the disc material.

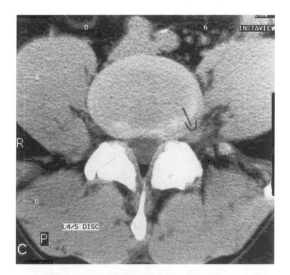

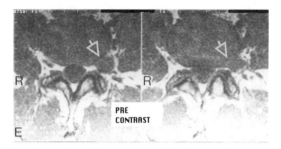

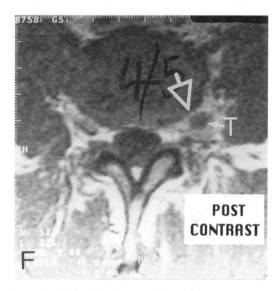

Figure 19.2 Caption is on previous page.

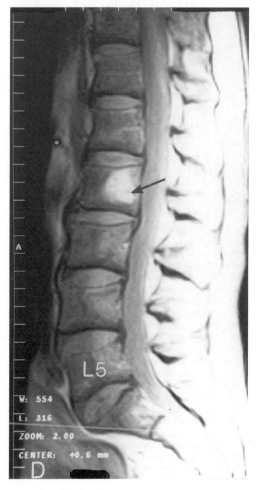

Figure 19.2 Caption is on previous page.

The CT report concluded: 'Possible left far lateral L4–5 disc protrusion. Differential diagnosis is a tumour of neural origin. CT myelography or MRI suggested for further evaluation. Disc degeneration L3–4, L4–5 and L5–S1 levels. L4–5 level mild canal stenosis' (Fig. 19.2C).

In order to differentiate between a possible left far lateral L4–5 disc protrusion and a tumour of neural origin, an MRI with and without contrast was performed; the sagittal T1-weighted image (Fig. 19.2D) was non-contributory but showed a lesion of increased signal intensity involving the L2 body posteriorly (arrow) which reduces in signal intensity on T2 images, the appearance favouring a haemangioma or an area of fatty deposition. The axial views through the L4–5 disc area showed the lesion

Box 19.1   Chemical pathology

		Units	Reference range
Sodium	138	mmol/l	(133–146)
Potassium	4.3	mmol/l	(3.3–4.5)
Chloride	106	mmol/l	(97–110)
Bicarbonate	28	mmol/l	(20–32)
Anion gap	**4**	mmol/l	(8–17)
Urea	3.9	mmol/l	(3.0–6.0)
Creatinine	0.11	mmol/l	(0.04–0.12)
AST (aspartate amino-transferase)	20	U/l	(10–40)
Protein (total)	67	g/l	(60–80)
Albumin	45	g/l	(35–50)
Globulin	22	g/l	
ALP (alkaline phosphatase)	52	U/l	(40–120)
Gamma-glutamyl transferase	22	U/l	(<60)
Serum ALT (alanine aminotransferase)	11	U/l	(5–60)
Bilirubin (total)	15	μmol/l	(<17)
Calcium	2.23	mmol/l	(2.10–2.60)
Calcium (corrected)	2.13	mmol/l	(2.10–2.60)
Phosphate	**0.77**	mmol/l	(0.80–1.40)

Box 19.2   Haematology

		Units	Reference range
Haemoglobin	151	g/l	(135–180)
White cell count	10.8	×10⁹/l	(4.0–11.0)
Platelets	341	×10⁹/l	(140–400)
Haematocrit	0.44		(0.39–0.52)
Red cell count	5.11	×10¹²/l	(4.50–6.00)
MCV (mean corpuscular volume)	86.1	fl	(80.0–98.0)
Neutrophils	**8.2**	×10⁹/l	(2.0–8.0)
Lymphocytes	1.6	×10⁹/l	(1.0–4.0)
Monocytes	**0.9**	×10⁹/l	(0.1–0.8)
Eosinophils	0.1	×10⁹/l	(<0.2)
Basophils	0.0	×10⁹/l	(<0.2)
ESR	10	mm/hr	(<15)

under investigation but the pre-contrast study (Fig. 19.2E) was not able to differentiate between a far lateral disc lesion and a neural tumour. However, the post-contrast view (Fig. 19.2F) demonstrated that there is no continuity between the lesion and the disc, therefore indicating a neural tumour, i.e. a neurofibroma or a Schwannoma.

A histopathology section cut in the horizontal plane is shown in Fig. 19.3. This indicates how there should be fatty tissue surrounding neural structures which should not normally touch disc material as the neural structures pass through the intervertebral foramen.

TREATMENT

This man's condition was explained to him and he was told that surgery would most likely not help because of the benign neural tumour. A NSAID was prescribed. He was asked to return should his condition not improve.

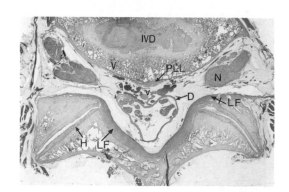

Figure 19.3 A 200-micron thick horizontal histopathological section through the lower lumbar spine of a 46-year-old male that serves to illustrate the principle involved in the above case. Note the intervertebral disc material (IVD), the posterior of the vertebral body (V) and the nerve root ganglion (N) within the intervertebral foramen. The space between the neural structures (N) and the posterior part of the vertebral body and disc and, for that matter, the anteromedial portion of the ligamentum flavum (LF tailed arrow) can be seen. Therefore, with contrast medium in the nerve root sleeve (sheath) it should be possible to see a space between the neural structures and the adjacent structures, due to contrast material being introduced, if the structures under investigation are adjacent to each other and not apart from each other. The dural tube (D) is shown containing some of the cauda equina nerve roots. Small blood vessels (v) are seen between the posterior longitudinal ligament (PLL) and the dural tube. The hyaline articular cartilage (H) on the articular facet surfaces can be seen. (Erhlich's haematoxylin and light green counterstain).

RESULTS

The administration of NSAIDs gave him adequate symptomatic relief.

Key point
Chronic recurring symptoms of low back pain and sciatica may be related to pathology other than nerve root pressure.

FURTHER READING

Cassidy J R, Ducker T B, Dienes E A 1997 Intradural tumors. In: Frymoyer JW (ed.) The adult spine: principles and practice, 2nd edn. Lippincott-Raven, Philadelphia, pp 1015–1029.
Haldeman S 1999 Differential diagnosis of low back pain. In: Kirkaldy-Willis WH, Bernard TN (eds) Managing low back pain, 4th edn. Churchill Livingstone, New York, pp 227–248.

Case 20 Perineural fibrosis

COMMENT
When spinal surgery is unsuccessful, thoroughly reinvestigate the patient.

PROFILE

A 45-year-old muscular male who does not smoke and only drinks alcohol socially.

PAST HISTORY

A history of low back pain which began while lifting heavy weights. Following this injury, left-sided sciatica had become so severe that he had to undergo a micro-discectomy at the L5–S1 level 2 years prior to this consultation; surgery temporarily relieved the low back pain and sciatica enabling him to walk better for several months.

PRESENTING COMPLAINT (Fig. 20.1)

Constant left-sided low back pain and sciatica which recurred after the micro-discectomy. He is unable to sit or stand for any length of time, lift more than approximately 5-kg weights, carry out any gardening (apart from simple hosing) and drive his car without low back pain and left sciatica. He has chronic sleep disturbance due to severe nocturnal back pain that does not occur at any particular time. The left leg feels 'numb and weak' and he has a 'sharp, deep and stabbing pain' across the low back. Coughing and sneezing aggravate the low back pain.

Physiotherapy has not been helpful and he has stopped taking NSAIDs and analgesics as they were not helpful.

He has not been able to work since the discectomy operation 2 years before this consultation.

AETIOLOGY

Carrying heavy objects at work over a 12-year period.

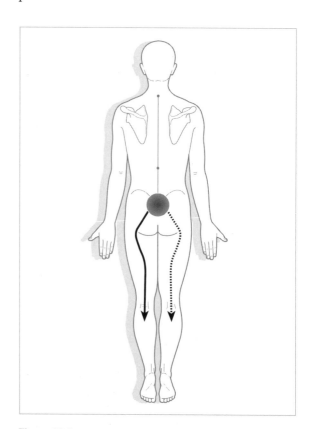

Figure 20.1

EXAMINATION

SLR was limited by low back pain to approximately 65° (right) and 20° (left). There was hypoaesthesia over the posterolateral aspect of the left leg and over the dorsum of the left foot. The left ankle jerk was absent and the plantar responses were normal. All lumbar spine active ranges of movement were very limited and painful and there was bilateral tenderness on deep palpation over the paraspinal muscles in the lower lumbosacral spine at approximately the L5–S1 level. There was L5 root motor weakness.

CLINICAL IMPRESSION

L5–S1 left-sided recurrent disc or perineural fibrosis.

IMAGING REVIEW

No post-surgical imaging had been performed to re-evaluate his condition.

WHAT ACTION SHOULD BE TAKEN?

A lumbar MRI was performed to see what his lumbosacral spine looked like following surgery. The sagittal scans showed disc space narrowing at the L5–S1 level (Fig. 20.2A). In addition there was a generalized anular bulge of the L5–S1 disc. The axial scans (Fig. 20.2B) showed a soft tissue structure in the left posterolateral aspect of the spinal canal adjacent to the left S1 nerve root which showed no evidence of enhancement with intravenous contrast. This was considered to be post-operative inflammatory tissue and the lack of enhancement was considered to be due to some problem with the contrast injection. Soft tissue was seen anterior to and investing the left nerve root and was considered to be disc material (see Fig. 20.3).

TREATMENT

He was referred for a further surgical opinion and subsequently underwent a laminectomy at the L5–S1 level. Further inferior L5 left lamina and part of the superior lamina of S1 were

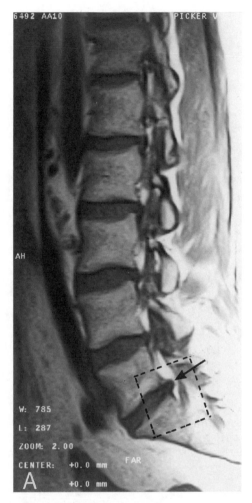

Figure 20.2 (A) Parasagittal left-sided T1-weighted MRI scan of the lumbosacral spine showing the generalized anular bulge of the L5–S1 disc (arrow). The area within the broken lines is represented histologically in Fig. 20.3.

removed to display the theca and ligamentum flavum. No free disc fragments were found but there was a 'grossly swollen' left S1 nerve root that was fully mobilized and the lateral recess was decompressed.

RESULTS

Unfortunately the patient continued to suffer from disabling low back pain and left-sided sciatica, so an L5 rhizolysis was performed but without success so, 18 months later a spinal cord stimulator was inserted with variable results.

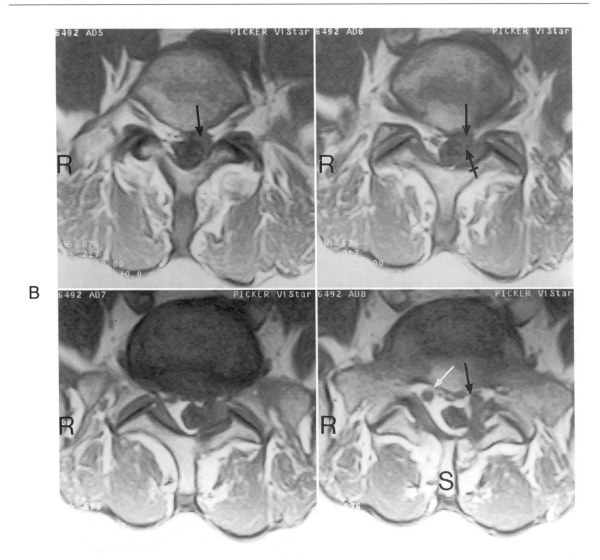

Figure 20.2 (B) Axial T1-weighted MRI scans (AD5 to AD8) of the L5–S1 disc. These show the soft tissue in the left lateral aspect of the spinal canal (top left axial scan AD5 see arrow) around the left S1 nerve root; this has the configuration of post-operative inflammatory tissue. This soft tissue is also seen anterior to and investing the left nerve root in the top right axial scan (tailed arrow). The bottom right axial scan shows a normal S1 nerve root on the right side (white arrow), and the swollen S1 nerve root on the left side (black arrow) surrounded by perineural fibrosis. R = right side of patient; S = spinous process.

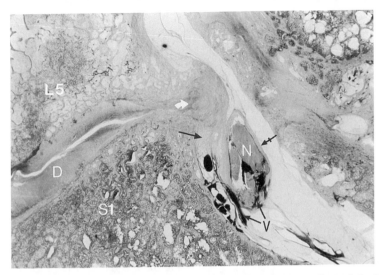

Figure 20.3   A 200-micron thick histopathology section, cut in the parasagittal plane through the lumbosacral inter-vertebral disc of a 59-year-old cadaver, showing a disc protrusion (small curved white arrow) with perineural adhesions (arrow) between it and the adjacent neural structures (N) in the dural sleeve (tailed arrow). D = intervertebral disc; L5 = fifth lumbar vertebral body; S1 = first sacral segment. Note the extensive vascularity (V) posterior to the sacrum and within and around the neural structures. This histological section represents a similar area to the area shown within the broken lines on Fig. 20.2A. (Erhlich's haematoxylin and light green counterstain.)

Key point(s)

1. Post surgical complaints need to be fully investigated to look for recurrent disc material and perineural fibrosis affecting the adjacent nerve root.
2. According to Loupasis et al (1999), the long-term results of standard lumbar discectomy are not very satisfying; micro-discectomy results can be disappointing too.

REFERENCE

Loupasis G A, Stamos D, Katonis P G, Sapkas G, Korres D S, Hartofilakidis G 1999 Seven- to-20-year outcome of lumbar discectomy. Spine 15: 2313–2317.

FURTHER READING

Boden S D, Lee R R, Herzog R J 1997 Magnetic resonance imaging of the spine. In: Frymoyer JW (ed.) The adult spine: principles and practice, 2nd edn. Lippincott-Raven, Philadelphia, pp 563–629.
Fan Y F, Chong V F, Tan S K 1995 Failed back surgery syndrome: differentiating epidural fibrosis and recurrent disc prolapse with Gd-DTPA enhanced MRI. Singapore Medical Journal 36: 153–156.
Vishteh A G, Dickman C A 2001 Anterior lumbar microdiscectomy and interbody fusion for the treatment of recurrent disc herniation. Neurosurgery 48: 334–337.

Case 21 Synovial cyst

COMMENT
More than one cause of low back pain with referred leg pain may be present requiring appropriate surgical intervention.

PROFILE

A 68-year-old retired builder who stopped smoking some 40 years ago and only drinks alcohol moderately. He has generalized osteoarthritic pains for which he takes a NSAID.

PAST HISTORY

He had prostatism diagnosed some years ago. Recently he was found to have hypertension (200/90).

PRESENTING COMPLAINT (Fig. 21.1)

Mild low back pain for approximately 5 years with periodic left or right lower limb radicular pain of 3 months duration. Two years ago he developed 'shooting' pains in the lateral aspect of the right leg but this completely resolved until 2 months ago when there was a recurrence of some pain in the right lower leg, particularly on getting up in the morning or on sitting for long periods of time.

Coughing and sneezing did not aggravate his low back pain and he said he could walk for long distances without any paraesthiae or weakness; he did not have any pain in the feet. Bowel and bladder function were normal.

AETIOLOGY

He could not recall any specific injury.

EXAMINATION

He had a good range of active lumbar spine movements. Supine SLR was limited to 80° on the right due to an increase in low back pain. There were no sensory or reflex changes and power was normal.

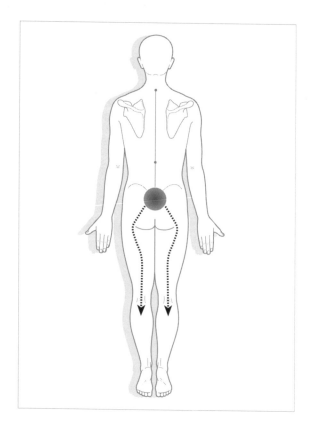

Figure 21.1

106

IMAGING REVIEW

Plain X-ray films showed a grade 1 spondylolisthesis of L4 on L5 due to osteoarthrotic degenerative changes of the L4–5 zygapophysial joint facets, i.e. degenerative spondylolisthesis. Disc thinning was present at both the L4–5 and L5–S1 levels with associated osteoarthrotic involvement of the zygapophysial facet joints. There were no pars interarticularis defects.

CLINICAL IMPRESSION

Low back pain and alternating left and right leg pains probably due to the degenerative grade 1 spondylolisthesis of L4 on L5.

WHAT ACTION SHOULD BE TAKEN?

In view of the patient's history and age, chemical pathology and haematology tests were performed (Boxes 21.1 and 21.2). Although there were minor variations from normal, these were considered to be unrelated to his presenting symptoms and signs and he was referred to his general medical practitioner for further consideration of the results.

As a precaution in view of the alternating left and right leg symptoms associated with his low back pain, a CT lumbar spine (L3–S1 levels) was performed; this confirmed the grade 1 spondylolisthesis at L4–5 and extensive degenerative changes in the 'facet' joints at this level which are responsible for the 'degenerative spondylolisthesis'. There was no evidence of

Box 21.1   Chemical pathology

		Units	Reference range
Sodium	139	mmol/l	(135–148)
Potassium	4.5	mmol/l	(3.2–5.0)
Chloride	109	mmol/l	(95–109)
Carbon dioxide	27	mmol/l	(23–32)
Urea	7.3	mmol/l	(2.5–7.5)
Creatinine	0.09	mmol/l	(0.04–0.12)
Prostate-specific antigen	0.2	ng/ml	(0.0–4.0)

Box 21.2   Haematology

		Units	Reference range
Haemoglobin	136	g/l	(125–175)
White cell count	9.6	×10^9/l	(4.0–11.0)
Platelets	243	×10^9/l	(150–400)
Haematocrit	**0.39**		(0.40–0.54)
Red cell count	4.12	×10^{12}/l	(4.20–6.50)
RBC distance width	**11**		(12–14)
MCV (mean corpuscular volume)	95	fl	(75–95)
MCH (mean corpuscular haemoglobin)	**33.1**	pg	(27.0–32.0)
MCHC (mean corpuscular haemoglobin concentration)	349	g/l	(310–350)
Neutrophils	5.0	×10^9/l	(2.0–7.5)
Lymphocytes	3.5	×10^9/l	(1.0–4.0)
Monocytes	**0.8**	×10^9/l	(0.0–0.8)
Eosinophils	0.2	×10^9/l	(0.0–0.4)
Basophils	0.1	×10^9/l	(0.0–0.1)

pars interarticularis defects. The spinal canal was reasonably spacious but was encroached upon to some extent at the upper border of L5 by a combination of the spondylolisthesis and pronounced ligamentum flavum thickening. This thickening had a nodular appearance on the left at the L4–5 joint level where it indents the theca (Fig. 21.2A). The extensive degenerative change in the facet joints shows osteoarthrotic changes and remodelling of the bone on the left and right sides of the spine. In order to give the reader an appreciation of this type of osteoarthrotic degenerative zygapophysial joint change, a histopathology section is shown in Fig. 21.2B.

An MRI scan of the lumbar spine was performed and showed a round area of soft tissue projecting into the spinal canal from the left L4–5 facet joint – this had the appearance of a synovial cyst and caused some spinal canal stenosis due to impingement of the thecal sac (Fig. 21.2C).

TREATMENT

The patient was referred for a surgical opinion regarding (i) his leg symptoms and (ii) the

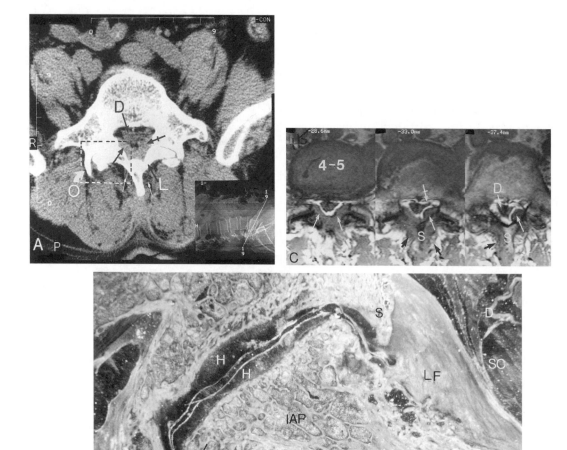

Figure 21.2 (A) Axial CT scan through the L4–5 zygapophysial joint 'facets'. Note the hypertrophy of the ligamentum flavum bilaterally (small arrow) and the nodular thickening of the ligamentum flavum on the left side opposite the L4–5 zygapophysial joint (tailed arrow). Note how the left side of the dural tube (D) is being indented by the nodular synovial cyst. L = lamina; O = osteophyte on the right superior articular process of the L5 vertebra. The rectangle shown between the broken lines represents an area shown histologically in (B) from postmortem material. Note in (A) the quite marked irregularity of the spinous process with thickening of the soft tissues adjacent to the laminae and the spinous process (small white arrows). P = posterior side of the patient's lumbar region. (B) A 200-micron thick horizontal histopathology section through the right zygapophysial facet joint of a 65-year-old postmortem specimen. Note the hyaline articular cartilage (H) on the facet surfaces and how it has developed around the lateral margins of the joint forming 'bumper-fibrocartilage' (black arrows) as a result of the development of the large osteophytic spur (O) beneath the fibrous joint capsule (F). D = part of the dural tube; IAP = inferior articular process; LF = ligamentum flavum; S = spur adjacent to the ligamentum flavum and projecting from the superior articular process of the vertebra below. SC = spinal canal. (C) Axial T1-weighted MRI views through the L4–5 zygapophysial joints at approximately the same level as shown in the CT scan (A). Note the thickening of the ligamentum flavum bilaterally (white arrows) and the synovial cyst on the left side that compresses the dural tube (D), and to some extent the left nerve root at this level (small tailed arrow). Note the abnormal tissue (small black arrows), tracking along the right lamina and the spinous process (S) suggesting an inflammatory or degenerative process.

abnormal tissue noted adjacent to and affecting the L4–5 facet joint and lamina on the left. It was decided by the surgeon that the right-sided nerve root entrapment at L4–5, due to a combination of thickened ligamentum flavum and zygapophysial joint arthropathy, indicated that surgery should be undertaken to decompress the right L5 nerve root in the lateral recess via an L4–5 fenestration; this was done, as well as removing a moderate-sized disc protrusion at that level. However, the left-sided synovial cyst was not removed as the surgeon considered that the synovial cyst was a completely incidental finding and did not warrant exposing the left side of the spine during surgery; he felt it was 'completely unnecessary' to do this.

RESULTS

The surgery produced good relief from the patient's right-sided sciatica. However, the patient presented again with symptoms of spinal stenosis, so a laminectomy and decompression was performed including the lower portion of L3 to L5, the spinouses and laminae being removed due to the 'significant central canal stenosis, particularly at L4–5' where there was a 'large synovial cyst' as originally noted.

The patient made an uneventful post-operative recovery.

Note

This raises the interesting question of whether, when two lesions are present at the same level of the spine, i.e. L4–5 in this case, both lesions should be removed at the time of initial surgery to minimize the risk to a patient having to undergo follow-up surgery, while also lessening the cost of surgery, hospitalization, etc.

Key point

When more than one spinal pathology is present it would appear to be wise to address both pathologies at the same time in order to maximally help the patient and to save the costs associated with re-admission to hospital and a second surgical procedure at the same level.

FURTHER READING

Gundry C R, Heithoff K B 1999 Lumbar spine imaging. In: Kirkaldy-Willis WH, Bernard TN (eds) Managing low back pain, 4th edn. Churchill Livingstone, New York, pp 176–205.

Postacchini F, Trasimeni G 1999 Differential diagnosis. I. Organic disease. In: Postacchini F (ed.) Lumbar disc herniation. Springer-Verlag, New York, pp 293–318.

Rowe L 1997 Imaging of mechanical and degenerative syndromes of the lumbar spine. In: Giles LGF, Singer KP (eds) Clinical anatomy and management of low back pain, Vol I. Butterworth-Heinemann, Oxford, pp 276–313.

Zinreich S J, Heithoff K B, Herzog R J 1997 Computed tomography of the spine. In: Frymoyer JW (ed.) The adult spine: principles and practice, 2nd edn. Lippincott-Raven, Philadelphia, pp 467–522.

Case 22   Internal disc disruption

COMMENT
Low back pain can arise from a variety of low
back structures.

PROFILE

A 49-year-old woman who does not smoke or drink
alcohol.

PAST HISTORY

Three years ago she had a cervical spine
discectomy and fusion for left arm pain but she
still experiences neck pain.

PRESENTING COMPLAINT (Fig. 22.1)

Three years of low back pain radiating into both
thighs anteriorly with a sensation like 'electric
shocks'. These attacks initially took place
approximately once a year and would last for
2–3 weeks. Her symptoms are now constant and
chronic, with a deep burning pain over the
lumbar area that radiates into both thighs and
groins. Over recent months, she has developed
right sciatica extending to halfway down her
right calf and a 'cold and burning' sensation in
the feet.

Her symtpoms are exacerbated by bending,
standing, sitting and housework but they are not
aggravated by coughing or sneezing.

She had tried physiotherapy, swimming
(including aqua-aerobics), acupuncture and
NSAIDs; the latter caused indigestion,
oesophageal reflux and oesophagitis, for which
she takes antacids.

She is often awakened by low back pain at
night but not at a particular time, so she takes an
analgesic to try to relieve the pain.

AETIOLOGY

Her low back pain syndrome began after
straightening up from being bent forwards, at
which time she also felt the 'electric shock' sensation across her lower back and it extended into
the thighs anteriorly.

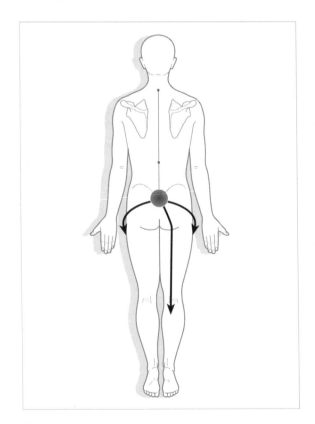

Figure 22.1

EXAMINATION

She was neurologically intact. Foot pulses were normal. She was tender on deep palpation of the paravertebral muscles of the lower lumbar spine. SLR was to 80º bilaterally and painless. Active ranges of lumbar spine movement were full with pain only on flexion.

IMAGING REVIEW

Plain lumbosacral spine films dating back 2 years were reported as showing 'slight degenerative changes present at the L4–5 and L5–S1 disc levels'. A CT scan through the lower three disc spaces found 'no disc herniation at any of the visualized levels, no spinal canal stenosis or paravertebral soft tissue mass'.

CLINICAL IMPRESSION

The symptoms suggested mechanical involvement of soft tissue structures in the lower lumbosacral spine as there was no abnormal neurology and SLR was painless, suggesting no large disc bulge posteriorly; internal disc disruption was considered likely. The 'cold and burning' sensation in the feet was considered to be due to autonomic involvement either via the paraspinal sympathetic nerve chain or the recurrent meningeal nerves (see Fig. ii, General Introduction).

WHAT ACTION SHOULD BE TAKEN?

In view of her presenting complaint the following laboratory tests were performed as a precaution: full blood count, urea and electrolytes, liver function tests and serum calcium; all were within the normal range except for a very slightly elevated ESR (Box 22.1).

A lumbar MRI study ordered concurrently showed:

Mild circumferential disc bulges at L4–5 and L5–S1 (Fig. 22.2A and B) and desiccation of the L4–5 and L5–S1 discs (Fig. 22.2B). Facet and ligamentum flavum hypertrophy at these levels causes mild lateral recess stenosis bilaterally. Paravertebral soft tissues

Box 22.1			
		Units	Reference range
ESR (erythrocyte sedimentation rate)	12	mm in 1 hr	(3–9)
Rheumatoid factor protein	<20	IU/ml	(<30)
Anti-nuclear antibody	Negative		

are within normal limits. An incidental finding of minor haemangiomas at L1 and L3 was noted.

TREATMENT

In view of her symptoms of an 'electric shock' type of pain going to the upper thighs anteriorly and the 'cold and burning' in the feet with a constant deep 'burning' low back pain, it was considered that she may have pain due to lower lumbar spine autonomic nervous system involvement, as well as pain from the changes within the L5–S1 disc. This disc had fairly large anterior bulging (Fig. 22.2A), probably affecting the autonomic chain, as well as some minor posterior bulging probably interfering with the recurrent meningeal nerves posteriorly. Therefore, a discogram (Fig. 22.2C) was ordered with a request that a local anaesthetic be injected into the disc if there were significant internal disc disruption. The discogram confirmed advanced internal disc disruption when 4 ml of contrast were injected into the disc under low pressure. This aggravated her chronic pain syndrome shortly after injection, the delay suggesting that the pain was coming from tissue structures adjacent to the disc that may have been irritated by the extravasated contrast anteriorly and laterally. The CT scan that followed (Fig. 22.2D) demonstrated total internal disc disruption at L5–S1 with contrast tracking freely across the endplates and extravasating anteriorly and to the right. The contrast coursed around the disc to the true posterior position beneath the posterior longitudinal ligament (see also Fig. 22.3).

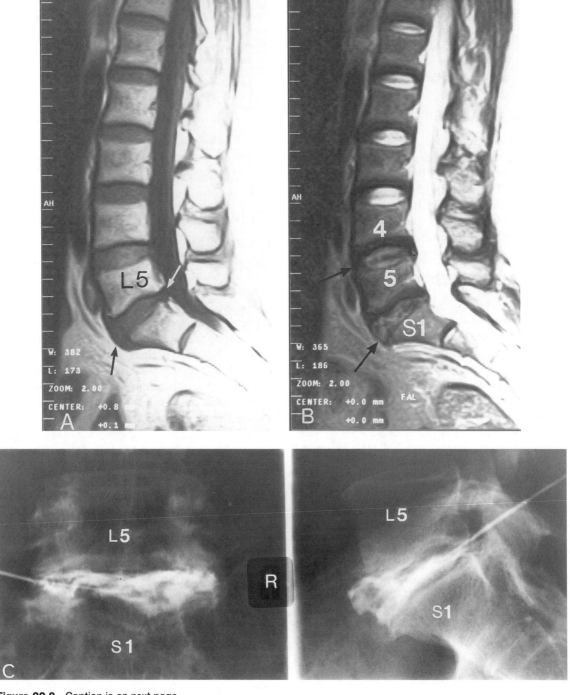

Figure 22.2 Caption is on next page.

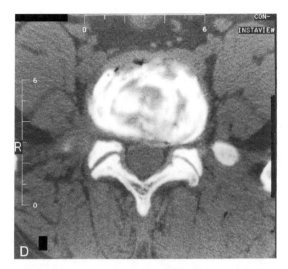

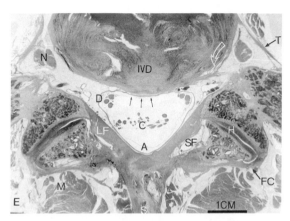

Figure 22.2 (A) A sagittal T1-weighted MRI image of the lumbosacral spine showing the large anterior (black arrow) and small posterior (white arrow) disc bulges at the L5–S1 level. (B) A sagittal T2-weighted MRI image of the lumbosacral spine showing considerable desiccation of the L4–5 and L5–S1 discs (arrows) which have become quite dark in colour compared to the discs above which have a normal grey colour with a normal black line through them, i.e. the intranuclear cleft. (C) Anteroposterior and lateral discograms of the lumbosacral disc (L5–S1) showing the internal disc disruption and extravasation of contrast material during injection. (D) A CT axial scan view of the L5–S1 intervertebral disc showing significant internal disc disruption with loss of the normal anular fibres and extravasation from the disc across the endplates and into the paravertebral soft tissues.

Figure 22.3 A 200-micron thick horizontal histological section from a 51-year-old female postmortem specimen. Note the internal disc disruption within the intervertebral disc (IVD) with some radial tears seen as white spaces and there is some disruption of the outer anulus fibrosus fibres (curved white arrow). There is some central posterior bulging of the disc which effaces (small black arrows) the anterior part of the dural tube (D) which contains the cauda equina (C) that is surrounded by cerebrospinal fluid and the arachnoid membrane (A). The neural structures (N) passing through the lateral part of the intervertebral foramen are in close proximity to transforaminal ligaments (T). S = remains of spinal process. SF = synovial fold adjacent to the ligamentum flavum (LF). H = hyaline articular cartilage surfaces on the facets of the zygapophysial joints. FC = fibrous joint capsule posterolaterally. M = multifidus muscle. (Erhlich's haematoxylin and light green counterstain.) See also colour plate section.

RESULTS

Following the discogram, 1 ml of local anaesthetic was injected into the disc. This abolished all her pain for 3 weeks, at which time she kept a pre-arranged appointment with a surgeon who said that the 'anaesthetic could not have helped the pain' and suggested that she should have some traction, although she was virtually pain free. Therefore, she had traction and her pain syndrome returned. However, she did not want to undergo the discogram procedure again 'with that big needle', so she decided that she would prefer to put up with her chronic low back pain syndrome now that she knew what was causing her problem and she opted to use one Indocid suppository at night as required.

Key point(s)

1. Low back pain associated with apparently bizarre symptoms such as 'cold and burning' in the feet should suggest possible involvement of the paraspinal sympathetic chain.
2. Paraspinal sympathetic chain involvement most likely suggests irritation due to an anterolateral disc herniation or a claw spondylophyte affecting the paraspinal sympathetic chain.
3. Freemont et al (1997) showed nerve fibres that express substance-P deep within diseased intervertebral discs. In chronic low back pain patients the nerves extended into the inner third of the anulus fibrosus and into the nucleus pulposus in 46% and 10% of samples, respectively. Therefore, it is reasonable to suggest that the pain cycle from such a disc may be broken by an intradiscal injection of anaesthetic and steroid or by thermal anular heating and coagulation.

REFERENCE

Freemont A J, Peacock T E, Goupille P, Hyland J A, O'Brien J O, Jayson M I V 1997 Nerve ingrowth into diseased intervertebral disc in chronic back pain. The Lancet 350: 178–181.

FURTHER READING

Kleinstueck F S, Diederich C J, Nau W H, Puttlitz C M, Smith J A, Bradford D S, Lotz J C 2001 Acute biomechanical and histological effects of intradiscal electothermal therapy on human lumbar discs. Spine 26: 2198–2207.

Postacchini F, Gualdi G 1999 Imaging Studies. In: Postacchini F (ed.) Lumbar disc herniation. Springer-Verlag, New York, pp 210–278.
Saal J S, Saal J A 2000 Management of chronic discogenic low back pain with a thermal intradiscal catheter. A preliminary report. Spine 25: 382–388.

Case 23   Intervertebral disc protrusion

COMMENT
Believe your patient until it is proven that the
complaint is not genuine! Rely upon your own
diagnostic acumen and not that of others.

PROFILE

A 53-year-old man who was depressed because of
his 4-year history of undiagnosed low back pain.
He does not smoke and only drinks one glass of
wine per day.

He only came for a consultation because his wife
was concerned about his suicidal ideation as he
had been told that there was 'nothing wrong' with
him following several specialists' consultations.
His wife made the appointment for him and
accompanied him to the consultation.

PAST HISTORY

A degree of asthma but otherwise unremarkable.

PRESENTING COMPLAINT (Fig. 23.1)

Approximately L3–4 level pain extending into
the left buttock with radiation to the lateral
aspect of the left thigh and some left testicular
pain. He was also experiencing urinary difficulties, with occasional hesitancy and poor stream,
but there was no burning/dysuria or urethral
discharge. He had also been constipated as he
was taking NSAIDs and analgesics.

The symptoms are worsened on sneezing.
Sitting causes a severe increase in his symptoms,
so he spends much of his time walking or standing when he is not resting on his bed.

AETIOLOGY

He was knocked over by a car and suffered severe
low back and left buttock and posterolateral

thigh pain for 1.5 years before his symptoms
settled to a 'tolerable' level. He then inad-
vertently twisted his low back causing an acute
exacerbation of his low back pain syndrome; following chiropractic treatment, his symptoms
settled over a 1-month period. He then had four

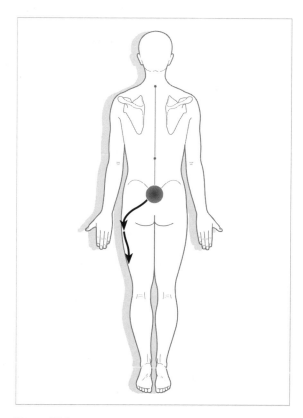

Figure 23.1

further acute episodes, the most recent being due to bending over to pick up a light weight at home, approximately 8 weeks ago; this caused such acute low back and left buttock and thigh pain that he had to stop working.

EXAMINATION

His blood pressure was 170/100 in the supine position with a pulse rate of 68 per minute. His chest was clear without any evidence of a wheeze. His abdomen was normal on auscultation and on palpation. On deep palpation of the paraspinal muscles he was tender over approximately the L3–L4 level of the lumbar spine. Supine SLR was limited by low back pain to 40° (left) and 60° (right). The left knee jerk was decreased. Muscle tone in both lower limbs was normal but there was a decrease in power in the left lower limb; this appeared to be due to his low back pain syndrome. The plantar response was normal as was sensation in the legs. The range of active lumbar spine movements was markedly reduced in all directions due to lower lumbar pain. The prostate was smooth but somewhat enlarged. There was normal sacral sensation and anal tone.

IMAGING REVIEW

A series of low back X-rays showed some mild disc narrowing from L2 to L5 with small marginal osteophytes and mild zygapophysial joint osteoarthrosis.

CLINICAL IMPRESSION

Possibly L3–4 or L4–5 disc protrusion.

WHAT ACTION SHOULD BE TAKEN?

In view of the history, laboratory tests were performed for chemical pathology and haematology (Boxes 23.1 and 23.2).

An MRI lumbar spine was ordered concurrently and this showed a spinal canal of normal dimension with a mild disc bulge present at L4–5 and quite a large L3–4 left-sided focal disc

Box 23.1 Chemical pathology

		Units	Reference range
Sodium	141	mmol/l	(135–148)
Potassium	4.8	mmol/l	(3.5–5.0)
Chloride	109	mmol/l	(95–109)
Carbon dioxide	31	mmol/l	(23–32)
Urea	5.9	mmol/l	(2.5–7.5)
Creatinine	0.10	mmol/l	(0.04–0.12)
Prostatic specific antigen	1.8	ng/ml	(0.0–4.0)

Box 23.2 Haematology

		Units	Reference range
Haemoglobin	175	g/l	(130–180)
Red cell count	5.69	$\times 10^{12}/l$	(4.50–6.50)
Red blood cell distance width	12		(12–14)
Haematocrit	0.52		(0.40–0.54)
MCV (mean corpuscular volume)	92	fl	(75–95)
MCH (mean corpuscular haemoglobin)	30.7	pg	(27.0–32.0)
MCHC (mean corpuscular haemoglobin concentration)	333	g/l	(310–350)
Platelet count	250	$\times 10^9/l$	(150–400)
White cell count	9.1	$\times 10^9/l$	(4.0–11.0)
Neutrophils	5.5	$\times 10^9/l$	(2.0–7.5)
Lymphocytes	2.8	$\times 10^9/l$	(1.0–4.0)
Monocytes	0.5	$\times 10^9/l$	(0.0–0.8)
Eosinophils	0.4	$\times 10^9/l$	(0.0–0.4)
Basophils	0.0	$\times 10^9/l$	(0.0–0.1)
Bands	0.0	$\times 10^9/l$	
Metamyelocytes	0.0	$\times 10^9/l$	
Myelocytes	0.0	$\times 10^9/l$	
ESR	6	mm/hr	(2–10)

protrusion outside the spinal canal in a far lateral position, i.e. partly extra-foraminally (see Fig. 23.2A and B). This protrusion displaced the left L3 nerve root as shown in the axial T1-weighted view (Fig. 23.2B). See also Fig. 23.3.

TREATMENT

When the patient came back to hear the results of his blood test and the MRI scan he was shown

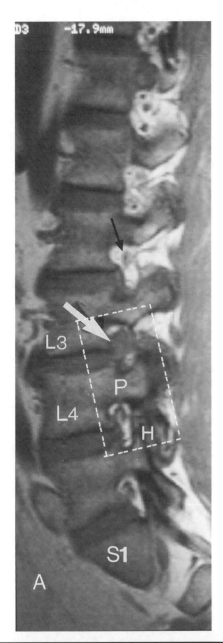

the large disc protrusion at the L3–4 level. He broke down and cried, then rushed out to the waiting room and called his wife in stating 'they have found out what is wrong with me – look a large disc protrusion! It's not in my head!'. He and his wife were delighted and he was referred for a surgical opinion and this lead to decompression of the left L3 nerve root with an extended fenestration and partial facetectomy to access the lateral disc protrusion and the intervertebral foramen; a single large sequestrated fragment of nucleus pulposus compressing the nerve was removed, freeing it. His post-operative course was unremarkable and he was discharged on the seventh post-operative day.

RESULTS

At 1 month after surgery he was doing well and he experienced good relief from his sciatica, although he still experienced some back discomfort by the end of the day. He was advised to gradually start swimming to strengthen his back muscles and he continues to do well some 5 years post-operatively. He was extremely grateful that his condition had, at last, been taken seriously and that a proper diagnostic work-up had led to a diagnosis and subsequent treatment.

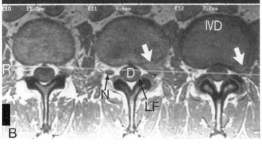

Figure 23.2 (A) A parasagittal left-sided T1-weighted MRI view showing the lumbosacral spine with a large L3–4 disc protrusion (white arrow) projecting into the intervertebral foramen and displacing the left L3 nerve root. Note the intervertebral foramina above and below the L3–4 level that show the normal position of the nerve within the foramen (small black arrow). L3 = third lumbar vertebral body; L4 = fourth lumbar vertebral body; S1 = first sacral segment; P = pedicle of the fourth lumbar vertebra. H = hyaline articular cartilage of the zygapophysial (facet) joint between the inferior articular process of the L4 vertebra and the superior articular process of the L5 vertebra. The area shown within the rectangle is represented in a histopathology section in Fig. 23.3. (B) A series of three consecutive axial T1-weighted MRI views at the L3–4 disc level. The white arrows show the far lateral partly extra-foraminal disc protrusion at the L3–4 level that compresses the nerve in the middle and right-hand scans. The right nerve root ganglion (N) is clearly shown in the middle scan but the left neural structures are severely compressed. The dural tube (D) is shown within the spinal canal adjacent to the ligamenta flava (LF). IVD = intervertebral disc; R = right side of the patient.

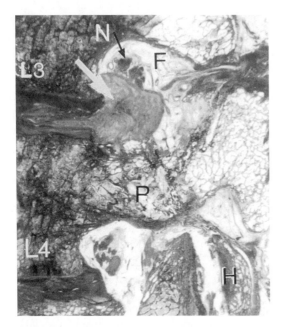

Figure 23.3 A 200-micron thick parasagittal histopathology section from a 69-year-old male postmortem specimen approximately corresponding to the rectangle in Fig. 23.2A. Note the disc protrusion (arrow) projecting into the intervertebral foramen (F) and how the neural structures (N) are being compromised. L3 = part of the third lumbar vertebral body; L4 = part of the fourth lumbar vertebral body; P = pedicle of the fourth lumbar vertebra; H = hyaline articular cartilage on the inferior articular process of the L4 vertebra. (Erhlich's haematoxylin and light green counterstain.)

Key point(s)

1. Never disbelieve your patient unless you have good evidence to do so.
2. A detailed history and careful physical examination, supplemented if necessary by MRI, can differentiate a herniated disc from other possible causes of similar symptoms.
3. Rely upon your own diagnostic acumen and not on that of others.

FURTHER READING

Cox M J 1999 Diagnosis of the low back and leg pain patient. In: Cox JM (ed.) Low back pain: mechanism, diagnosis, and treatment. Williams & Wilkins, Baltimore, pp 377–507.

Hoppenfeld S 1976 Physical examination of the spine and extremities. Appleton-Century-Crofts, New York.

Hoppenfeld S 1977 Orthopaedic neurology: A diagnostic guide to neurologic levels. J B Lippincott, Philadelphia.

Patten J 1996 Neurological differential diagnosis, 2nd edn. Springer-Verlag, Berlin, pp 282.

Postacchini F 1999 Lumbar disc herniation. Springer-Verlag, New York.

Rickenbacher J, Landolt A M, Theiler K 1982 Applied anatomy of the back. Springer-Verlag, Berlin.

Weinstein J N, Rydevik B L, Sonntag V K H 1995 Essentials of the spine. Raven Press, New York.

Case 24 Intervertebral disc dysfunction

COMMENT
Erect posture functional imaging of the lumbar
spine can be very useful.

PROFILE

A 39-year-old married man who does not drink
alcohol or smoke cigarettes and who worked as a
patient carer.

PAST HISTORY

Suffers from high blood pressure and oesophageal
ulcers for which he takes medication.

PRESENTING COMPLAINT (Fig. 24.1)

Low back pain at the L4–5 level, which sometimes radiates to his right buttock and into the
posterior aspect of his right thigh.

The low back pain improves with lying down
but he has to be cautious as he moves about
because he can suddenly get 'twinges of pain'. If
he sits on the floor to play with his children, he
has to gradually get up and slowly straighten
his low back as it becomes very stiff. Sometimes
he can bend forwards without pain but bending
backwards is always painful.

The only medication that he takes is an analgesic as he is wary of taking medication.

He had to resign from work as he was unable
to manage with the physical demands of his
work due to his chronic low back pain. He
had been told by orthopaedic consultants that
there was nothing wrong with his back and
that he should return to his carer work and one
orthopaedic surgeon stated that the patient
should be placed under the surveillance of a

Field Officer. Fortunately, one orthopaedic
surgeon agreed that he could have internal disc
disruption, as did a specialist in rehabilitation
medicine.

Unfortunately, anti-inflammatory medication,
physiotherapy treatment, facet block injections,

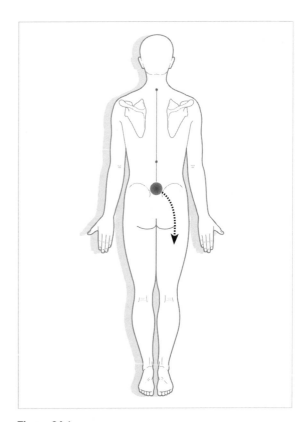

Figure 24.1

medical acupuncture and a paravertebral muscle injection of anaesthetic and cortisone did not provide long-lasting relief. He had had manipulation on two occasions but this apparently aggravated the low back pain. He had tried swimming but it did not help, so he was currently performing hydrotherapy exercises with some benefit.

AETIOLOGY

While helping a large disabled man from a car into a wheelchair the disabled man suddenly slipped and this strained the carer's low back, resulting in immediate and acute low back pain as he took the weight of the patient. While sitting in the car after the incident, he momentarily felt a 'sharp jab like an electric shock' in the low back. The pain radiated from the lower back to both testicles.

EXAMINATION

The knee and ankle jerk deep tendon reflexes were normal, as was the case with pinprick sensation of the lower extremities. His thigh circumference was 50 cm bilaterally, 18 cm above the patella. In the erect posture, there was no evidence of pelvic obliquity on palpation of the posterior superior iliac spines.

Active lumbar spine ranges of movement were as follows:

1. Flexion – he was able to bend forwards to within 2 cm of the floor but he was very cautious as he flexed his spine due to pain at the L4–5 level and also as he unrolled, i.e. extended his spine to the normal erect posture.
2. Extension was limited by approximately 70% due to pain at the L4–5 level.
3. Left and right lateral bending were painless.
4. Right rotation was painless.
5. Left rotation was limited by about 15% due to L4–5 pain.

Palpation over the L4 and L5 spinous processes and the interspinous ligament elicited localized pain. Deep palpation of the lumbar paraspinal muscles elicited pain bilaterally from

L4 to S1. He was able to toe and heel walk without difficulty. He had normal power in the lower extremities. Upon getting onto the examination table he did so cautiously. In the supine position, SLR was limited to approximately 75° (right) and 80° (left) due to 'tightness' of the hamstring muscles. Bilateral hip flexion caused considerable low back pain at approximately 80° elevation of the thighs from the examination table. Cervical spine flexion caused only very slight low back pain and compression of the jugular veins while he coughed (Naffziger test) did not reproduce the low back pain. The pulses in the feet were normal. Hoover's sign for malingering was normal, i.e. it did not indicate any malingering. He was hardly able to raise both his legs simultaneously (Milgram's test) due to an increase in low back pain. In the seated position, the slump test did not aggravate his low back pain.

IMAGING REVIEW

An MRI scan taken approximately 12 months prior to his present consultation reported the following: 'There is no evidence of disc herniation or nerve root compression. Normal marrow signals are observed. The conus ends at L1 and is of normal size and configuration. No evidence of spinal stenosis'.

CLINICAL IMPRESSION

Soft tissue injury at L4–5 level – probably internal disc disruption.

WHAT ACTION SHOULD BE TAKEN?

Because the patient was considered to be entirely genuine in his low back pain complaint, in spite of an apparently normal MRI examination, lumbosacral erect posture anteroposterior and left and right lateral bending functional radiographs were taken. A plumb line was used as a reference point for measuring the angle between the inferior endplate of the L4 vertebra and the plumb line in order to determine whether he had L4–5 joint dysfunction. In the neutral erect posture anteroposterior view there was minor wedging of the L4–5 intervertebral disc that was narrower on the left and wider on the right (Fig. 24.2A).

Although the superior endplate of the L5 vertebral body remained essentially at an angle of 90° to the vertical plumb line in the erect posture neutral position, it can be seen that on left and right lateral bending there is a significant difference between the angle made by the inferior endplate of L4 and the plumb line, as shown by the broken line drawn along the inferior endplate of the L4 vertebral body (Fig. 24.2A, B and C).

In left lateral bending (Fig. 24.2B) the intervertebral joints at the L4–5 level allow bending in conformity with the normal lateral bending posture, i.e. the disc spaces become narrower on the left and wider on the right. However, on right lateral bending, the L4–5 joint refuses to allow normal movement between the vertebral bodies L4 and L5, preventing normal wedging of the disc space. This finding indicates that he has a spinal functional problem at L4–5.

Because this man had a claim for injuries at work, the question arose of whether he should have a discogram performed to confirm that he had internal disc disruption. However, the risks were explained to him and he did not wish to take the risk. He went to court to settle his injury claim based on the non-invasive functional plain X-ray films; the court found in his favour in view of the abnormal functioning of the L4–5 intervertebral disc, as shown by the L4 vertebral body movement with respect to the plumb line.

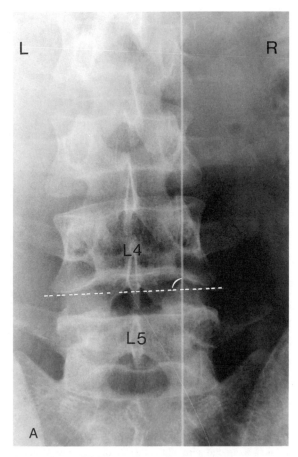

Figure 24.2 (A) Erect posture anteroposterior plain X-ray of the lumbosacral spine (L2–S1). Note the minor wedging of the L4–5 intervertebral disc which is slightly narrower on the left (L) as shown between the broken line across the inferior endplate of L4 and the superior endplate of L5. The angle between the broken line showing the inferior endplate of L4 and the vertical plumb line measures 93°. R = right side of patient.

TREATMENT

Facet block injections, acupuncture and paraspinal muscle blocks had not given him lasting relief, and anti-inflammatory medication gave him gastric problems. As surgery was not indicated, he was advised not to perform any heavy manual work but to continue with water aerobics and then to swim as frequently as possible. He was also advised to perform back exercises (see exercises presented in Case 10).

In addition, he was advised to undergo retraining so that he could perform light duties only.

RESULTS

The main issues that helped him were that he was taken seriously and that an explanation was provided as to why he had chronic low back pain. In addition, he was grateful that an exercise programme was established for him so that he could control his pain levels, which he did satisfactorily over a period of some months.

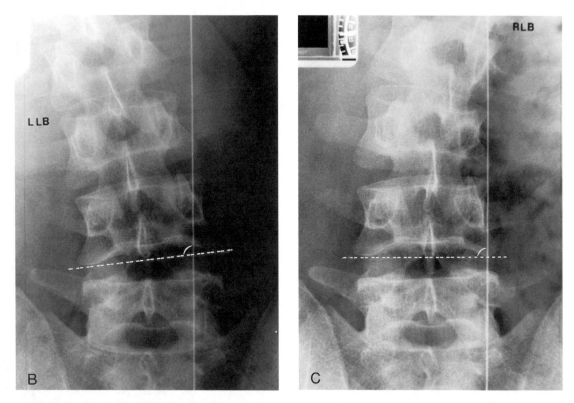

Figure 24.2 (B) Erect posture left lateral bending (LLB) plain X-ray of the lumbosacral spine showing normal wedging of the L4–5 intervertebral disc (which is narrower on the left) and the discs above, i.e. all disc spaces are narrower on the left side and wider on the right. The angle between the L4 inferior endplate line and the plumb line measures 97°. (C) Erect posture right lateral bending (RLB) plain X-ray of the lumbosacral spine showing the L4–5 intervertebral disc which refuses to wedge normally, i.e. to become narrower on the right and wider on the left; the discs above L4 do wedge normally, i.e. become narrower on the right side and wider on the left. The angle between the endplate line and the plumb line measured 91°, i.e. only approximately 2° less than in the neutral anteroposterior view shown in (A).

Key point

The value of plain film anteroposterior erect posture radiography of the lumbar, including functional left and right lateral bending views, should not be underestimated.

Ohnmeiss D D, Vanharanta H, Ekholm J 1997 Degree of disc disruption and lower extremity pain. Spine 22: 1600–1605.

Schwarzer A C, Aprill C N, Derby R, Fortin J, Line G, Bogduk N 1995 The prevalence and clinical features of internal disc disruption in patients with chronic low back pain. Spine 20: 1878–1883.

FURTHER READING

Brightbill T C, Pile N, Eichelberger R P, Whitman M 1994 Normal magnetic resonance imaging and abnormal discography in lumbar disc disruption. Spine 19: 1075–1077.

Case 25   Leg length inequality

COMMENT
Radiographic erect posture examination for leg length inequality is essential when leg length inequality is suspected.

PROFILE

A 37-year-old male of muscular build who does not smoke and only drinks alcohol occasionally.

PAST HISTORY

No recollection of unusual illnesses or of trauma of any kind and has always been fit and healthy.

PRESENTING COMPLAINT (Fig. 25.1)

Low back pain of insiduous onset of several years duration. The pain does not awaken him at night and he feels better of a morning. There is no radiation to the lower extremities.

Coughing and sneezing do not aggravate his symptoms. NSAIDs have not been helpful nor have analgesics. He had seen three medical practitioners regarding his chronic low back pain and presented with three sets of good quality lumbosacral spine radiographs taken in the anteroposterior, lateral and oblique views while in the recumbent position.

AETIOLOGY

Unknown.

EXAMINATION

The deep reflexes in the lower extremities were normal as was the case with pinprick sensation and vibration sensation at the ankles. Power and tone were normal and the plantar response was normal. Deep palpation of the paraspinal muscles elicited pain at the lumbosacral level. The circumference of the thighs and calves was equal on both sides. Bearing down did not increase his

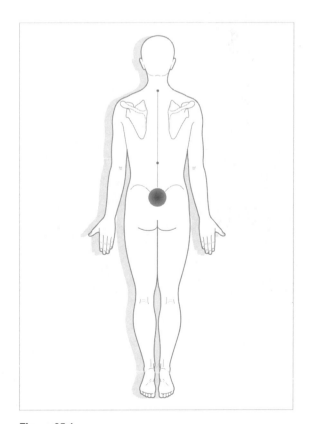

Figure 25.1

123

low back pain. SLR did not aggravate his low back pain. Erect posture examination indicated pelvic obliquity, with the posterior superior iliac spine lower on the right side, with a postural scoliosis.

IMAGING REVIEW

All the previous imaging had been performed in the recumbent position and, although the imaging was of good quality (see Fig. 25.2A), there was no indication of his underlying pelvic obliquity.

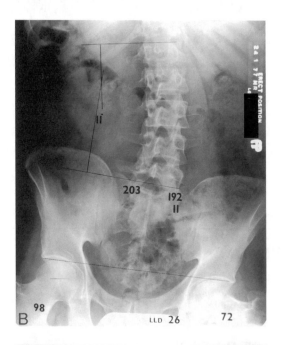

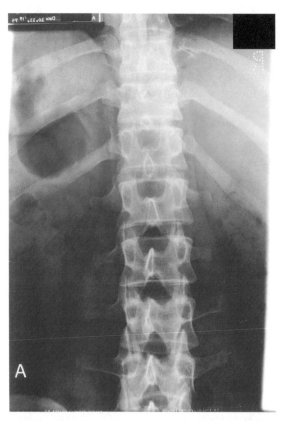

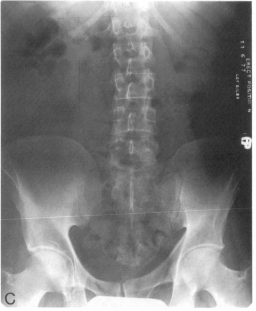

Figure 25.2 (A) A recumbent lumbosacral spine anteroposterior radiograph shows that the lumbar spine is almost straight and gives no indication of the pelvic obliquity and postural scoliosis seen in (B). (B) An erect posture pelvis and lumbar spine anteroposterior radiograph. Note the right leg length discrepancy of 26 mm, the sacral obliquity of 11 mm when measured across the left and right superior sacral notches, and the superimposed lumbar postural scoliosis of 11° measured using the Cobb (1948) method. In addition, the following can be noted: (i) the L3–4 facets on the concave side of the postural scoliosis are apparently more closely apposed than on the convex side; (ii) the L4–5 facets appear to be more closely apposed on the convex side with less apposition of the facets on the concave side; and (iii) the concavity in the inferior surface of the L4 vertebral body is asymmetrical – the concavity is nearer to the convex side of the postural scoliosis. (C) An erect posture pelvis and lumbar spine anteroposterior radiograph taken with the patient standing on a right foot-raise of 26 mm; this raise virtually eliminated the pelvic obliquity and the postural scoliosis.

CLINICAL IMPRESSION

Low back pain due to leg length inequality, pelvic obliquity and postural scoliosis.

WHAT ACTION SHOULD BE TAKEN?

An erect posture pelvis and lumbar spine anteroposterior radiograph was taken with him standing on a horizontal steel platform and with the film in a horizontal bucky and touching the inside bottom of the X-ray cassette. This showed a significant leg length inequality of 26 mm on the right side (Fig. 25.2B). The antero-posterior pelvis and lumbar spine radiograph was repeated with the patient standing on a right foot-raise of 26 mm and this eliminated the pelvic obliquity and the postural scoliosis (Fig. 25.2C).

TREATMENT

This man was advised to always wear a right shoe raise of 26 mm and was given a lum-bosacral and right sacroiliac joint manipulation with him lying on his left side. He was asked to return in one week following building up of his shoes, sandals and slippers.

RESULTS

At the time of his follow-up consultation he said his low back pain had virtually gone. He was delighted that this simple approach should pro-vide him with such dramatic relief; he was advised always to wear built up footwear. He was not seen for 2 years at which time he returned and stated that he was experiencing some recurrence of his low back pain. He was asked whether he was still wearing built up shoes, to which he replied: 'No, because my back was feeling so good!' He was reminded that he would always have to wear built up footwear under the right foot and to wear one thicker thong (equivalent to approxi-mately 26 mm) on his right foot when he showered. He promised to remember to have all new shoes built up and he was not seen again. A relative stated that his back pain had

completely disappeared since wearing the built up shoes.

Note

As a precaution, it should be noted that there may be a leg length inequality but virtually no pelvic obliquity on comparing the left and right superior sacral notches on an erect posture anteroposterior X-ray film. Therefore, this should always be taken into account when measuring for leg length inequality (see Fig. 25.3).

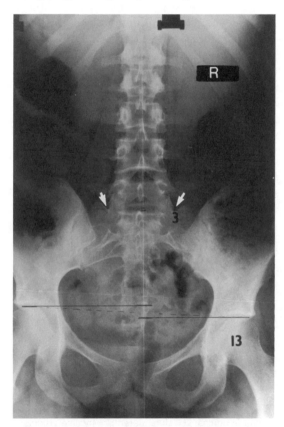

Figure 25.3 An erect posture pelvis and lumbar spine anteroposterior radiograph of a 20-year-old female show-ing a right leg length discrepancy of 13 mm on drawing a horizontal line from the left femur head to the vertical plumb line and a similar line from the right femur head. The broken line shows the inclination between the left and right femur heads. Note that there is no postural scoliosis as the left and right superior sacral notches (white arrows) are almost at the same height (within 3 mm) as measured to the plumb line. As there is no significant sacral base obliquity, this patient would not require a shoe-raise. (Modified from Giles 1984.)

When considering what structures may contribute to low back pain in cases of leg length inequality and pelvic obliquity, apart from the difference in EMG muscle activity between the left and right sides of the spine that is known to occur with patients with a 1-cm or more leg length discrepancy (Vink & Kamphuisen 1989), there are many other possible sources of low back pain. For example, the sacroiliac joints and the lower lumbar spine zygapophysial joints could be sources of pain. A postmortem histological section is shown in Fig. 25.4 which shows some soft tissue structures that may be affected in cases of pelvic obliquity and postural scoliosis. For example, the fibrous joint capsule may be subjected to different stresses between the left and right sides of the spine and the intra-articular synovial fold may become more vulnerable to pinching. In addition it is possible that the outermost layers of the anulus fibrosus are subjected to abnormal stresses leading to disc injuries.

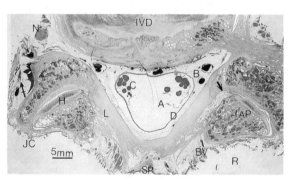

Figure 25.4 A 100-micron thick slightly oblique horizontal histopathology section of the lumbosacral zygapophysial joints at the level of the inferior joint recesses from a 54-year-old male. A = arachnoid membrane; B = Batson's venous plexus; BV = blood vessel; C = cauda equina; D = dura mater; H = hyaline articular cartilage; IVD = intervertebral disc; JC = posterolateral fibrous joint capsule; L = ligamentum flavum; N = spinal ganglion; R = right side; S = sacrum; SP = spinous process. The intra-articular synovial fold is shown by the black arrow. A neurovascular bundle close to the zygapophysial joint is shown by the tailed arrow. (Erhlich's haematoxylin stain with light green counterstain). (Reproduced with permission from Giles L G F, Taylor J R 1982 Intra-articular synovial protrusion in the lower lumbar apophyseal joints. *Bulletin of the Hospital for Joint Diseases Orthopaedic Institute* 42(2): 248–255.) See also colour plate section.

Key point(s)

1. The relationship between low back pain and leg length inequality of greater than 9 mm has been noted by many authors over the years. These authors have come from many different backgrounds as indicated by the further reading list.
2. Erect posture estimation of leg length inequality using the method described by Giles and Taylor (1981) is very useful for accurately determining leg length inequality.

REFERENCES

Cobb J R 1948 Outline for the study of scoliosis. Instructional course lectures. American Academy of Orthopedic Surgeons 5: 261–275.
Giles L G F 1984 Letter to the Editor (re: Clinical symptoms and biomechanics of lumbar spine and hip joint in leg length inequality; Friberg, O, Spine 1983; 8: 643–651) Spine 9: 842.
Giles L G F, Taylor J R 1981 Low-back pain associated with leg length inequality. Spine 6: 510–521.
Vink P, Kamphuisen H A C 1989 Leg length inequality, pelvic tilt and lumbar back muscle activity during standing. Clinical Biomechanics 4: 115–117.

FURTHER READING

Edeen J, Sharkey P F, Alexander A H 1995 Clinical significance of leg-length inequality after total hip arthroplasty. American Journal of Orthopedics 25: 347–351.
Friberg O 1987 The statics of postural pelvic tilt scoliosis; a radiographic study on 288 consecutive chronic LBP patients. Clinical Biomechanics 2: 211–219.
Giles L G F 1981 Lumbosacral facetal 'joint angles' associated with leg length inequality. Rheumatology and Rehabilitation 20: 233–238.
Gofton J P, Trueman G E 1967 Unilateral idiopathic osteoarthritis of the hip. Canadian Medical Association Journal 87: 1129–1132.
Harcke H T, Mandell G A 1993 Scintigraphic evaluation of the growth plate. Seminars in Nuclear Medicine 23: 266–273.
Hazleman B, Bulgen D 1981 Low back pain. International Medicine. Rheumatic Disorders 1: 486–491.
Hoffman K S, Hoffman L L 1994 Effects of adding sacral base leveling to osteopathic manipulative treatment of back pain: a pilot study. Journal of the American Osteopathic Association 94: 217–220, 223–226.
Lawrence D 1984 Lateralization of weight in the presence of structural short leg: a preliminary report. Journal of Manipulative and Physiological Therapy 7: 105–108.
Lawrence D 1984 Chiropractic concepts of the short leg: a critical review. Journal of Manipulative and Physiological Therapy 8: 157–161.

Mattassi R 1993 Differential diagnosis in congenital vascular–bone syndromes. Seminars in Vascular Surgery 6: 233–244.

Parry C B W 1994 The failed back. In: Wall PD, Melzack R (eds) Textbook of Pain, 3rd edn. Churchill Livingstone, Edinburgh, pp 1075–1094.

Reid D C, Smith B 1984 Leg length inequality: a review of etiology and management. Physiotherapy Canada 36: 177–182.

Rush W A, Steiner H A 1946 A study of lower extremity length inequality. American Journal of Roentgenology 56: 616–623.

Subotnick S I 1981 Limb length discrepancies of the lower extremities (the short leg syndrome). Journal of Orthopaedic and Sports Physical Therapy 3: 11–16.

Tjernstrom B, Rehnberg L 1994 Back pain and arthralgia before and after lengthening. 75 patients questioned after 6 (1–11) years. Acta Orthopaedica Scandinavica 65: 328–332.

Tjernstrom B, Olerud S, Karlstrom G 1993 Direct leg lengthening. Journal of Orthopaedic Trauma 7: 543–551.

Williams P C 1974 Low back and neck pain. Charles C Thomas, Springfield, p 52.

Case 26   Discitis and osteomyelitis

COMMENT
This case highlights complications that may occur in intravenous drug users.

PROFILE
An 18-year-old thin, tall man.

PAST HISTORY
A history of intravenous drug use. No history of trauma.

PRESENTING COMPLAINT (Fig. 26.1)
A feeling of being generally unwell and feverish with various spinal aches and pains and hip joint pains. He was immediately hospitalized and seen by a specialist physician.

AETIOLOGY
Intravenous drug addiction.

CLINICAL IMPRESSION
Possibly septicaemia/osteomyelitis.

EXAMINATION AND ACTION TAKEN
A comprehensive diagnostic work-up resulted in a diagnosis of bacterial endocarditis and spinal osteomyelitis secondary to septicaemia. He was found to have positive cultures for the following organisms: methycillin-sensitive *Staphylococcus aureus*, *Staphylococcus epidermidis* and *Bacillus cereus*. His ESR was 130 mm/hr (normal 1–10) and his blood pressure was 90/60.

An initial transthoracic echocardiogram showed some tricuspid regurgitation but no vegetations. Transoesophageal echocardiogram showed vegetations consistent with endocarditis of the tricuspid valve. An initial bone scan showed probable abnormalities in his clavicle,

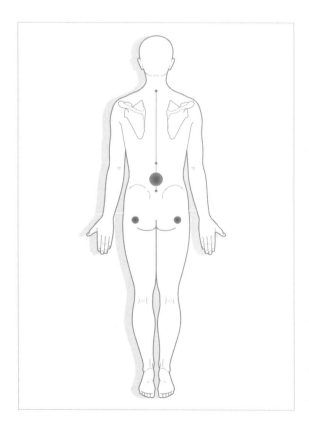

Figure 26.1

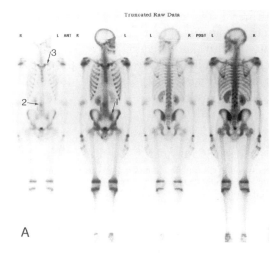

A

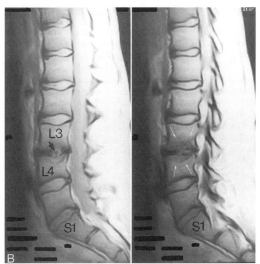

B

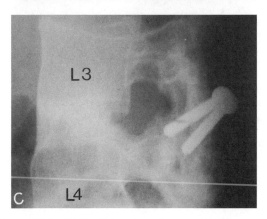

C

mid-lumbar vertebral region and in the sacro-iliac joints.

He was hospitalized for 8 weeks while undergoing intravenous antibiotic drug therapy. Following 8 weeks of antibiotic treatment a three phase bone scan with SPECT and an echocardiogram were repeated. The echocardiogram showed lesser residual vegetations on the tricuspid valve and the bone scan showed:

Increased blood pool activity in the left sacroilic joint and a slight increase in blood pool activity in the right side of the mid lumbar spine, approximately in the region of the L3–4 body consistent with hyper-aemia. SPECT tomographic images have confirmed increased tracer uptake in the left sacroiliac joint and at the L3–4 level of the lumbar spine on the right. Relatively increased tracer uptake in both shoulders is symmetrical and almost certainly represents activity in incompletely fused epiphyses. Increased tracer uptake is noted in the medial aspect of the left clavicle. Tracer distribution elsewhere in the skeleton is otherwise unremarkable. Comments: appearance on bone scan suggests a sacroiliitis, some focus in the medial end of the left clavicle and a further focus of probable infection in the L3–4 region of the lumbar spine (Fig. 26.2A).

He was referred for a CT scan that showed lytic lesions in the L3 and L4 lumbar vertebrae where he still had pain. Therefore, although all organisms were reported sensitive to the antibiotic used, this obviously did not eliminate the infection, perhaps because the antibiotic has brief peaks of high serum concentration and then washed out very quickly and the sporing

Figure 26.2 (A) The three phase bone scan with SPECT truncated raw data view shows 'activity in the left sacroiliac joint (arrow 1) and a slight increase in activity in the right side of the mid lumbar spine in the region of L3/L4 (arrow 2). Relatively increased tracer uptake in both shoulders is symmetrical and almost certainly represents activity in incompletely fused epiphyses. Increased tracer uptake is noted in the medial aspect of the left clavicle' (arrow 3). The 'hot spot' (arrow 2) at the L3–4 level is where surgery was later performed. (B) A sagittal STIR MRI view of the lumbar spine showing discitis of the L3–4 disc with destruction of the adjacent vertebral body endplates and associated marrow oedema (arrows). There is a small degree of enhancement of this disc posteriorly (black arrow). The remaining discs appear normal. L3 = third lumbar vertebral body; L4 = fourth lumbar vertebral body; S1 = first sacral segment. (C) A lateral plain X-ray view of the L3 and L4 bodies showing an anterior interbody fusion with posterior fixation (using two screws).

nature of the bacillus cerus allows some organisms to resist the peaks. Antibiotic treatment was changed and he was referred for an orthopaedic opinion regarding his L3–4 discitis secondary to infection.

An MRI scan was performed (Fig. 26.2B) and found: 'There is discitis of the L3–4 disc with destruction of the endplates and associated marrow oedema. There is a small degree of enhancement of this disc posteriorly. No epidural extension seen. The other discs appear normal'.

TREATMENT

With the intention of eradicating the infective discitis, surgery was then performed to remove the L3–4 disc and adjacent endplates, followed by fusion of the levels involved by simple fixation (Fig. 26.2C).

RESULTS

Following the above treatment that involved prompt referral for care by several specialists, this young man recovered in due course. His blood pressure was 110/65, he was afebrile at 36.5°C, there was no evidence of an enlarged pulsatile liver and no swelling of his ankles. Heart sounds indicated a soft pan systolic murmer at the left sternal edge consistent with tricuspid regurgitation. ECG showed normal sinus rhythm and a chest X-ray did not reveal any abnormalities. He was left with a mild to moderate tricuspid regurgitation and he has periodic re-evaluations.

> **Key point**
>
> Intravenous drug users with spinal and other pains may present with life-threatening infections that require immediate referral for specialized medical care.

FURTHER READING

Fortun J, Navas E, Martinez-Beltran J, Perez-Molina J, Martin-Davila P, Guerrero A, Moreno S 2001 Short-course therapy for right-sided endocarditis due to *Staphylococcus aureus* in drug abusers: cloxacillin versus glycopeptides in combination with gentamicin. Clinical Infectious Diseases 33: 120–125.

Hopkinson N, Stevenson J, Benjamin S 2001 A case ascertainment study of septic discitis: clinical, microbiological and radiological features. Quarterly Journal of Medicine 94: 465–470.

Lopez-Majano V, Miskew D B 1980 Sacro-iliac joint disease in drug abusers: the role of bone scintigraphy. European Journal of Nuclear Medicine 5: 459–463.

Lopez-Majano V, Miskew D, Sansi P 1981 Bone scintigraphy in drug addiction. European Journal of Nuclear Medicine 6: 17–21.

Cervical spine cases

INTRODUCTION

Before presenting the cervical spine cases it is important to consider the following summary of some possible causes of cervical spine pain with or without radiculopathy (Table v).

Table vi summarizes some possible causes of pain referred into the arm from the neck and thorax. In addition, pain arising in the brachial plexus and peripheral nerves is included, as also are lesions at the shoulder, elbow, wrist and hand, which specifically or characteristically affect the upper limb (Keat 1996).

Table v Some possible causes of cervical spine pain

Acute spinal pain
  Febrile disorders
  Injury

Chronic spinal pain

Traumatic, mechanical or degenerative:
  Cervical spine strain; 'whiplash'
  Injuries of bone, joint, intervertebral disc or ligaments; clay
    shoveler's avulsion fracture of C6 or C7 spinous process
  Degenerative or traumatic changes of the spine
    (osteoarthrosis; spondylosis)
  Cervical spine instability syndromes, e.g. spondylolisthesis
  Scoliosis: primary and secondary
  Spinal or intervertebral canal stenosis
  Cervical rib
  Upper brachial plexus avulsion

Joint dysfunction:
  Zygapophysial
  Intervertebral disc

Metabolic:
  Osteoporosis
  Osteomalacia
  Hyper- and hypo-parathyroidism
  Ochronosis
  Fluorosis

Unknown causes:
  Inflammatory arthropathies of the spine, such as
    ankylosing spondylitis and the spondylitis of Reiter's
    (Brodie's) disease, psoriasis, rheumatoid arthritis,
    polymyalgia rheumatica

Infective conditions of bone, joint and theca of the spine:
  Osteomyelitis
  Tuberculosis
  Melioidosis
  Undulant fever (abortus and melitensis)
  Typhoid and paratyphoid fever and other *Salmonella*
    infections
  Syphilis

continued

Table v Continued

Yaws
Very rarely, Weil's disease (leptospirosis
  icterohaemorrhagica)
Spinal pachymeningitis
Chronic meningitis
Subarachnoid or spinal abscess
Herpes zoster
Cervical adenitis
Poliomyelitis
Tetanus
Febrile states – meningism
Malaria

Psychogenic:
  Anxiety
  Depression
  Hysteria
  'Compensation neurosis'
  Malingering

Neoplastic – benign or malignant, primary or secondary:
  Osteoid osteoma
  Eosinophilic granuloma
  Metastatic carcinomatosis
  Bronchial carcinoma
  Oesophageal carcinoma
  Sarcoma
  Myeloma
  Primary and secondary tumours of spinal canal and nerve
    roots: ependymoma; neurofibroma; glioma; angioma;
    meningioma; lipoma; rarely cordoma
  Reticuloses, e.g. Hodgkin's disease

Cardiac and vascular:
  Subarachnoid or spinal haemorrhage
  Aneurysm
  Vertebral artery tortuosity causing bony erosion
  Visceral referral – heart, oesophagus and lung
    carcinoma

Blood disorders:
  Acute haemolytic states

Modified from Hart (1985) and Patten (1996).

PHYSICAL EXAMINATION

The physical examination should be orderly and systematic and should include the following cervical spine examinations, as indicated by the patient's presenting complaint(s) (Table vii).

It is essential to remember that the signs and symptoms caused by a herniated cervical disc depend on the location of the herniation:

- Figure vii shows the clinical features of a *posterolateral* cervical disc herniation that

Table vi Some possible causes of arm pain specific to the neck

Lesions in the neck
  Disc prolapse
  Spondylosis
  Syringomyelia
  Fracture dislocations
  Post-herpetic neuralgia
  Radiculitis – paralytic/viral (neurologic amyotrophy)
  Spinal abscess
    Tuberculous
    Brucella
    Pyogenic

  Epidural abscess
  Pachymeningitis cervicalis
  Tumours
    Spinal cord
    Meninges
    Nerve roots
    Vertebrae – primary, secondary
    Metastatic carcinoma in deep cervical nodes

Lesions of the brachial plexus
  Cervical rib
  Malignant infiltration, e.g. Pancoast tumour
  Costoclavicular compression
  Subclavian aneurysm
  Scalenus anterior syndrome

Lesions of the thorax and thoracic spine
  Cardiac ischaemia
  Syphilitic aortitis
  Thoracic disc
  Oesophagitis

Lesions at the shoulder
  Periarthritis/capsulitis
  Subacromial bursitis
  Calcific tendonitis
  Bicipital tendonitis
  Shoulder–hand syndrome

Lesions at the elbow
  Epicondylitis
  Olecranon bursitis

Lesions of the forearm, wrist and hand
  Carpal tunnel syndrome
  Tenosynovitis
  Ulnar neuritis
  Trigger finger
  Algodystrophy (reflex sympathetic dystrophy, RSD)
  Hypertrophic osteoarthropathy
  Pachydermoperiostitis
  Repetitive strain injury (RSI)

Lesions which may arise from skin disease are excluded.

Modified from Keat (1996) and Patten (1996).

Table vii Some elements of the cervical spine physical examination

Erect posture examination
Observe for:
  Fluidity of movement
  Body build
  Skin markings – café-au-lait spots
  Posture
Observe gait:
  Steady or unsteady

Seated
Test cervical spine motion, with caution and bearing in mind possible injury to the vertebral arteries, for:
  Flexion
  Extension
  Side bending
  Rotation
  Cervical rotation plus extension

Bony palpation:
  Anterior aspect
    Hyoid bone
    Thyroid cartilage
    First cricoid ring
    Carotid tubercle

  Posterior aspect
    Occiput
    Inion
    Superior nuchal line
    Mastoid processes
    Spinous processes of the cervical vertebrae
    Facet joints

Special tests:
  Naffziger test*
  Valsalva manoeuvre*
  Compression test*
  Swallowing test*
  Adson's test*

Palpate for:
  Muscle spasm
  Myofascial trigger points
  Supraspinous and interspinous ligament tenderness
  Adjacent muscle tenderness

Neurological tests:
  Biceps reflex
  Triceps reflex
  Brachioradialis reflex
  Muscle power testing
  Pinprick sensation upper extremities
  Vibration sensation at elbows

Test major peripheral nerves:
  Wrist extension
  Thumb extension
  Thumb abduction
  Thumb pinch
  Apposition of thumb and index finger
  Deltoid

Test for upper motor neuron lesion:
  Hoffmann's sign
  Plantar response (Babinski test)

Measure
  Arm/forearm circumference bilaterally

(Adapted from Hoppenfield 1976, Mackenzie 1985, Keim & Kirkaldy-Willis 1987.)
*See Abbreviations and Definitions chapter.

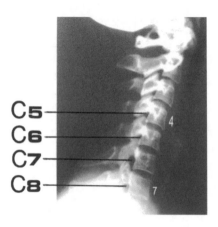

HERNIATION NERVE ROOT	C4-5	C5-6	C6-7	C7-T1
	C5	C6	C7	C8
SENSORY SUPPLY				
PAIN	Lateral arm, medial scapula	Lateral forearm ▶ thumb and index finger	Triceps, front and back of mid-forearm ▶ middle finger; Medial border of scapula	Medial forearm ▶ ring and little finger
MOTOR WEAKNESS	Deltoid Supraspinatus Infraspinatus Rhomboids	Wrist extensors (C6) Biceps (C5,6) Forearm pronators & supinators	Triceps Wrist extensors & flexors Pectoralis major Latissimus dorsi	Finger flexors Hand intrinsic muscles
SCREENING EXAM	Shoulder abduction, Shoulder internal & external rotation Elbow flexion	Elbow flexion Wrist extension Forearm pronation & supination	Finger extension Elbow extension Shoulder adduction Wrist flexion	Finger flexion Thumb & forefinger pinching
REFLEXES	Biceps	Brachioradialis	Triceps	-

Figure vii   The clinical features of a posterolateral cervical disc herniation that may cause nerve root impingement. C5–C8 shows nerve root level. Adapted from Hoppenfeld (1976, 1977), Patten (1996) and Wilkinson (1986).

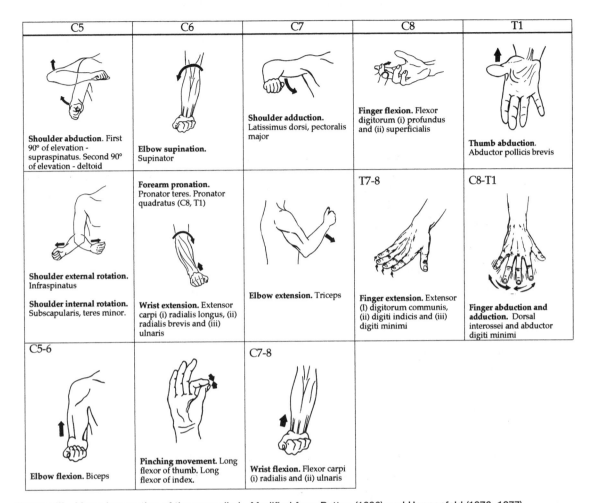

Figure viii Motor innervation of the upper limb. Modified from Patten (1996) and Hoppenfeld (1976, 1977).

may cause nerve root impingement, as summarized in Fig. vii.

• *Midline* herniation may cause symptoms in the arm, upper thoracic region and/or in the legs.

The motor innervation of the upper limb is shown in Fig. viii.

REFERENCES

Hart F D 1985 Back, pain in. In: Hart FD (ed.) French's index of differential diagnosis, 12th edn. Butterworth & Co. Ltd, Oxford, pp 72–73.

Hoppenfeld S 1976 Physical examination of the spine and extremities. Appleton-Century-Crofts, New York.

Hoppenfeld S 1977 Orthopaedic neurology: A diagnostic guide to neurologic levels. J. B. Lippincott, Philadelphia.

Keat A 1996 Arm, pain in. In: Hart FD (ed.) French's index of differential diagnosis. Butterworth-Heinemann, Oxford, p 34.

Keim H A, Kirkaldy-Willis W H 1987 Clinical symposia. Low back pain, vol 39. Ciba-Geigy, Jersey.

Mackenzie I 1985 Spine, tenderness of. In: Hart FD (ed.) French's index of differential diagnosis, 12th edn. Butterworth & Co. Ltd, Oxford, p 788.

Patten J 1996 Neurological differential diagnosis, 2nd edn. Springer-Verlag, Berlin, pp 282.

Wilkinson J L 1986 Neuroanatomy of medical students. John Wright and Sons, Bristol, p 290.

Case 27 Post motor vehicle accident intervertebral disc injuries

COMMENT
In addition to routine cervical spine radiographs, functional cervical spine radiographs are essential following neck trauma unless there is a risk to the vertebral/carotid arteries and/or cord with neck flexion and extension.

PROFILE

A 44-year-old female who does not smoke and only drinks alcohol socially.

PAST HISTORY

No past history of neck pain, headaches or arm symptoms before a motor vehicle accident approximately 4 weeks prior to consultation.

PRESENTING COMPLAINT (Fig. 27.1)

A 'deep and intense pain' bilaterally in the cervical spine and extending to the T5 level with radiation of pain to the left arm, forearm, thumb, index and middle finger (C6). Her neck is very painful on arising from bed and she finds that heat from the hot shower helps temporarily. She experiences significant bilateral occipital headaches which she says are 'different' to very occasional headaches from which she had suffered previously. She had no history of migraine.

She had had two analgesic injections for the pain and depended on analgesic medication to help with her neck and arm pain.

AETIOLOGY

She had been driving her car, with her seat belt in place, and had almost stopped behind a line of cars when her vehicle was hit by a large vehicle from behind. Her car was then pushed into a vehicle in front of hers. She was looking straight ahead during the impact. She immediately felt neck pain and 'numbness' in her left arm; the numbness persisted for a few days. Initially, she experienced a severe headache.

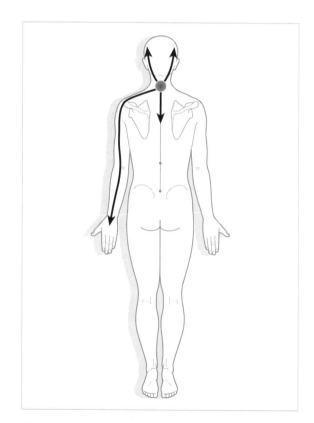

Figure 27.1

136

EXAMINATION

The deep reflexes in the upper extremities were normal but the left patella reflex was diminished to one plus, as compared to the right which was two plus, i.e. normal. The ankle reflexes were normal. Pinprick sensation elicited hypoaesthesia in the left thumb (C6) and in the left middle finger (C7). Light touch in the left hand was diminished. Vibration sensation in the legs and arms was normal. Power appeared to be approximately equal and normal for the upper and lower extremities. Eye movements and visual fields appeared to be normal, as was the case with the consensual light and accommodation reflexes. The optic discs were normal. She was able to perform the finger to nose test normally. In the seated position, the blood pressure in the arms was 129/87 (right) and 129/85 (left). The Valsalva manoeuvre was normal, as were foot plantar responses.

Deep palpation of the paravertebral muscles of the cervical spine elicited tenderness bilaterally as far as C7; the thoracic spine was tender to T4.

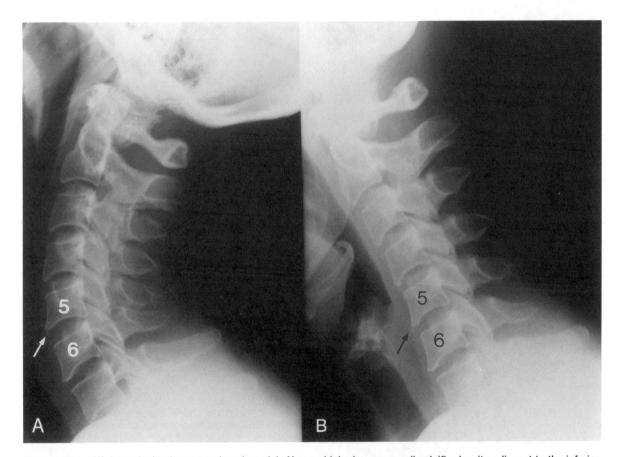

Figure 27.2 (A) A cervical spine extension view plain X-ray which shows a small calcific density adjacent to the inferior endplate of C5 anteriorly (white arrow). Also, the disc height is increased anteriorly at C5–6 compared to the discs at C4–5 and C6–7 levels, suggesting weakness of the anterior anular fibres and perhaps an injury to the anterior longitudinal ligament at C5–6. The disc height posteriorly at C6–7 is greater than the disc height anteriorly, raising the possibility of injury posteriorly to the intervertebral disc and the posterior longitudinal ligament at this level. In addition, note the slight retrolisthesis of the C3 body on the C4 body. (B) Cervical spine flexion view showing the calcific density described above (black arrow). Note how this structure changes its position on extension and flexion. Also, note that there is an angulation at the C4–5 level with the vertebral bodies below this level aligned in an almost straight line, particularly from C5 to C7, indicating limited movement below the C4 level.

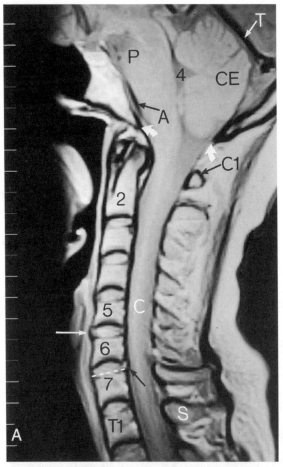

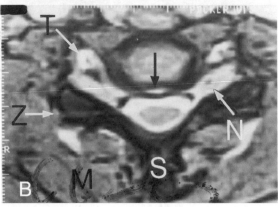

Figure 27.3 (A) Sagittal T1-weighted MRI scan slice showing the small posterior disc protrusion at the C6–7 disc (black arrow) and the anterior disc bulge at C5–6 (white arrow). 2 = body of the second cervical vertebra; 5, 6 and 7 show the bodies of the fifth, sixth and seventh cervical vertebrae; T1 = body of first thoracic vertebra; C = spinal cord; S = spinous process of T1 vertebra;

Box 27.1

	Normal range	Measured range	Comments
Flexion	50°	37°	Caused centrally located neck pain
Extension	60°	48°	Limited due to 'neck stiffness'
Left & right lateral bending	45°	23°	Caused pain on the contralateral side at the C5 to T1 levels
Left rotation	80°	64°	Caused a 'pulling' sensation on the right of C5
Right rotation	80°	64°	Caused pain in the left cervico-shoulder region

Cervical spine active ranges of movement were measured using a Cervical Range of Motion instrument (CROM product of Performance Attainment Associates, St Paul, MN, USA), as shown in Box 27.1.

Both sternocleidomastoideus muscles were very tender to palpation and when she tried to perform various neck movements. Percussion of the thoracic and lumbar spines was painless.

IMAGING REVIEW

A cervical spine X-ray study, including cervical spine flexion and extension functional views reported a small bony fragment adjacent to the

---

C1 = posterior tubercle of the first cervical vertebra; CE = cerebellum; 4 = fourth ventricle; P = pons; T = tentorium cerebelli; A = basilar artery; curved white arrows show the anterior (clivus) and the posterior (or occiput) margins of the foramen magnum. The approximate level for the axial scan shown in (B) is represented by the white broken line that gives the plane of the axial section. (B) Axial T2-weighted MRI scan at the C6–7 level (see A). M = muscles adjacent to the spinous process (S); T = transverse foramen (containing the vertebral artery, vertebral vein and the sympathetic plexus on the vertebral artery); Z = zygapophysial joint with superior and inferior articular facets opposite each other; N = nerve root ganglion in the left intervertebral foramen; black arrow shows the disc protrusion posterior to the C6–7 intervertebral disc.

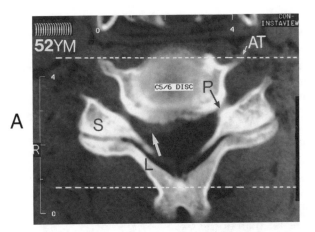

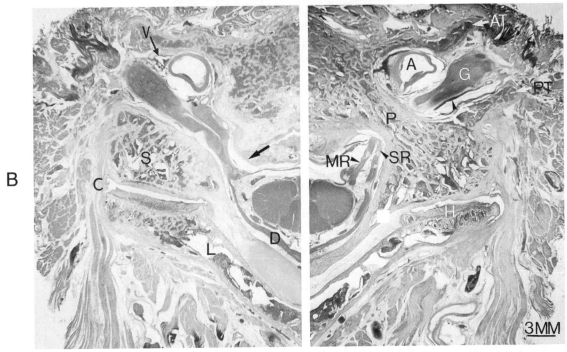

Figures 27.4 (A) An example of an axial (horizontal) cervical spine CT scan from a 52-year-old man and a histopathological section in a similar plane from postmortem material (B). The axial CT scan (A) at the C5–6 level shows the
approximate area (between the broken lines) of the histopathological sections in (B). The CT scan also shows some
posterior spondylosis of the vertebral body with some disc herniation on the right side (white arrow), both of which
cause some narrowing of the spinal canal and the right intervertebral foramen. The montage represents two
histopathological sections from the mid-cervical spine of a middle-aged postmortem specimen. Note how osteophytosis
of the posterolateral region of the uncovertebral joint (black arrow) can deform the nerve roots. AT = anterior tubercle;
C = capsule of the zygapophysial joint; D = dural tube; G = spinal ganglion (highly vascular) and intermediate neural
branch blood vessel (arrowhead); H = hyaline articular cartilage on the facet of the inferior articular process; L = lamina;
MR = motor root; P = pedicle; PT = posterior tubercle; S = superior articular process; SR = sensory root; V = thin-walled
vein adjacent to the vertebral artery. Note the spinal cord lying within the dural tube and how the motor (MR) and
sensory (SR) roots pass into the intervertebral foramen beneath the pedicle on the right side of the histopathology
section. It is important to realize that imaging has limited resolution when compared to actual anatomy and histology, so
histopathological changes cannot be visualized on imaging until they become advanced. (Reproduced with permission
from: Giles LGF (2000) Mechanisms of neurovascular compression within the spinal and intervertebral canals. *Journal of
Manipulative and Physiological Therapeutics* 23: 107–111.) See also colour plate section.

inferior endplate of the C5 body anteriorly and described this as being 'consistent with a limbus vertebra, i.e. a normal variant'.

However, further findings were noted on reviewing the films themselves (Fig. 27.2A and B). Note how the 'limbus' bone moves between the extension and flexion views, raising the possibility that this structure is, in fact, calcification in the anterior fibres of this disc, or in the anterior longitudinal ligament, due to injury having caused bleeding followed by calcification. The cervical spine extension view (Fig. 27.2A) shows some widening of the C5–6 intervertebral disc space anteriorly that is greater than at the C4–5 and C6–7 levels, suggesting that the anterior fibres of the intervertebral disc have been torn as well as some fibres of the anterior longitudinal ligament. On cervical spine flexion (Fig. 27.2B) the C5–6 intervertebral disc space is narrower anteriorly. In addition, there is some widening of the C6–5 intervertebral disc space posteriorly. These findings suggest that there has been some tearing of the posterior fibres of the intervertebral disc at C5–6 and perhaps some tearing of the posterior longitudinal ligament. Furthermore, the flexion view (Fig. 27.2B) shows that there is limited movement below the C4 vertebral level.

CLINICAL IMPRESSION

Soft tissue injuries to various parts of the cervical spine, but most likely to the C5–6 and C6–7 intervertebral discs, with possible tearing of the anterior fibres at C5–6 and the posterior fibres at C6–7; i.e. a cervical spine 'whiplash'-type injury.

WHAT ACTION SHOULD BE TAKEN?

In view of the plain X-ray film findings a cervical spine MRI was ordered. The MRI report noted a 'small disc protrusion at the C6–7 disc posteriorly' (Fig. 27.3A). However, no mention was made of the anterior disc bulge at C5–6. The small disc protrusion posteriorly at C6–7 was confirmed on the axial views (Fig. 27.3B).

Approximately 1 year later a further MRI was performed which showed similar findings to the previous MRI but with clearer visualization of the posterior anular tearing on the axial scans.

A C4 to C7 cervical spine discogram, followed by a CT examination, was performed. This showed the following:

C5–6 level: there is a full thickness left posterolateral tear in the anular fibres with contrast extravasating adjacent to the posterior margin of the left uncovertebral joint; C6–7 level: there is a full thickness posterior tear in the anular fibres with extravasation of contrast material beneath the posterior longitudinal ligament.

TREATMENT

In view of persisting deep and intense pain in the cervical spine and the associated referred pain, the patient was referred to a neurosurgeon who performed a C6–7 anterior cervical discectomy and fusion (Cloward procedure) using a right iliac crest graft and metallic plate fixation.

RESULTS

Unfortunately, surgery did not resolve the left upper limb symptoms. However, the bilateral occipital headaches resolved.

Note

In order to fully appreciate the soft tissue anatomy surrounding the cervical spine, see Fig. 27.4A and B. A parasagittal histopathology section of the cervical spine is shown in Case 31 (Fig. 31.2B).

Key point(s)

The value of cervical spine flexion and extension functional views has been well documented in the literature and this case indicates how important it is to look at lateral view functional plain film radiographs to determine:

(a) the overall contour of the cervical spine,
(b) the disc space height for any possible disc thinning, suggesting injury,

(c) disc space height anteriorly and posteriorly which may suggest tearing of the anterior and/or posterior fibres of the intervertebral disc and the associated ligaments,
(d) whether any segmental instability is present.

FURTHER READING

An H S 1998 Cervical spine trauma. Spine 23: 2729–2731.
Dai L 1998 Disc degeneration and cervical instability. Correlation of magnetic resonance imaging with radiography. Spine 23: 1734–1738.
Gunzburg R, Szpalski M 1998 Whiplash injuries: current concepts in prevention, diagnosis and treatment of the cervical whiplash syndrome. Lippincott-Raven, Philadelphia.
Jackson R 1977 The cervical syndrome, 4th edn. Charles C. Thomas, Springfield, IL.
Noakes J 1998 The spine. In: Anderson J, Read JW, Steinweg J (eds) Atlas of imaging in sports medicine. McGraw-Hill, Sydney, pp 317–373.

Case 28 Vertebral artery dissection

COMMENT
Always look carefully for abnormal anatomy.

PROFILE

A 34-year-old man of muscular build who smokes 12–15 cigarettes per day and consumes only a modest amount of alcohol.

PAST HISTORY

Healthy apart from having had surgery for an appendectomy many years ago.

PRESENTING COMPLAINT (Fig. 28.1)

Constant and significant neck pain with severe headaches and intermittent 'blackouts'; some symptoms of 'weakness' in his legs. He recently experienced two blackouts from which it took him several minutes to recover. His symptoms caused him major depression as he had previously been fit and able to lead a perfectly normal and very active life. He had been diagnosed as having a minor 'cervical whiplash injury' due to a 'low-speed impact' and was referred by his medical practitioner for a further opinion.

Sneezing causes a significant increase in neck pain as does lifting relatively minor weights, e.g. 10–12 kg. The neck pain increases severely with all movements of the neck which are extremely limited by pain.

NSAIDs provide only limited relief. Panadeine Forte, Capadex and Valium in large doses, as well as Endone, only provide minor relief. He was also on an antidepressant medication for major depression that resulted from his significant cervical spine syndrome.

Physiotherapy treatment was of no benefit. He had consulted a number of general medical practitioners including several specialists. One neurologist had found the fundi were clear, the cranial nerves were intact and examination of his limbs revealed no focal signs; his pulse was regular and he was normotensive and there

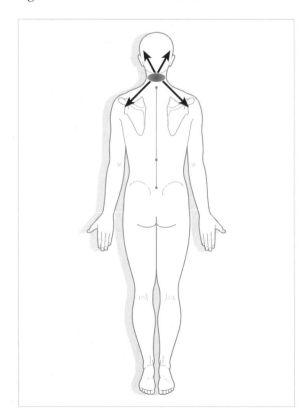

Figure 28.1

were no cardiac murmurs or cervical bruits. He said a plain X-ray examination of his neck and a CT scan had both been reported as normal.

he experienced a 'burning' pain posteriorly in the neck. Three days later the pain became so bad that he required Pethidine injections.

AETIOLOGY

Three years ago, while being driven during his work, he was a seat-belted passenger in a motor vehicle that rear-ended the vehicle in front at approximately 50 km/hr. At the time of impact his head was turned to one side. Within 15 minutes

EXAMINATION

All cervical spine ranges of neck movement were severely restricted due to a significant increase in pain. Neurological examination appeared to be normal. Abduction of the arms beyond 90° aggravated his neck pain.

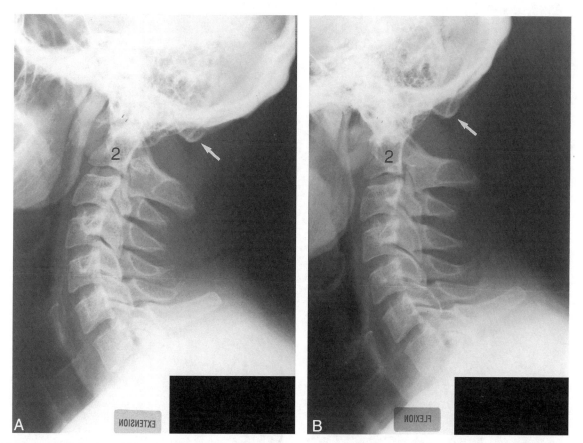

Figure 28.2 Lateral cervical spine extension (A) and flexion views (B), respectively. Note the posterior arch of atlas is missing apart from the posterior tubercle (white arrows) that is assimilated into the occiput. Also note the very limited range of cervical spine extension and flexion as well as very limited skull/cervical spine movements.

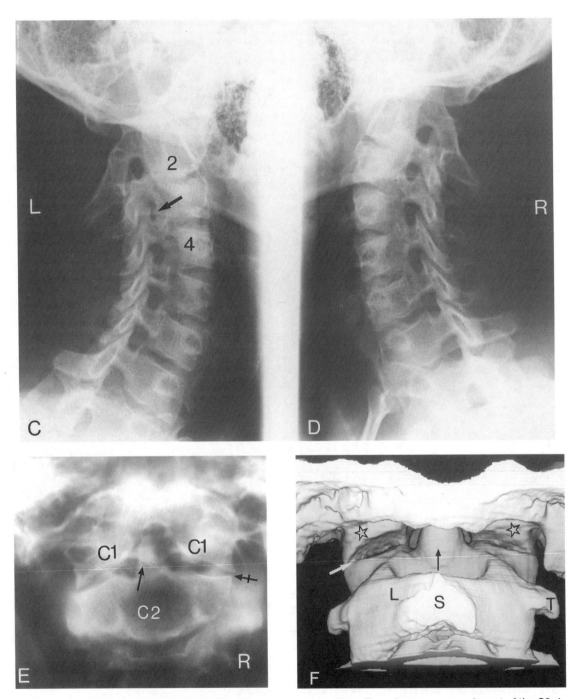

Figure 28.2 Cervical spine left (C) and right (D) oblique views, respectively. There is some encroachment of the C3–4 intervertebral foramen in (C) (arrow) due to osteophytic encroachment from the uncovertebral joint. (E) A cervical spine open mouth tomogram view that shows the C1 lateral masses (C1). The odontoid peg of C2 is seen (arrow) and the zygapophysial joints are normal between the assimilated atlas lateral masses and the lateral masses of C2 (tailed arrow). R = right side of patient. (F) CT cervical spine reconstruction showing complete incorporation of the C1 lateral masses (*) into the base of the skull. Black arrow = odontoid peg; white arrow = superior articular facet of the C2 vertebra. L = lamina of C2 vertebra; S = spine of C2; T = transverse process of C2.

IMAGING REVIEW

Plain X-ray anteroposterior, lateral and oblique views were reported as showing a 'normal examination'. However, on reviewing these films it was noted that there was assimilation of the atlas within the skull base. Because of the severity of his neck pain with restriction of all active ranges of movement, a delayed whole body bone scan with SPECT of the cervical spine had been performed. This was reported as a 'normal examination'.

CLINICAL IMPRESSION

Cervical spine soft tissue injuries including a vascular component that causes the 'blackouts' – query vertebral artery injury.

WHAT ACTION SHOULD BE TAKEN?

Plain X-ray films, including cervical spine extension and flexion functional views, were ordered (Fig. 28.2A–E). The functional views (Fig. 28.2A and B) showed assimilation of the atlas within

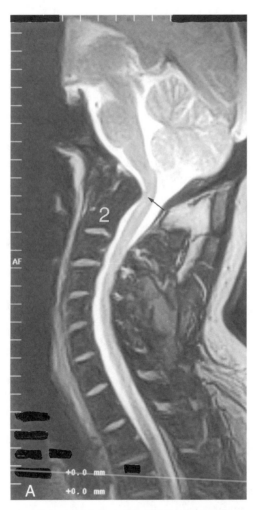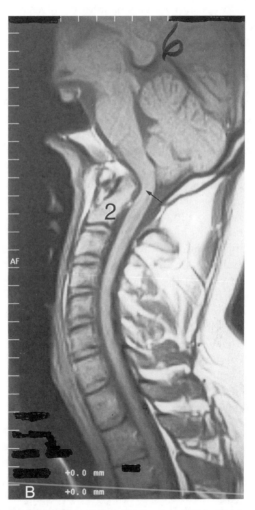

Figure 28.3 (A) A sagittal T2-weighted MRI scan of the cervical spine. The second cervical vertebra (2) is shown with its odontoid peg impressing upon the anterior aspect of the brain stem/cord that is sharply angulated (small black arrow). (B) A sagittal T1-weighted MRI scan of the cervical spine. The second cervical vertebra (2) is shown with its odontoid peg impressing upon the anterior aspect of the brain stem/cord that is sharply angulated (small black arrow).

the skull base, with no obvious widening of the gap between the anomalous C1 posterior tubercle and the spinous process of C2 detected between these films; pain permitted only limited extension and flexion. The open mouth view showed incorporation of the atlas within the skull base (Fig. 28.2E), as did a CT reconstruction view (Fig. 28.2F).

A cervical spine MRI was ordered and this showed that the vertebral bodies from C2 to T3 and the intervening disc spaces appeared intact. There was no disc herniation and the cord appeared normal in diameter with no syrinx. However, there was posterior impression of the odontoid peg on the anterior aspect of the brain stem, with early flattening at the C1–2 level and effacement of the CSF with impingement on the anterior aspect of the cervicomedullary junction where the cord/brain stem was sharply angulated at the level of the foramen magnum (Fig. 28.3A and B, small black arrows).

In view of his severe symptoms, a carotid duplex ultrasound study was performed to ascertain whether there was basilar or vertebral artery stenosis. However, the examination was reported as being 'normal'. Therefore, an angiogram was ordered to look for vertebral artery injury but this procedure was denied by the radiologist on the grounds of being 'too risky'. In view of the patient's significant symptoms and depression he was referred to a psychiatrist for support while further steps were taken to have an angiogram performed elsewhere; this was arranged and showed dissection of both vertebral arteries.

TREATMENT

There is no treatment for vertebral artery dissection other than psychological support, analgesics, relaxation techniques and advice to avoid performing head and neck movements that would aggravate his condition. Having provided a diagnosis for the patient this, in itself, was of great therapeutic value as he previously had been labelled as a malingerer.

RESULTS

Unfortunately, his chronic neck pain syndrome persisted but he was grateful that he had been taken seriously, at last, and that a diagnosis of organic pathology was confirmed and that he would no longer be considered a malingerer.

Note

It seems unlikely that the low-speed impact would have caused any instability of the ligaments attached to the odontoid process. Therefore, it is possible that the posterior impression of the odontoid peg on the anterior aspect of the brain stem was apparently asymptomatic before the motor vehicle accident but it now may have affected the anterior spinal artery on the anterior surface of the spinal cord. Furthermore, the blackouts most likely relate to injury of the vertebral arteries (dissection) and their associated sympathetic nerve plexus.

As Professor Ruth Jackson (1977) pointed out, when a neck injury occurs with the head and neck rotated to one side, the injury will be more severe.

Key point(s)

1. This again emphasizes how important it is for the clinician to look at the films and not only at the imaging report.
2. To miss the obvious C1 osseous anomaly could lead to disastrous consequences if the spine were considered to be normal and then manipulated. Hence, the wisdom of first looking at spinal structures to examine their integrity before providing manipulative therapy.
3. The vulnerability of the vertebral arteries to rotational movements should always be remembered.
4. When a clinician requests a particular type of imaging, it behoves the radiologist to discuss with the referring clinician the issue of whether the imaging should proceed. To summarily dismiss the request is tantamount to malpractice.

REFERENCE

Jackson R 1977 The cervical syndrome, 4th edn. Charles C. Thomas, Springfield, IL.

FURTHER READING

Ahmad H A, Gerraty R P, Davis S M, Cameron P A 1999
Cervicocerebral artery dissections. Journal of Accident
and Emergency Medicine 16: 422–424.

Giles L G F, Baker P G 1998 Introduction. In: Giles L G F,
Baker P G (eds) Clinical anatomy and management of
cervical spine pain. Butterworth-Heinemann, Oxford,
pp 3–19.

Klufas R A, Hsu L, Barnes P D, Patel M R, Schwartz R B
1995 Dissection of the carotid and vertebral arteries:
imaging with MR angiography. American Journal of
Roentgenology 164: 673–677.

Vernon H 2001 The cranio-cervical syndrome: mechanisms,
assessment and treatment. Butterworth-Heinemann,
Oxford.

Case 29 Vertebral artery tortuosity

COMMENT
When a patient presents with unexplained headaches with apparent sympathetic nervous system involvement, consider intracranial and extracranial causes.

PROFILE

A 41-year-old man who does not smoke cigarettes and only drinks a small amount of alcohol.

PAST HISTORY

Suffered from 'cluster' headaches as a teenager until his late 20s.

PRESENTING COMPLAINT (Fig. 29.1)

Thirteen-year history of suboccipital neck pain that radiates bilaterally to cause frontal headaches which occur mainly at weekends and can last all day. These are associated with nausea and dizziness. He does not suffer from photophobia or eye problems. The neck pain is worse when he is tired. All neck movements may increase the pain. His general health is very good.

Physiotherapy, traction, acupuncture and chiropractic manipulation had not given any long lasting benefit but NSAIDs provide some relief. He said plain X-ray films of his neck and a CT scan were normal.

AETIOLOGY

Unknown.

EXAMINATION

He had undergone a full neurological examination that showed no obvious deficit; he had also had a neurosurgical opinion but a diagnosis was not made. Deep palpation of the upper cervical spine paravertebral muscles elicited bilateral tenderness. The blood pressure in the seated posture was essentially normal at 120/85.

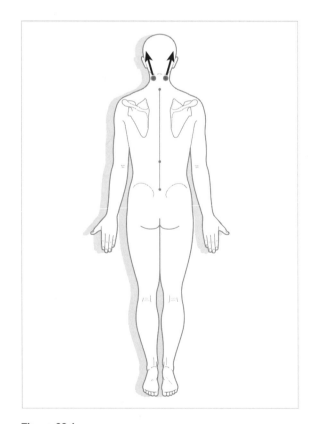

Figure 29.1

IMAGING REVIEW

The plain X-ray report stated: 'Disc spaces and neural foramina are normal. No fracture, bony infiltration or soft tissue abnormalities seen. No instability with flexion or extension, although there is some reduction in the range of flexion'. A review of the plain X-ray films that had essentially been reported as 'normal', showed a curvilinear line, indicating bone erosion, on the left side at C2 (Fig. 29.2) that had not been reported. This represented a tortuosity of the vertebral artery.

The CT scan from C3 to T1 showed no evidence of disc herniation and was reported as a normal study. Unfortunately, the CT scan did not include the area of his main pain, i.e. the upper cervical spine.

CLINICAL IMPRESSION

Vertebral artery tortuosity at C2 with sympathetic plexus involvement.

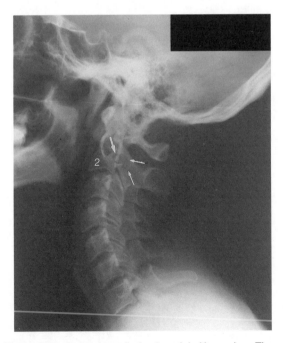

Figure 29.2   Lateral cervical spine plain X-ray view. The large arrow shows the C2 foramen transversarium and the two small arrows indicate the smooth curvilinear line caused by the vertebral artery tortuosity.

WHAT ACTION SHOULD BE TAKEN?

The patient was told that there were early sclerotic changes in the C2–3 and C3–4 zygapophysial joints but that the most likely cause for his headaches was irritation of the sympathetic nervous plexus on the vertebral artery at the area of the tortuosity.

TREATMENT

An explanation was given for his condition and he was grateful to know that a probable cause had been found, as he was concerned about various types of significant disease processes that may previously have been overlooked.

RESULTS

He was greatly relieved by the diagnosis and managed well on over-the-counter anti-inflammatory medication as required.

Note

It should be noted that the cervicothoracic (stellate) ganglion sends grey rami communicantes to various structures, including the seventh and eighth cervical and first thoracic spinal nerves and the vertebral arteries before extending to the basilar artery and as far as the posterior cerebral arteries, where they meet a plexus from the internal carotid (Harati 1993). Therefore, interference with the vertebral arteries may cause symptoms of vascular insufficiency of the posterior portion of the brain (Jackson 1977). Symptoms due to pressure upon the sympathetic nerve plexus surrounding the vertebral artery constitute a bizarre and confusing clinical picture – the Barre–Lieou syndrome (including headache, nausea, vertigo, nystagmus and suboccipital tenderness) (Hadley 1964).

Key point

When a patient presents with autonomic nervous system symptoms, such as nausea and dizziness, there may be several causes, one of which is vertebral artery tortuosity.

REFERENCES

Hadley L A 1964 Anatomico-roentgenographic studies of the spine. Charles C Thomas, Springfield, pp 158–171.

Harati Y 1993 Anatomy of the spinal and peripheral autonomic nervous system. In: Low PA (ed.) Clinical autonomic disorders: evaluation and management. Little, Brown and Company, Boston, pp 17–37.

Jackson R 1977 The cervical syndrome, 4th edn. Charles C. Thomas, Springfield, IL, p 148.

FURTHER READING

Brahee D D, Gueber G M 2000 Tortuosity of the vertebral artery resulting in vertebral erosion. Journal of Manipulative and Physiological Therapy 23: 48–51.

Giles L G F 1997 Vertebral-basilar artery insufficiency. Journal of the Canadian Chiropractic Association 21: 112–115.

Giles L G F, Baker P G 1998 Introduction. In: Giles L G F, Singer K P (eds) Clinical anatomy and management of cervical spine pain. Butterworth-Heinemann, Oxford, pp 3–19.

Yunten N, Alper H, Calli C, Selcuki D, Ustun E E 1998 Cervical osseous changes associated with vertebral artery tortuosity. Journal of Neuroradiology 25: 136–139.

Case 30   Cervical cord ependymoma

PROFILE

A 56-year-old male manual worker who does not
smoke or drink alcohol.

PAST HISTORY

Cervical spine pain causing headaches since a
motor vehicle accident 20 years ago. Two years
ago he underwent a laminectomy and fusion at L5
for sciatica; this gave him relief from his sciatica.
A 20-year history of mid-thoracic spine pain since
the motor vehicle accident.

PRESENTING COMPLAINT (Fig. 30.1)

1. Frontal headache with some narrowing of
   the lateral visual fields.
2. A general feeling of being unwell.
3. Some 'weakness' of his right leg during the
   last month or so.
4. Right thumb slight weakness making it
   difficult for him to hold his pen.
5. Some mid-thoracic spine pain during the last
   20 years.

There was no history of night pain apart from
headaches awakening him during the night.

AETIOLOGY

Unknown.

EXAMINATION

The deep reflexes, pinprick sensation and vibration sensation were normal in the upper and
lower limbs. There was decreased power (4/5)
in right (a) shoulder abduction (C5), (b) finger
flexion (C8) and extension (C7), (c) hand grip
strength, and (d) his right leg. There was some
narrowing of the left and right visual fields.

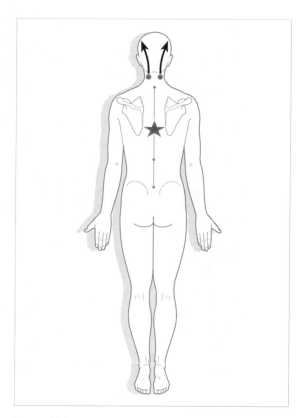

Figure 30.1

151

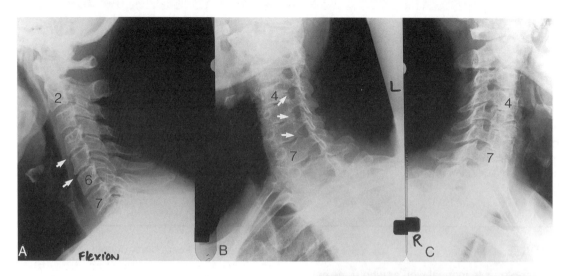

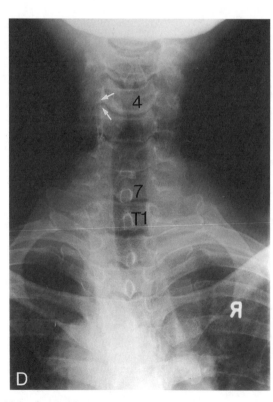

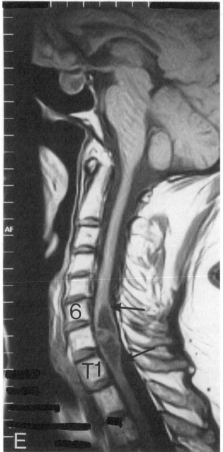

Figure 30.2 Caption is on next page.

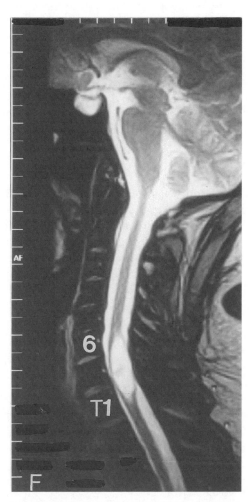 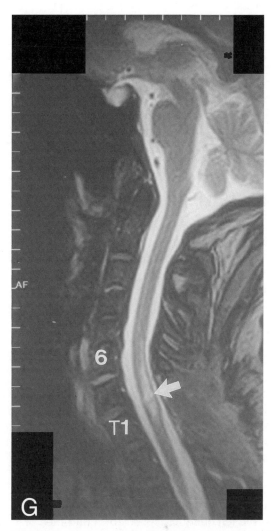

Figure 30.2   (A) A cervical spine flexion plain X-ray view showing the abnormal cervical spine contour, restriction in the range of flexion and loss of disc height at C4–5 and C5–6 (arrows). (B, C) Cervical spine oblique views showing only minor joint of von Luschka (uncovertebral joint) osteophytic lipping at the C4–5, C5–6 and C6–7 levels on the left side in particular (arrows). (D) A cervical spine anteroposterior view X-ray which shows the osteophytic lipping of the joints of von Luschka at the C4–5 (arrows) and C5–6 levels on the left. The lung apices appear to be within normal limits and there are no cervical ribs. 7 = seventh cervical vertebra; T1 = first thoracic vertebra. (E) A sagittal T1-weighted MRI scan of the cervical spine that shows the large ependymoma extending from C6 to T1 (arrows) in the cervical spinal cord. (F) A sagittal T2-weighted MRI scan of the cervical spine that shows the ependymoma. (G) A sagittal T2-weighted MRI post-operative scan showing the change in the tumour 4.5 months following surgery.

Cervical spine active ranges of movement were decreased by approximately 50% due to 'stiffness'. Thoracic spine active ranges of movement were decreased by approximately 25% on extension due to localized mid-thoracic spine pain.

IMAGING REVIEW

Cervical spine and thoracic spine plain X-ray films and a cervical CT scan taken approximately 2.5 years ago showed decreased C4–5 and C5–6 disc height and T6 body anterior wedging with associated anterior osteophytes. A recent CT of his brain and pituitary fossa showed a pituitary tumour protruding into the suprasella cistern, most probably causing some pressure effect on the adjacent optic chiasm. A MRI brain scan confirmed the pituitary tumour as most likely being a macroadenoma. A MRI thoracic spine examination showed a small disc protrusion at the T5–6 level.

CLINICAL IMPRESSION

1. Pituitary tumour causing headaches and diminished lateral visual fields.
2. ? Cervical cord tumour causing slight weakness of the right thumb and of the right leg.
3. ? Mid-thoracic spine disc causing local pain.

WHAT ACTION SHOULD BE TAKEN?

1. Referral to the neurosurgeon who was to operate on the pituitary tumour.
2. Laboratory tests: these showed an ESR of 26 (normal range <15 mm/hr).
3. Request for new cervical spine X-ray films; these showed the previously known C4–5 and C5–6 decreased disc height (Fig. 30.2A) with only minor joint of von Luschka (uncovertebral joint) osteophytic lipping at the C4–5, C5–6 and C6–7 levels, particularly on the left oblique (Fig. 30.2B,C) and the anteroposterior view (Fig. 30.2D).
4. The patient was advised to ask the neurosurgeon who was to remove the pituitary tumour to have a cervical spine MRI performed in view of the right thumb and leg weakness. However, this was denied as being unnecessary. Therefore, a cervical spine MRI study was arranged via an orthopaedic surgeon 3 months later when the patient said his right thumb weakness was progressively

becoming worse. The MRI showed a large primary neoplasm (an ependymoma or a cystic astrocytoma) extending from C6 to T1 (Fig. 30.2E, F), thus explaining his right thumb and right leg weakness.

TREATMENT

The patient was referred for urgent surgery for his cervical cord tumour.

RESULTS

The tumour was found to be an ependymoma on histopathology examination.

The cervical cord tumour surgery gave him very good results over some months with an almost complete return to normal strength of his right thumb and leg (Fig. 30.2G). Unfortunately, the tumour recurred 2.5 years later.

Key point

Never think a patient is a malingerer just because more and more symptoms develop. Thoroughly review the history and consider all new symptoms before performing imaging and laboratory tests otherwise the patient will be disadvantaged.

FURTHER READING

Akutsu H, Shibata Y, Okazaki M, Hyodo A, Matsumura A 2000 Intramedullary clear cell ependymoma in the cervical spine cord: case report. Neurosurgery 47: 1434–1437.

Cassidy J R, Ducker T B, Dienes E A 1997 Intradual tumors. In: Frymoyer JW (ed.) The adult spine: principles and practice, 2nd edn. Lippincott-Raven, Philadelphia, pp 1015–1029.

Yochum T R, Barry M S 1996 Diagnostic imaging of the musculoskeletal system. In: Yochum TR, Rowe LJ (eds) Essentials of skeletal radiology, 2nd edn. Williams & Wilkins, Baltimore, pp 373–545.

Case 31 Post motor vehicle accident soft tissue injuries

COMMENT

Cervical spine flexion and extension functional views are essential to properly evaluate the cervical spine following a neck injury, as long as the patient feels comfortable in these positions and does not feel 'dizzy' or nauseous during the examination.

PROFILE

A 29-year-old married woman of cheerful disposition who is somewhat overweight. She does not smoke or drink alcohol. She is very concerned about having lost her job, which she really enjoyed, due to her motor vehicle accident.

PAST HISTORY

The patient had always been healthy and her only surgical history was that of an operation on her left ear drum about 6 years ago.

PRESENTING COMPLAINT (Fig. 31.1)

She was referred by her general medical practitioner regarding her chronic neck and upper thoracic spine pain. Her main complaint was the neck pain that radiates to both arms variably and sometimes has a 'burning' sensation. She also experiences some intermittent pain radiating around her rib cage at approximately the breast level.

She found that physiotherapy treatment made her neck and upper thoracic spine feel worse, so she decided to stop this form of treatment. She felt that one of the mobilizing manoeuvres had caused some 'numbness in the hands'.

She was referred to a neurologist where a MRI study was ordered. She has tried many different types of medication without lasting relief. The neurologist advised her to go back to work but this caused an increase in her neck and arm pains so she had to take Endone.

She saw many specialists including a psychiatrist and a clinical psychologist as she was severely depressed and tearful about her condition.

In an attempt to help her stop the increasing medication, she had been advised to try a

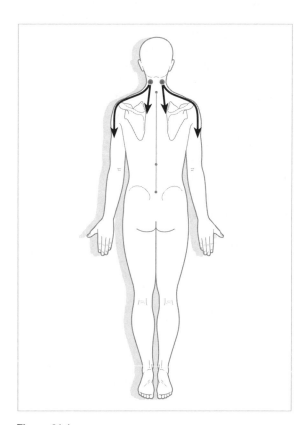

Figure 31.1

transcutaneous electrical nerve stimulator (TENS) machine for her chronic neck and arm pains; this was of considerable help, although she still could not wear a shoulder bag or a necklace as these items aggravate her neck pain. She feels a 'squishey' sensation at times on moving her neck.

She has trouble falling asleep and is awakened by the pain during the night, but at no particular time; she has to get up and walk around before trying to go to sleep again.

She uses a 'really hot' shower on her cervicothoracic region and this gives her some temporary relief. However, she cannot understand why the water feels hot on her arms and hands but not when it is directed onto her cervicothoracic region.

AETIOLOGY

A motor vehicle accident 16 months ago. She was the seat-belted driver of her truck waiting at a red traffic light and, just as the light turned green, her truck was suddenly hit from the rear, with considerable impact, by a motor car which pushed her truck several metres across the intersection. Her head 'jerked backwards and forwards' but she does not recall it hitting anything in the truck, although it may have hit a bar behind the headrest. She felt severe neck pain a few minutes after the accident so was taken to the hospital where she was examined and allowed to go home.

EXAMINATION

The biceps (C5,6) and radial (C5,6,7) deep reflexes were normal, as was the right triceps (C7) reflex. However, it was not possible to elicit the left triceps reflex. The knee jerk (L2,3,4) and ankle jerk (S1,2) deep tendon reflexes were normal.

Resisted tests for shoulder movement:

1. Abduction (C5–6) appeared normal bilaterally.
2. Shoulder shrug (spinal accessory and C3, 4 ± C5 nerves) appeared bilaterally equal but possibly diminished in strength and caused cervical spine pain bilaterally.

3. Tensioning the left and right brachial plexus nerves (C5–T1) caused ipsilateral brachial plexus pain.

Adson's manoeuvre caused contralateral cervical spine pain but no obliteration of the radial pulse.

Eye movements were normal, as were the optic fundi and discs. Auscultation of the heart and lungs was normal and the blood pressure in the right arm (seated position) was 118/82. The circumference of the forearms, 8 cm below the elbow joint, was 28.3 cm (left) and 28.8 cm (right). Pinprick sensation to the upper and lower extremities was normal, except for a subjective decrease in sensation in the C6 dermatome bilaterally between the thumb and index finger. Deep palpation of the paraspinal muscles of the neck elicited bilateral pain, particularly at the C1, 2 and C4–6 levels. There was also minor tenderness at approximately the T4, T12 and lumbosacral levels.

Cervical spine active ranges of movements were measured using a Cervical Range of Motion instrument (CROM product of Performance Attainment Associates, St Paul, MN, USA), as shown in Box 31.1.

Left and right SLR were limited at 70° elevation due to minor low back pain.

Box 31.1			
	Normal range	Measured range	Comments
Flexion	50°	40°	Caused pain to extend from C1 to C7 with a bilateral 'pulling' sensation in the back of the neck.
Extension	60°	54°	Caused pain in the right cervico-shoulder region.
Left & right lateral bending	45°	40.5°	Caused cervico-shoulder pain on the contralateral side.
Left & right rotation	80°	72°	Caused pain in the ipsilateral cervico-shoulder region.

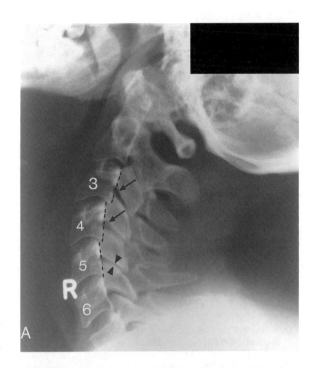

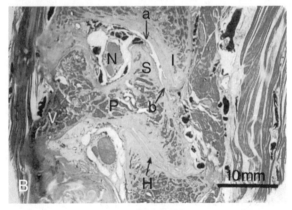

IMAGING REVIEW

The cervical spine plain X-ray films had been reported as 'normal' but did not include functional views.

CLINICAL IMPRESSION

Whiplash-type syndrome due to soft tissue injuries particularly at the C1–2 and C4–6 levels.

WHAT ACTION SHOULD BE TAKEN?

Cervical spine flexion and extension views to augment the previous imaging; the report stated: 'Normal examination'. When the patient returned with the X-ray films she was in tears and said that 'nothing was found on the X-ray films'. She was shown the flexion and extension views and a long discussion ensued regarding particularly the extension view (Fig. 31.2A). The patient was told:

There is some backward displacement of C3 vertebra on C4 and of the C4 vertebra on C5. The zygapophysial facet joint planes are parallel except at the C3–4 and C4–5 levels where the zygapophysial joints 'gap' anteriorly in keeping with the slight retrolisthesis of C3 on C4 and of C4 on C5.

She was told how certain soft tissue structures (Fig. 31.2B) may be injured.

TREATMENT

The patient was delighted to find that there was indeed some evidence of soft tissue injuries to

Figure 31.2   (A) Lateral cervical spine extension (functional) plain X-ray view. Note the: (i) backward displacement (retrolisthesis) of the C3 vertebral body on the C4 body (as shown by the dotted line on the posterior aspect of the vertebral bodies) suggesting instability due to soft tissue injuries; (ii) backward displacement of C4 vertebral body on C5; and (iii) zygapophysial facet joint planes are parallel (for example, see arrowheads at the C5–6 facets) except at the C3–4 and C4–5 levels of instability where the zygapophysial joints 'gap' anteriorly (arrows). The soft tissues associated with the cervical spine are partly represented in (B). (B) Parasagittal section from a cervical spine showing part of the anterolateral aspect of the vertebral body (V) and the superior (S) and inferior (I) articular processes of the zygapophysial joint. Note the superior (a) and inferior (b) highly vascular synovial folds which can be nipped between joint surfaces during injury. H = hyaline articular cartilage on the lower joint's facet surfaces which is essentially normal. Note that the cartilage on the upper joint facets one level above has almost worn away on the superior articular process (S). N = neural structures in the intervertebral foramen which are surrounded by fatty tissue and many blood vessels. P = pedicle joining the vertebral body and the posterior spinal elements, i.e. superior and inferior articular processes, etc. The darkly stained muscle groups anteriorly and posteriorly are illustrated. (Reproduced with permission from Giles L G F 1986 Lumbosacral and cervical zygapophyseal joint inclusions. *Manual Medicine* **2** 89–92.)

her neck and that she was not 'imagining the pain'; she was referred back to her general medical practitioner with an explanation of the functional X-ray findings. Her medical practitioner then referred her back for ongoing psychological support and treatment which consisted of needle acupuncture.

RESULTS

The needle acupuncture gave her significant relief, as long as it was performed in the seated position so that hyperextension of the cervical spine was not introduced (which would occur were she to lie prone).

Note

Cervical spine joint dysfunction may be completely missed if flexion and extension functional views are not ordered as suggested by Davis (1945), when no contraindication exists. Flexion/extension radiographs are able to detect disco-ligamentous instability in patients with otherwise normal radiographs. Normal plain radiographs should also be taken prior to obtaining the dynamic motion study (Chapman & Anderson 1997). The dynamic functional techniques should not be performed in the acute post injury phase (Chapman & Anderson 1997).

According to Jackson (1977), when there is no disorder of the cervical spine, flexion and extension result in a smooth curve. The stature of the cervical spine should not be interpreted on CT or MRI examinations because these are performed with the patient supine (Van Goethem et al 1998).

Key point(s)

1. Flexion and extension functional views should always be taken to determine whether there is any cervical spine instability, unless there is a contraindication such as suspected vertebral artery injury with dizziness and nausea, or joint dislocation.
2. Patients receiving needle acupuncture for cervical spine injuries should preferably be treated in the seated position to eliminate hyperextension of the cervical spine unless the patient is comfortable lying on their side. (NB Ensure the patient cannot fall of the chair.)

REFERENCES

Chapman J R, Anderson P A 1997 Cervical spine trauma. In: Frymoyer JW (ed.) The adult spine: principles and practice, 2nd edn. Lippincott-Raven, Philadelphia, pp 1245–1295.

Davis A G 1945 Injuries of the cervical spine. Journal of the American Medical Association 127: 149–156, 936.

Jackson R 1977 The cervical syndrome, 4th edn. Charles C. Thomas, Springfield, IL, p 212.

Van Goethem J W M, Widelec J, de Moor J, Hauwe L, Parizel P M, Petroons P, De Schepper A M A 1998 Normal imaging of the cervical spine: roentgen anatomy, variants, and pitfalls. In: Gunzburg R, Szpalski M (eds) Whiplash injuries: current concepts in prevention, diagnosis and treatment of the cervical whiplash syndrome. Lippincott-Raven, Philadelphia, pp 21–30.

FURTHER READING

Giles LGF, Singer KP (eds) 1998 The clinical anatomy and management of back pain series. Volume 3: Clinical anatomy and management of cervical spine pain. Butterworth-Heinemann, Edinburgh, 1998.

See Case 27 for a further histological understanding of the cervical spine.

Case 32 Intervertebral disc protrusion

COMMENT
This case demonstrates how important it is for clinicians treating spinal pain syndromes to be well versed in the anatomy, symptoms and signs related to a particular part of the spine.

PROFILE

A 46-year-old married man who has always been involved in manual activities. He does not smoke and only drinks beer socially.

PAST HISTORY

Following a motor vehicle accident 10 years ago he developed left upper limb radicular symptoms of pain with 'tingling' in the middle finger (C7). Symptoms came on immediately following the motor vehicle accident and for three years he saw several specialists who gave him the impression that the pain was psychosomatic. Eventually, he was referred to a psychiatrist by an orthopaedic surgeon, which the patient told me was 'the best advice he had ever been given'. During the psychiatric evaluation the psychiatrist told the patient that he knew exactly what was wrong, so the patient asked the psychiatrist how he knew this. The reply was that the psychiatrist had also had a motor vehicle accident and ruptured a disc in the lower part of his neck and been told that he was imagining his problem, having seen various specialists until he found an orthopaedic surgeon who examined him with MRI and found a disc prolapse in his neck! The patient was referred by the psychiatrist to his orthopaedic surgeon who performed a Cloward procedure at the C6–7 level which very successfully resolved the left-sided neck pain, radicular symptoms and the tingling in the middle finger.

PRESENTING COMPLAINT (Fig. 32.1)

Right-sided neck pain with some left-sided neck pain.

He had been referred from interstate with a request that an 'appropriate diagnosis be made without the patient going through the 3 years of indecision that occurred previously' when the symptoms were on the left side.

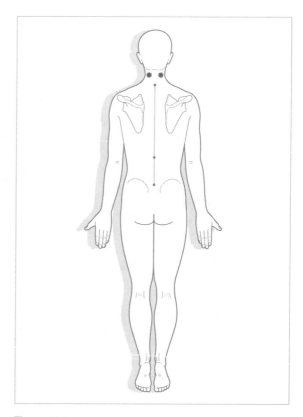

Figure 32.1

159

AETIOLOGY

A motor vehicle accident 10 years ago when a sedan approaching from the opposite direction hit the patient's four-wheel-drive vehicle head on with such force that the four-wheel-drive's chassis was severely damaged. He immediately felt neck pain with pain extending into his left shoulder/arm.

EXAMINATION

Deep palpation of the paravertebral muscles of the cervical spine elicited pain on the right side at the occiput–C1 level and bilaterally at the C4–7 levels. Toe walking power (S1) and heel walking power (L5) were normal. The deep reflexes in the upper extremities were normal but the ankle jerks (S1) were somewhat diminished bilaterally at one plus (two plus being normal). Pinprick sensation of the upper and lower extremities was normal. Vibration sensation at the elbows and ankles was normal. Power in the upper and lower extremities appeared to be normal.

All cervical spine active ranges of movement were restricted by approximately 50%. Cervical traction and compression did not aggravate his neck pain. The circumference of the forearm, 12 cm below the elbow, was 33.5 cm bilaterally.

IMAGING REVIEW

His previous MRI imaging was reviewed and this showed a large disc protrusion at the C6–7 level prior to surgery (Fig. 32.2A).

CLINICAL IMPRESSION

Central disc protrusion above the spinal fusion level at C6–7 (as there are no unilateral radicular symptoms).

WHAT ACTION SHOULD BE TAKEN?

A new MRI was ordered and this showed protrusions at the C5–6 and C3–4 levels, both of

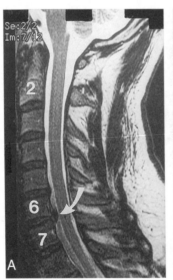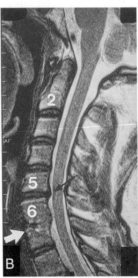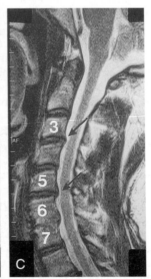

Figure 32.2 (A) Cervical spine sagittal T2-weighted MRI scan. The numbers represent the vertebral body level and the curved arrow shows the large C6–7 disc protrusion that considerably indents the pain-sensitive anterior surface of the dural tube and almost touches the spinal cord itself. (B, C) Cervical spine sagittal T2-weighted MRI scans. The numbers represent the vertebral bodies and the white arrow shows where surgery was performed at the C6–7 level. The black arrows show the disc protrusions at the C3–4 and C5–6 levels, respectively. Note how the disc protrusions indent the pain-sensitive anterior surface of the dural tube.

which impinge upon the pain-sensitive anterior part of the dural tube (Fig. 32.2B and C).

TREATMENT

The patient was advised not to perform any activities that would aggravate his neck pain. He was also advised to sleep with a pillow of appropriate thickness, to fill the gap between his shoulder and the side of his neck when he lies on his side in bed. He was told that he should consider consulting the orthopaedic surgeon who had operated on his C6–7 level should his symptoms reach a stage where he required a surgical opinion. Having shown him his MRI images, and explained that prevention was better than cure, he went home satisfied that he knew what was wrong with his neck and he was determined to protect it by not performing activities that could worsen the disc lesions at the C3–4 and C5–6 levels.

RESULTS

Some months post consultation he continues to be active while being careful not to strain or jar his neck.

Note

It is interesting to note that on the slice shown in Fig. 32.2B, the C3–4 disc looks almost normal, whereas in Fig. 32.2C the protrusion is clearly shown. This variation is because the slices are through different sections of the spine and this example shows why sagittal plane scans begin

on one side of the spine and finish on the other side of the spine so that any protrusions between the left and right sides can be seen, as not all protrusions are central.

Key point(s)

1. Bearing in mind the issue of dermatomal and dynatomal pain patterns (Slipman et al 1998) discussed in the Introduction, it should be possible to make a clinical diagnosis of central or posterolateral cervical disc protrusion. MRI is a very useful tool for suspected cervical spine disc protrusion.
2. The clinical examination and the pain pattern should make it possible for the spinal level responsible for symptoms and signs to be established with a considerable degree of certainty.
3. MRI imaging can be used for confirmation of disc bulges and protrusions but may well miss tears in the anular fibres (Schellhas et al 1996).

REFERENCES

Schellhas K P, Smith M D, Gundry C R, Pollei S R 1996 Cervical discogenic pain. Prospective correlation of magnetic resonance imaging and discography in asymptomatic subjects and pain sufferers. Spine 21: 300–312.
Slipman C W, Plastaras C T, Palmitier R A, Huston C W, Sterenfeld E B 1998 Symptom provocation of fluoroscopically guided cervical nerve root stimulation. Are dynatomal maps identical to dermatomal maps? Spine 23: 2235–2242.

FURTHER READING

Gunzburg R, Szpalski M 1998 Whiplash injuries: current concepts in prevention, diagnosis, and treatment of the cervical whiplash syndrome. Lippincott-Raven, Philadelphia.

COMMENT
Surgical errors occur and should be considered when a patient's symptoms do not improve after surgery.

PROFILE

A 41-year-old tall, well-built married man who did not smoke and only drinks alcohol socially.

PAST HISTORY

Nothing relevant in his history. He had essentially been fit and active. Three months prior to consultation he had undergone a Cloward procedure at the C5–6 intervertebral disc level for a right-sided osteophyte and a disc herniation that followed a work injury.

PRESENTING COMPLAINT (Fig. 33.1)

Neck pain that shoots up to the occipital area of his skull, especially on the right side, and to the shoulder blade and across his shoulders and upper thoracic region. The neck pain particularly radiates to his right arm as far as his hand and he feels a 'stabbing' pain in the right arm. The arm pain goes along the posterior aspect of the arm then crosses to the front of the forearm then radiates along the ulnar distribution to the last three fingers of his right hand. He complained of almost complete 'numbness' and some pins and needles in the fourth and fifth fingers of his right hand.

He was referred by his general medical practitioner because neither the doctor nor the patient could understand why the patient's symptoms felt 'exactly the same before and after surgery'. No one had been able to answer this question.

AETIOLOGY

Work-related injury approximately three and a half months prior to consultation.

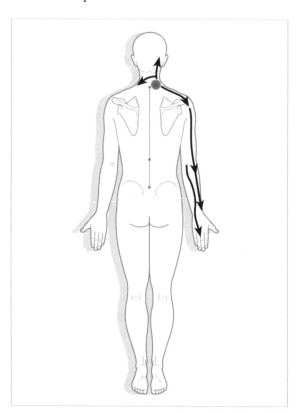

Figure 33.1

EXAMINATION

The right biceps (C5–6) reflex was diminished at one plus (two plus being normal) as was the case with the right triceps (C7) reflex. Pinprick sensation of the upper and lower extremities was normal, apart from hypoaesthesia of the right middle finger (C7) and no sensation for the right fourth and fifth fingers (C8). There was decreased pinprick sensation on the posterior aspect of the right shoulder in the C5 dermatome. There was also an area of no sensation on the lateral aspect of the right leg, approximately 15 cm above the ankle (L5). The circumference of the arms, 10 cm above the elbow joint, was 34 cm (left) and 32 cm (right) showing a 2 cm difference; presumably due to muscle wasting. Vibration sensation was reported as being significantly less when a tuning fork was applied to the right elbow as compared to the left (perhaps indicating some injury to the posterior columns of the spinal cord, although vibration sensation at the ankles appeared to be normal).

Cervical spine active ranges of movement in the seated position were as follows:

1. Flexion – limited by approximately 40% due to pain radiating to the right mid-forearm.
2. Extension – limited by approximately 80% due to slight pain at approximately the C5 level.
3. Left rotation – limited by approximately 80% due to pain on the left side of the cervical spine.
4. Right rotation – limited by approximately 80% due to cervico-shoulder pain on the right side radiating to the right scapula as far as its inferior aspect.

Deep palpation of the cervical paravertebral muscles elicited considerable tenderness, particularly on the right side at approximately the C5 level.

IMAGING REVIEW

The C5–6 disc protrusion was clearly seen on the sagittal and axial views of a MRI scan performed prior to surgery (Fig. 33.2A and insert).

CLINICAL IMPRESSION

? C5–6 or C6–7 right-sided posterolateral disc protrusion.

WHAT ACTION SHOULD BE TAKEN?

In view of the patient's obvious pain, which caused him to keep moving his arm and hand about in order to minimize the pain during the consultation, even though he was taking analgesics, a CT scan was ordered which

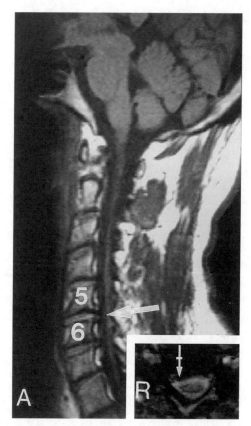

Figure 33.2 (A) A parasagittal T1-weighted MRI scan of the cervical spine showing osteophyte/disc herniation at C5–6 (white arrow). This right-sided posterolateral disc herniation is shown in the axial insert (tailed arrow). R = right side of patient. The MRI report read: There is some osteophyte/disc distortion of the cord at C5–6 level. Disc herniation extends into the intervertebral foramen. There also appears to be a right-sided posterolateral osteophyte at C6–7 but it does not impinge upon the right intervertebral foramen.

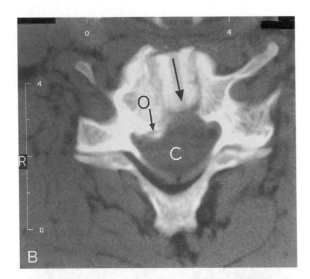

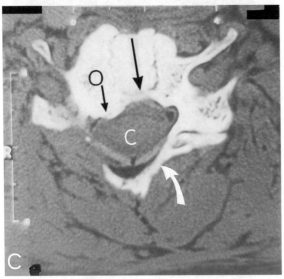

Figure 33.2 (B) A cervical spine axial CT scan of the C5–6 level following the Cloward procedure (performed 3 months previously) to remove the right-sided posterolateral disc herniation and osteophyte seen by MRI as being present at C5–6. Note that the *left* side was decompressed instead of the right side which still shows the disc osteophyte (O) complex on the patient's right side (R); this compresses the anterolateral portion of the dural tube. The surgical approach (large black arrow) was directed to the patient's left side. C = spinal cord within the spinal canal. (C) A cervical spine axial CT scan showing the laminectomy that was performed on the right side in an attempt to remove pressure from the disc/osteophyte complex projecting against the pain-sensitive dural

showed: 'C5–6 anterior interbody fusion. Right posterolateral osteophyte formation at this level with some bony narrowing of the right C6 nerve root exit foramen' (Fig. 33.2B).

TREATMENT

The patient and his referring medical practitioner were advised that surgery apparently had been directed to the patient's *left* side as demonstrated by the CT scan (Fig. 33.2B).

The patient was referred to another surgeon who performed a right-sided laminectomy (Fig. 33.2C). This was done in an attempt to decompress the neural structures on the right side, as it was now impossible to get to the right posterolateral osteophyte to remove it and any associated disc material because the previous Cloward procedure (Fig. 33.2B) apparently prevented access for a further anterior approach.

RESULTS

The further surgery was unsuccessful and resulted in perineural fibrosis. Unfortunately, the patient developed increasing right upper limb symptoms that led to severe depression and large doses of analgesics. He then began to develop leg symptoms due to cervical spondylosis and early myelopathy at the C5–6 level.

Note

In order to consider similar histopathology at this level in a postmortem specimen, please see Case 27, Fig. 27.4.

tube anteriorly. O = osteophyte; the large arrow indicates the original surgical approach which is directed to the patient's left side. The left lamina is shown by the curved white arrow and the corresponding lamina on the right side has been surgically removed. C = spinal cord within the spinal canal.

Key point(s)

1. Errors do occur with surgery, as they do in any branch of the healing profession. Therefore, it is important to carefully listen to the patient's description of post-surgical symptoms then to perform a thorough clinical and appropriate imaging investigation in order to re-evaluate the patient.
2. Cervical myelopathy is clearly related to spinal cord ischaemia and compression and stretching and compression of spinal cord tissue will result in a great spectrum of variability in the clinical symptoms (Bland 1987).

REFERENCE

Bland J H 1987 Disorders of the cervical spine: diagnosis and medical management. W.B. Saunders Company, Philadelphia, pp 186–235.

FURTHER READING

Benini A 1996 Die zervikale myelopathie: anatomopathologie, klinik und therapie. Schweizerische Rundschau Für Medizin Praxis 85: 1383–1386.

Giles LGF, Singer KP (eds) 1998 The clinical anatomy and management of back pain series. Volume 3: Clinical anatomy and management of cervical spine pain. Butterworth-Heinemann, Edinburgh.

Patten J 1996 Neurological differential diagnosis. Springer-Verlag, New York, pp 226–227.

Case 34   Uncovertebral joint osteoarthrosis

COMMENT
It is well known that there are many causes of headaches – all should be considered in the differential diagnosis.

PROFILE

A 48-year-old married woman of thin build who does not smoke or drink alcohol.

PAST HISTORY

She had a left C2 neurectomy performed approximately 18 years ago for left-sided headaches, without any relief but with resulting numbness involving the entire left occipital region ever since. The neurectomy specimen consisted of a fragment of 'pale tissue measuring 50 cm in length at macroscopic investigation and microscopic sections confirmed the presence of nerve trunks with no evidence of malignancy'. Narcotic injections and migraine prophylaxis had been to no avail for the left-sided headaches. She had had an appendectomy and a cholecystectomy performed some years ago.

PRESENTING COMPLAINT (Fig. 34.1)

Chronic left-sided neck pain and headaches that had flared up during the last few months, having begun 18 months ago. Although she has a history of headaches since her early teens, with multiple investigations and treatments over the years, the present headaches and left-sided neck-pain feel 'different'. These headaches appear to be severe vascular/tension type headaches due to severe left-sided cervicogenic pain.

She experiences left-sided neck symptoms of feeling 'hot'; these are then followed by pain radiating from approximately the left side of C5 vertebra to the upper neck then to behind the left eye, causing severe headaches. She believes that these neck symptoms are precipitated by various neck movements that cause the 'hot' sensation on the left side at approximately the C5 spinal level.

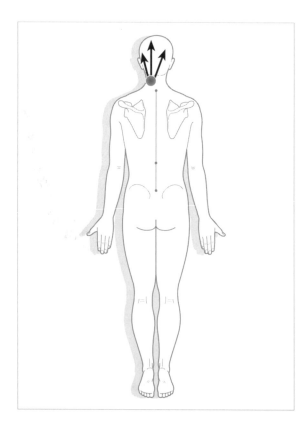

Figure 34.1

166

She had been taking analgesics, anti-inflammatory medication and an antidepressant for her chronic neck pain syndrome but had recently ceased all medication as she found that none helped, apart from periodic narcotic injections into the suboccipital region. She had also tried steroid and local anaesthetic injections in the paravertebral muscles which provided temporary relief. Spinal manipulation did not help.

AETIOLOGY

Unknown. Apparently suspected of being psychosomatic by previous clinicians.

EXAMINATION

The deep reflexes in the upper and lower extremities were normal as was the case with pinprick sensation and vibration sensation. Power in the upper and lower extremities was normal apart from slight (4/5) diminished power on flexion (C5–6) and extension (C7) at the elbows. All cervical spine ranges of movement were limited by neck pain, particularly extension. She was normotensive.

IMAGING REVIEW

A CT scan of her head and an angiogram had been performed but failed to reveal an aneurysm or any other intracranial pathology. Her plain film radiographs were reported as follows: 'A slight loss of disc space at the C6–7 level. No other bone or joint lesion seen' (Fig. 34.2). However, a review of the plain X-ray films showed a large osteophyte projecting from the left uncovertebral joint inferiorly on C5 vertebra toward the left vertebral artery (Fig. 34.2A). There were also osteophytes involving the C6–7 uncovertebral joints on both sides.

CLINICAL IMPRESSION

1. ? Left vertebral artery sympathetic plexus compromise due to encroachment by the C5

uncovertebral joint osteophyte upon the sympathetic plexus (suggested by the autonomic symptom of feeling 'hot' on the left side of the neck).
2. ? Neurofibroma at the site of the left-sided C2 neurectomy.

WHAT ACTION SHOULD BE TAKEN?

In view of the large left-sided uncovertebral joint osteophyte at C5, a CT cervical spine was performed with contrast which showed 'osteophytic encroachment on the medial aspect of the left transverse foramen at the C5 level with associated reduction in the calibre of the vertebral artery at this level' (Fig. 34.2E). The contrast showed that the vertebral arteries entered the transverse foramen at the C6 level bilaterally.

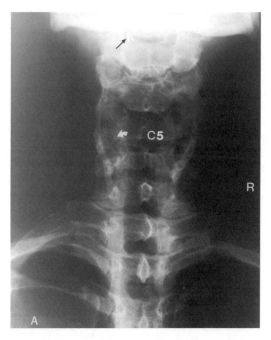

Figure 34.2 (A) An anteroposterior cervical spine plain X-ray view showing the clip (black arrow) in the left suboccipital region where the C2 neurectomy was performed and the C2 nerve was clipped and divided. C5 = fifth vertebra. White curved arrow shows the osteophyte projecting from the left uncovertebral joint toward the vertebral artery in the transverse foramen. R = right side of patient.

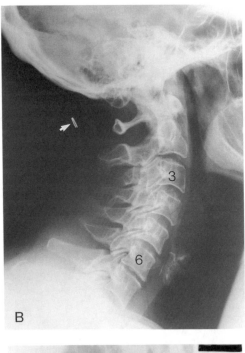

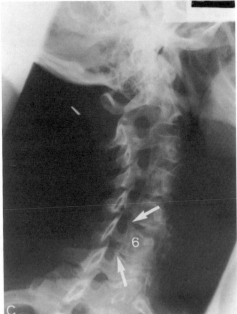

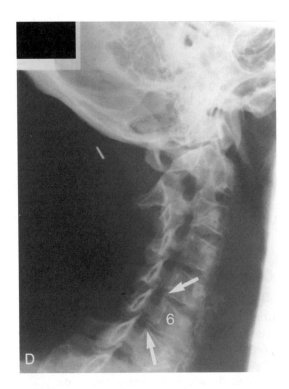

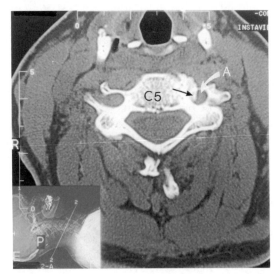

Figure 34.2   (B) A neutral lateral cervical spine plain X-ray view showing thinning at the C5–6 disc level and particularly at the C6–7 level. Note the neurectomy clip (white arrow). 3 = third vertebral body; 6 = sixth vertebral body. (C,D) Right and left oblique cervical spine plain X-ray views. The white arrows indicate osteophytic hypertrophy of the uncovertebral joints at C5–6 and C6–7 although the left uncovertebral joint osteophytosis at C5–6 is best visualized on the anteroposterior radiograph (A). (E) Axial cervical spine CT scan of the C5 vertebral body showing how the uncovertebral joint osteophytic encroachment (black arrow) at the medial aspect of the left C5 transverse foramen causes reduction in the calibre of the adjacent vertebral artery (A) within the transverse foramen. What cannot be seen is, of course, the effect that this osteophytic hypertrophy has on the sympathetic plexus on the vertebral artery.

TREATMENT

A change in her very active lifestyle to minimize her activities, psychological support, relaxation techniques and referral to yet another neurologist, a pain management anaesthetist and another neurosurgeon. These consultations resulted in the prescription of Epilim (400 mg twice per day with gradual increase for the neuralgic pain), Valium (2.5–5 mg three times per day as required for tension headaches), and Zomig (2.5 mg twice per day plus or minus Stemetil for migraine headaches). The most helpful of these medications was Epilim and her neurologist suggested that she should gradually increase this to a level where her pain control was manageable – she was not to exceed a maximum dose of 1 g twice per day in her particular case.

RESULTS

The Epilim medication initially gave some relief, so an uncectomy was not considered at the time. However, she developed an adverse reaction to the Epilim (nausea, diarrhoea and anaemia) and, because of the difficulty associated with performing an uncectomy, Neurontin (Gabapentin) was considered with surgery being reserved as a last resort measure should Neurontin fail. She manages to cope on four 400 mg tablets per day but also uses Mersyndol and Zomig as required. Full haematology, serum biochemistry and serum Gabapentin levels are monitored in case any abnormalities should occur over time.

Note

It is highly likely that irritation of the sympathetic nerve plexus on the vertebral artery is causing a vascular response that, in turn, causes her incapacitating vascular-type headaches. It is possible that this lady has two types of headaches: a headache with a neurovascular component due to irritation of the left vertebral artery and its sympathetic plexus, and a headache due to a neuroma that may have developed at the site of the C2 neurectomy. Because of the symptoms of feeling 'hot' on the left side of approximately the C5 level, precipitated by various neck movements, irritation of the sympathetic plexus appears to be the most likely cause.

Look at Case 27, Fig. 27.4B, to review the vertebral artery and vein anatomy and location in the transverse foramen in a histological cross-sectional view of the cervical spine. The intricate sympathetic nerve plexus is not shown at this magnification.

Key point

The issue of irritation of the vertebral artery's sympathetic plexus due to vertebral artery tortuosity has been discussed in Case 29. This case highlights how the sympathetic plexus on the vertebral artery may be irritated by uncovertebral joint osteoarthrosis.

FURTHER READING

Johnson J P, Filler A G, McBride D Q, Batzdorf U 2000 Anterior cervical foraminotomy for unilateral radicular disease. Spine 25: 905–909.

Nagashima C 1970 Surgical treatment of vertebral artery insufficiency caused by cervical spondylosis. Journal of Neurosurgery 12: 512–521.

Case 35 Cervical cord myelopathy

COMMENT
Beware of neck, arm and leg symptoms as they may be indicative of cervical cord myelopathy.

PROFILE

A 57-year-old man who smokes cigarettes.

PAST HISTORY

His past history was that he was involved in a motor vehicle accident approximately 7 years ago when the stationary vehicle in which he was sitting was rear-ended. Even though he wore a seat belt, he felt that his neck was 'whipped backwards and forwards' and that his head hit the headrest with enough impact to require stitching to the left and right occipital regions. He had been awarded an out of court settlement but still had to wear a soft cervical spine collar, in the reversed position, so as not to hyperextend his neck as that caused pain. He said he had always been healthy as a child but required a tonsillectomy at approximately 38 years of age due to chronic tonsillitis that developed in adulthood. He suffered from hypertension that was well controlled by medication.

PRESENTING COMPLAINT (Fig. 35.1)

His main complaints were of neck pain, especially at the C4–7 level, particularly on the left side and which radiated to the left elbow, as well as up to the occipital region causing headaches. He also had some 'foot drop' on the left side.

A minor secondary complaint was of slight low back pain extending to the left buttock and to the lateral aspect of the left thigh and calf, occasionally as far as his foot.

He said his neck and left leg problems were 'completely depressing' in spite of taking an antidepressant, as he could 'not see the light at the end of the tunnel'.

He had seen orthopaedic surgeons, neurosurgeons and a psychiatrist without help.

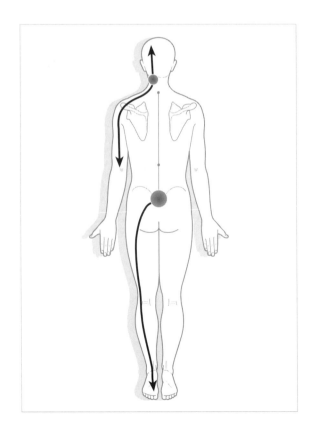

Figure 35.1

AETIOLOGY

Motor vehicle accident 7 years ago.

EXAMINATION

The deep reflexes in the arms and legs were normal. Pinprick sensation of the upper and lower extremities was normal apart from the left calf laterally (L5) where there was some hyperaesthesia. Vibration sensation at the elbows and ankles was normal. The circumference of the left thigh, 15 cm above the patella, was 1 cm less than on the right side (i.e. just within normal limits); the left calf, 12 cm below the patella, was 2 cm less than on the right side. Both seated and supine SLR indicated limitation to approximately 40° due to slight low back pain and hamstring 'pulling' on elevation of the left leg. Bilateral hip flexion caused minor low back pain at approximately 100° elevation of the thighs from the examination table. Power in the legs appeared to be normal apart from some weakness (4/5) on dorsiflexion (L4, 5) of the left foot. There was some weakness in his left hand on making a fist. The plantar responses appeared to be normal. The foot pulses were normal.

IMAGING REVIEW

Plain X-ray films of the cervical spine showed disc narrowing at the C4–5 and C5–6 levels with moderate degenerative changes in the associated lateral mass articulations and in the uncovertebral joints, with some narrowing of the left C4–5 nerve root foramen. Plain X-ray films of the lumbar spine showed minor degenerative osteophytic changes throughout the lumbar spine and extending into the lower thoracic region. A CT scan of the lumbar spine showed some degenerative change in the zygapophysial joints and at the vertebral body margins but no compromise of the spinal canal or exiting foraminae.

CLINICAL IMPRESSION

Cervical myelopathy in view of the left-sided arm symptoms and the left-sided 'foot drop'.

Differential diagnosis of cervical nerve root impingement with a concomitant and separate condition of left-sided L5 nerve root irritation.

WHAT ACTION SHOULD BE TAKEN?

A CT scan was performed of the cervical spine to evaluate the spinal canal. This showed, at the C4–5 level, a 'diffuse anular bulging of the disc and a large left posterolateral osteophyte formation indenting the thecal sac anteriorly with moderate spinal canal stenosis and left C4–5 intervertebral foramen stenosis' (Fig. 35.2A).

TREATMENT

He was referred for a neurosurgical opinion in view of the developing cervical cord myelopathy.

RESULTS

Surgical decompression at the C4–5 level provided relief from his neck and left arm pain and his foot drop.

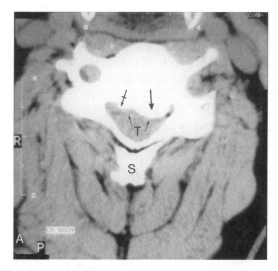

Figure 35.2 (A) CT scan showing the C4–5 disc diffuse anular bulge and large left posterolateral osteophyte formation (large black arrow) indenting the thecal sac (T) anteriorly (small black arrows) with moderate spinal canal stenosis and left intervertebral foramen stenosis. There is some bony narrowing of the right C4–5 neural foramen due to degenerative changes in the adjacent uncovertebral joint (tailed arrow). R = right side of patient; S = spinous process.

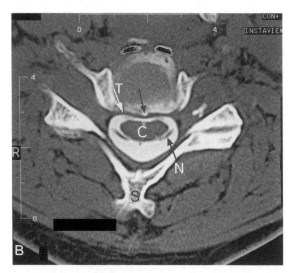

Figure 35.2   (B) CT myelogram from another patient showing how even a small posterior osteophyte (black arrow) will indent the anterior pain-sensitive part of the thecal sac (T) which contains the spinal cord (C) and nerve roots (N). Therefore, a large posterolateral osteophyte with diffuse anular bulging of the disc, causing left canal stenosis, would affect the tracts within the spinal cord with symptoms in the legs due to cervical cord myelopathy. R = right side of patient; S = spinous process.

Note

A relatively normal CT myelogram scan to demonstrate the radiological anatomy of the cervical spine in the axial view is shown in Fig. 35.2B for comparison with the stenotic spinal canal shown in Fig. 35.2A.

Key point(s)

1. It is important to remember that cervical spondylitic myelopathy has a diverse clinical presentation without any pathognomonic signs or symptoms (Shelokov 1991, Simeone & Rothman 1982).
2. The myelopathic patient has a mixture of abnormalities of both upper and lower extremities with possible subtle gait disturbance with upper motor neuron dysfunction (Shelokov 1991).

REFERENCES

Shelokov A P 1991 Evaluation, diagnosis and initial treatment of cervical disc disease. SPINE: State of the Art Reviews 5: 167–176.
Simeone F A, Rothman R H 1982 Cervical disc disease. In: Rothman RH, Simeone FA (eds) The spine. W.B. Saunders, Philadelphia, pp 440–476.

FURTHER READING

Ebersold M J, Pare M C, Quast L M 1995 Surgical treatment for cervical spondylitic myelopathy. Journal of Neurosurgery 82: 745–751.
Muhle C, Metzner J, Weinert D, Falliner A, Brinkmann G, Mehdorn M H, Heller M, Resnick D 1998 Classification system based on kinematic MR imaging in cervical spondylitic myelopathy. American Journal of Neuroradiology 19: 1763–1771.
O'Duffy J D 1997 Spinal stenosis: Development of the lesion, clinical classification, and presentation. In: Frymoyer JW (ed.) The adult spine: principles and practice, 2nd edn. Lippincott-Raven, Philadelphia, pp 769–779.
Ross J S 1995 Myelopathy. Neuroimaging Clinics of North America 5: 367–384.

Case 36   Advanced osteoarthrosis

COMMENT
The effects of appropriate needle acupuncture
should not be ignored.

PROFILE

A 69-year-old man who is a non-smoker and only
rarely drinks alcohol.

PAST HISTORY

He suffers from hypertension that is well
controlled by medication. He had undergone a
prostatectomy because of malignancy within the
last 5 months.

PRESENTING COMPLAINT (Fig. 36.1)

Bilateral neck pain particularly in the suboccipital region and in the lower neck; the latter
radiates to the right arm, almost to the elbow.
The neck pain also causes headaches.

   The neck pain and headaches do not awaken
him at a particular time at night but his neck
becomes stiff during the night. He can sit and
watch the television without neck pain.
Coughing and sneezing do not aggravate his
symptoms. Periodic prostate-specific antigen
(PSA) tests weeks before the consultation had
shown that the PSA level had decreased significantly since his surgery 5 months prior to
consultation.

AETIOLOGY

Working with a shovel in his garden had caused
neck pain and headaches approximately 2 weeks
before the consultation.

EXAMINATION

The blood pressure was 130/80 in the right
arm in the seated position. All cervical spine
movements were limited and caused some
mid to lower cervical spine pain in particular.

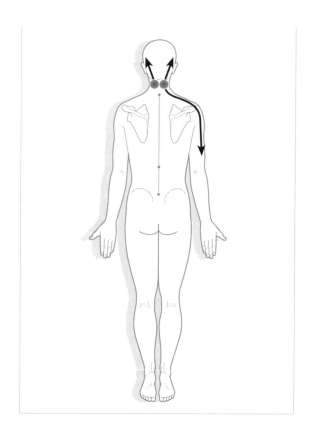

Figure 36.1

Neurologically he was intact with power in the upper and lower extremities being normal. The plantar response was normal.

IMAGING REVIEW

No imaging had been performed.

CLINICAL IMPRESSION

Osteoarthrotic changes in the cervical spine with a differential diagnosis of possible metastatic disease in view of his history.

WHAT ACTION SHOULD BE TAKEN?

A PSA blood test was performed and found to be 5.3 (i.e. normal for 61–70 years of age: range = 4 to 5.3 ng/ml). Cervical spine radiographs were ordered and these showed 'widespread degenerative changes involving the intervertebral discs, neurocentral and zygapophysial joints. No other bony lesion seen' (Fig. 36.2A, B, C). In view of his history, a bone scan was performed as a precaution to look for any possible bony metastatic disease and this was reported as being normal.

In view of the advanced osteoarthrotic changes in the cervical spine, he was advised to have a trial of needle acupuncture.

TREATMENT

Because of his neck pain and the considerable osteoarthrotic changes in his cervical spine, needle acupuncture was performed with him in the seated position so that he did not strain his neck, or injure the vertebral arteries, by lying prone. Acupuncture needles were placed in various places where deep palpation of the paraspinal muscles elicited tenderness. Up to 12 needles were used at each visit.

RESULTS

He responded well to acupuncture treatment for his neck pain, headaches and pain radiating to the right arm. After six visits he reported that, since the last visit, he had only experienced one headache, so he was advised to come in as required should his neck pain and headache symptoms recur. Periodically he comes for four to six acupuncture treatments when his neck

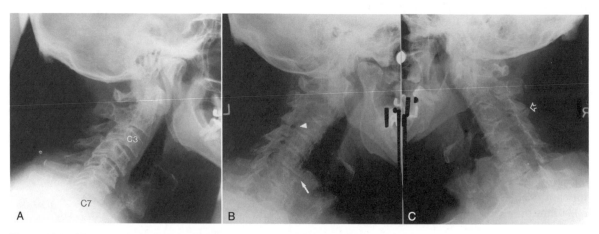

Figure 36.2 (A) A lateral cervical spine plain X-ray view showing the widespread osteoarthrotic degenerative changes involving the intervertebral and zygapophysial joints with disc space narrowing at C4–5, C5–6 and C6–7. Left (B) and right (C) oblique cervical spine plain X-ray views showing the widespread osteoarthrotic changes involving the intervertebral joints (white arrows), the zygapophysial joints (open arrow), and the uncovertebral joints with osteophytic encroachment upon some intervertebral foraminae (arrowhead).

pain and headaches trouble him but he goes for considerable periods of time (up to 2 years) without symptoms.

Key point

The value of needle acupuncture treatment for mechanical spinal pain in cases where manipulation is contraindicated should not be underestimated. Naturally, strict hygiene measures need to be used including the use of 'sharps' containers for appropriate disposal of needles.

FURTHER READING

Filshie J, White A 1998 Medical acupuncture. A Western scientific approach. Churchill Livingstone, Edinburgh.

Irnich D, Behrens N, Molzen H, Konig A, Gleditsch J, Krauss M, Natalis M, Senn E, Beyer A, Schops P 2001 Randomised trial of acupuncture compared with conventional massage and 'sham' laser acupuncture for treatment of chronic neck pain. British Medical Journal 322: 1–6.

Silvert M 2000 Acupuncture wins BMA approval. British Medical Journal 321: 11.

Vincent C 2001 The safety of acupuncture. British Medical Journal 323: 467–468.

Case 37 Intervertebral disc herniation

COMMENT
The usefulness of cervical spine functional (flexion and extension) views for evaluating neck pain due to a motor vehicle accident has already been described. However, the importance of this issue warrants a further case presentation.

PROFILE

A 30-year-old married woman who occasionally smokes cigarettes and rarely drinks alcohol. Her work involves light duty activities.

PAST HISTORY

Her past history has been one of excellent health apart from having an infected lymph gland removed from her left groin at approximately 16 years of age.

PRESENTING COMPLAINT (Fig. 37.1)

Constant and considerable lower neck pain radiating to the back of the head and particularly to the frontal regions causing bilateral headaches. The severity of the neck pain and headaches is activity related; i.e. increasing her activities causes an increase in symptoms. Considerable pain radiates to the left cervico-shoulder region and to the posterolateral aspect of the left arm (C5 dermatome), the left forearm (C6) and to the middle (C7) and fourth and fifth fingers (C8). She said the last three fingers of her left hand 'feel cold'.

She stated that she was depressed because of the protracted symtoms (4.5 years) and because various X-ray examinations had stated 'no osseous or articular abnormality seen' and her pain syndrome remained undiagnosed.

AETIOLOGY

The symptoms had resulted from a motor vehicle accident 4.5 years earlier when, as a seat-belted driver, she was approaching an intersection when a car turned in front of her motor vehicle causing a significant impact on the right side of her car. She could not remember the precise details of what happened to her but she remembers that an ambulance took her to

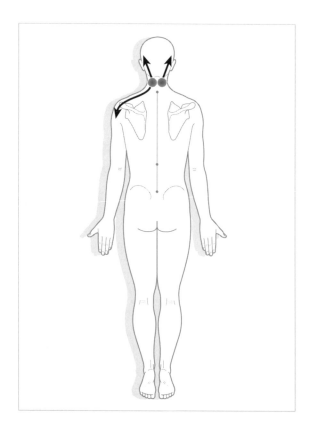

Figure 37.1

hospital where plain X-ray films were taken and she was advised to wear a soft collar. She was discharged home then, after resting for 2 days, went to see her general medical practitioner.

EXAMINATION

Deep palpation of the paravertebral muscles of the cervical spine elicited tenderness bilaterally at the C5–T1 level and midway between the neck and the left shoulder (in the left cervico-shoulder region) where there was a painful trapezius muscle trigger point.

Cervical spine active ranges of movement were measured using a Cervical Range of Motion instrument (CROM product of Performance Attainment Associates, St Paul, MN, USA), as shown in Box 37.1.

Resisted shoulder movements to test for pain and weakness were normal on the right side for flexion, extension, abduction and adduction. However, on the left side all these movements caused pain in the left cervico-shoulder region and there appeared to be some weakness in the left arm. When asked to put her hands behind her back (internal rotation and adduction of the shoulder), there was some restriction of left shoulder movement due to left cervico-shoulder arm pain. Resisted movements of the right wrist were normal but resisted movements for the left wrist appeared to be weaker and aggravated the pain in her left arm. Resisted finger abduction, and thumb flexion and extension, were normal on the right but appeared to be weaker on the left

and aggravated her left arm pain; the pain may have made the power appear weaker on the left.

Pinprick sensation of the right cervico-shoulder region, forearm and fingers was normal. However, there was some hypoaesthesia of the left arm laterally (C5), on the ulnar surface of the forearm (T1 and C8) and for the third to fifth fingers of the left hand (C7 and C8). Palpation of the two hands to compare their temperature indicated an objective finding of the left third to fifth fingers, and the lateral region of the left hand, being considerably cooler than the right (suggesting autonomic nerve involvement). The circumference of the arms, 8 cm above the elbow, was 32 cm (right) and 31 cm (left), while the circumference of the forearms, 10 cm below the elbow, was 24.5 cm (right) and 23.5 cm (left). These findings are just within normal limits, particularly in view of her right arm being dominant. The deep tendon reflexes in the arms and legs appeared to be normal. The plantar response was normal.

IMAGING REVIEW

Four sets of plain film radiographs were reviewed that had been reported as being normal. However, none of the examinations had included functional views of the cervical spine, a serious omission when it comes to investigating a patient's chronic neck pain following a motor vehicle accident as there was no radiological evaluation of cervical spine *function*. Two cervical spine MRI examinations were reported as normal.

CLINICAL IMPRESSION

- Cervicogenic headaches due to cervical spine soft tissue injuries.
- ? Disc bulge/protrusion at C5–6 or C6–7.

WHAT ACTION SHOULD BE TAKEN?

Cervical spine neutral, and flexion and extension functional views were taken to augment the previous imaging. The report stated: 'some limitation of motion on flexion and extension. No fracture or dislocation identified. Mild degenerative changes'. The neutral lateral view showed

Box 37.1			
	Normal range	Measured range	Comments
Flexion	50°	8°	Caused neck pain
Extension	60°	12°	Caused neck pain
Left lateral bending	45°	6°	Caused neck pain
Right lateral bending	45°	10°	Caused neck pain
Left rotation	80°	22°	Caused neck pain
Right rotation	80°	16°	Caused neck pain

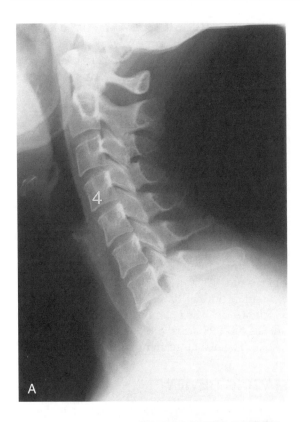

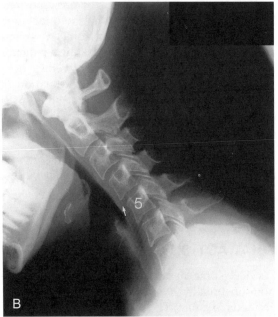

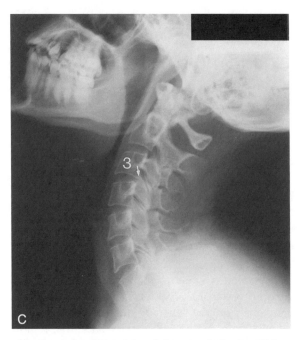

of motion below C5 and the slight anterolisthesis of C4 vertebra on C5 (white arrow), with an 'angulation' at the C5–6 level; (C) extension view showing limitation of motion and slight retrolisthesis of the C3 vertebra on C4 (white arrow). (D) A CT cervical spine scan at the C6–7 disc level showing a small central to left-sided disc herniation (black arrow). The rectangle within the broken lines is similar to the postmortem histological section (E). (E) A 100-micron thick horizontal histological section from a post-mortem specimen that shows the approximate area indicated in the rectangle on (D). Arrowhead shows an osteophyte compromising the root sleeve as it comes off from the dural tube (D) which surrounds the spinal cord (C); arrows = some of the blood vessels in the vicinity of the ganglion and nerve roots; F = zygapophysial (facet) joint; L = lamina; LF = ligamentum flavum; R = motor and sensory nerve roots, respectively; S = highly vascular spinal nerve ganglion. Only some of the anatomical structures can be seen on the CT scan in (D); this clearly indicates the principle that *imaging only provides a shadow of the truth*. (F) A cervical spine post-myelogram CT view showing the indentation of the anterior area of the dural tube (black arrow) due to the C6–7 level small central disc herniation. Blood vessels between the herniation and the pain-sensitive dural tube will be compressed, likely causing pain of ischaemic origin. In addition, the recurrent meningeal nerves will probably also be subjected to some pressure, resulting in pain. F = facet (zygapophysial) joint; L = lamina; P = pedicle; S = spinous process; U = uncinate or neurocentral process; black-headed white-tailed arrow indicates the sensory nerve root of the spinal cord passing through the cerebrospinal fluid.

Figure 37.2 Cervical spine plain X-ray views: (A) neutral lateral view showing a slight loss of normal cervical spine lordosis below C4; (B) flexion view showing the limitation

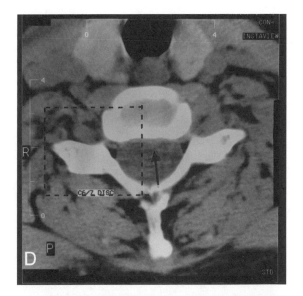

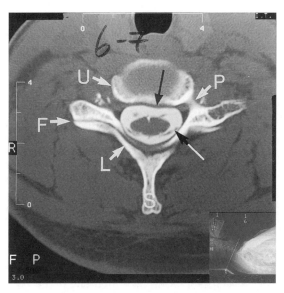

Figure 37.2   Continued.

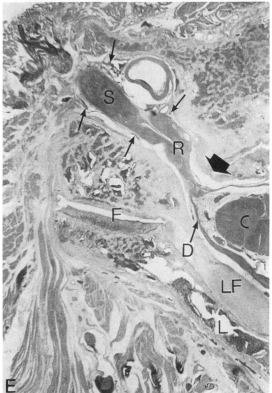

Figure 37.2   Continued.

a loss of the normal lordosis (Fig. 37.2A). The cervical spine did not function correctly on flexion and extension (Fig. 37.2B and C). In view of her symptoms of neck pain with headaches and some radiation to the left upper extremity, a CT examination of the cervical spine was performed from C3 to T1. This showed 'at the C6–7 level a very small central to left-sided disc herniation' (Fig. 37.2D). Figure 37.2E is a histopathology section of an area similar to that shown in the rectangle in Fig. 37.2D. In view of her considerable neck pain and left arm symptoms a myelogram was recommended to further evaluate the C6–7 disc level and this confirmed a small posterior disc herniation of the C6–7 disc; this was further demonstrated by a CT cervical spine post-myelography view (Fig. 37.2F).

TREATMENT

This women was told that a cause had been found for her symptoms and this provided her with great relief. She was told that the small disc herniation was not a lesion that warranted surgery and that she should be careful not to irritate her neck symptoms. She was also advised to minimize her intake of medication as this was causing nausea and gastric distress. She was advised to trial a course of needle acupuncture treatment.

RESULTS

The acupuncture treatment gave her acceptable relief but the main issue for her was that a thorough investigation had shown that she did have cervical spine dysfunction with a demonstrable small disc herniation at the C6–7 level, so she no longer had to find a reason for her symptoms. She said that she was pleased that this course had been taken as she knew the symptoms were 'not in my head'. She rapidly overcame her depression as she now knew that she had a reason for her pain; she said that she simply had not been able to convince anyone that further tests should be performed in order to search for the cause of her symptoms.

Key point(s)

The value of cervical spine flexion and extension functional views has been well documented in the literature and this case indicates how important it is to look at lateral view functional plain film radiographs to determine:

- the overall contour of the cervical spine
- the disc space height for any possible disc thinning, suggesting injury
- disc space height anteriorly and posteriorly which may suggest tearing of the anterior and/or posterior fibres of the intervertebral disc and the associated ligaments
- whether any segmental instability is present.

FURTHER READING

An H 1998 Cervical spine trauma. Spine 23: 2713–2729.
Anderson J, Read J W, Steinweg J 1998 Atlas of imaging in sports medicine. McGraw-Hill, Sydney.
Jackson R 1977 The cervical syndrome, 4th edn. Charles C Thomas, Springfield.

Case 38   Block vertebrae

COMMENT
Beware of cervical block vertebrae; i.e. fusion of
adjacent vertebrae.

PROFILE

A 48-year-old married woman who does not smoke
and only drinks alcohol socially.

PAST HISTORY

She has a past history of 15 years of a cervical
spine pain syndrome that led to chronic anxiety.

PRESENTING COMPLAINT (Fig. 38.1)

Mid to lower cervical spine pain that radiates to
the left and right cervico-shoulder regions and
was of gradual onset over an approximately
15-year period; the pain is now severe. This has
led to some disability regarding neck movements as she is frustrated because she is unable
to perform her housework. Her complaint is
steadily worsening.

She occasionally experiences 'dizziness' but
has no history of fits. Occasionally, she experiences occipital headaches which she believes
come from the neck and are increasing in frequency. Bowel and bladder function are normal.

Coughing may aggravate her neck pain. She
requires a contoured pillow for supporting her
neck at night.

She had previously tried physiotherapy treatment, spinal manipulation and anti-inflammatory medication, without success.

AETIOLOGY

Unknown, but no history whatsoever of trauma.

EXAMINATION

All cervical spine ranges of movement were limited by approximately 50% due to mid to lower
neck pain except for extension which was limited by approximately 75% for the same reason.
The reflexes in the upper and lower extremities

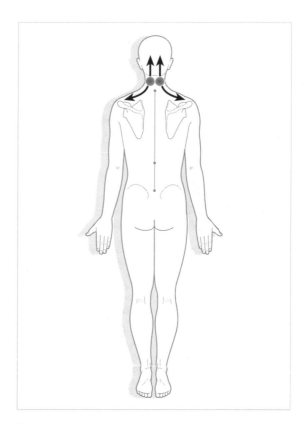

Figure 38.1

were slightly hyper-reflexic. Sensation to pin-prick was normal as was vibration sensation. Muscle strength was normal. The plantar response was normal. Deep palpation of the paraspinal muscles of the cervical spine elicited tenderness over the mid to lower cervical spine but particularly at the C5–6 level.

IMAGING REVIEW

Previous plain film imaging was reviewed and this showed a partial congenital block vertebra at the C6–7 vertebral level.

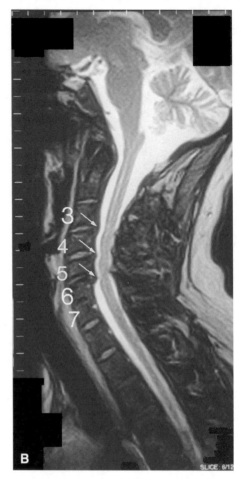

Figure 38.2 Continued.

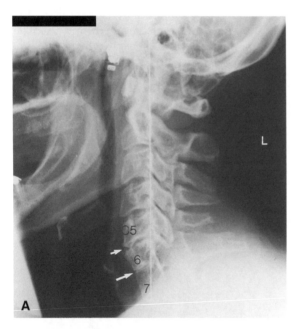

Figure 38.2 (A) Lateral cervical spine plain film X-ray showing the disc space narrowing at C5–6 (small white arrow) and the partial congenital 'block vertebra' at C6–7 (large white arrow). Note the angulation in the cervical spine contour at the C5–6 level which is clearly shown in relation to the vertical plumb line. L shows that the left side of the patient was against the X-ray bucky. (B) Sagittal T2-weighted MRI scan of the cervical spine showing degenerative changes at the C3–4, C4–5 and C5–6 levels (particularly at the C5–6 level) (arrows) with disc/osteophyte impression on the thecal sac at these levels with borderline canal stenosis at the C5–6 level. The vertebral bodies have been labelled 3, 4, 5, 6, 7 (just to their left side) so as not to obliterate the vertebral body with a numeral. Note the partial developmental fusion of the C6 and 7 vertebral bodies.

CLINICAL IMPRESSION

Cervical spine pain syndrome due to degenerative changes involving the C5–6 level.

WHAT ACTION SHOULD BE TAKEN?

Updated cervical spine radiographs were ordered and these showed 'disc space narrowing at C5–6 and C6–7 (Fig. 38.2A) with large posterior osteophytes at the C5–6 level. There is uncinate process hypertrophy with prominent osteophytes encroaching into the right neural foramen at C5–6 level. There is partial congenital block vertebra at C6–7 level'. In view of the plain film findings, a MRI examination was performed of the cervical spine. This showed:

Partial developmental fusion of C6 and C7 vertebral bodies. Degenerative changes at the C3–4, C4–5 and C5–6 levels, most marked at the C5–6 level. There are disc/osteophyte impressions on the thecal sac at these levels, most marked at C5–6 level. This causes borderline canal stenosis at the C5–6 level but the canal appears adequate at other levels' (Fig. 38.2B). There is also moderate osteophytic narrowing of the C5–6 intervertebral foramina bilaterally with the remaining foramina appearing adequate.

TREATMENT

She was given the option of medication or acupuncture treatment and she said that, as medication had previously not helped, she would prefer to try needle acupuncture. She did not want a surgical opinion until she had tried acupuncture.

RESULTS

She had 15 acupuncture treatments and reported at that time that she had obtained 'good relief' from her neck pain syndrome. She returned 2 months later and had a further course of 10 acupuncture treatments, again with good results. She then came occasionally, thereafter, during a 4-year period, whenever she experienced a recurrence of symptoms. When seen 4 years later she had experienced a recurrence of her symptoms due to having fallen but again responded well to acupuncture treatment.

Note

This case provides an example of how a congenital 'block vertebra' can cause excessive wear at levels above the congenital fusion when there is no history of trauma.

Key point(s)

1. This case, with no history whatsoever of trauma, indicates how considerable disc wear and tear changes can occur above the fused level.
2. When a patient has a congenital block vertebra, it is prudent to realize that there may be associated considerable soft tissue changes.
3. In block vertebra cases, plain X-ray films may not adequately indicate the soft tissue changes, so an MRI study may be necessary, depending on a patient's age, history, symptoms and signs.

FURTHER READING

Banki Z 1980 Partielle Blockbildung an der Halswirbelsaule. Fortschritte auf dem Gebiete der Roentgenstrahlen und der Nuklearmedizin 133: 637–640.
Bullough P G, Boachie-Adjei O 1988 Atlas of spinal diseases. JB Lippincott, Philadelphia, p 121.
Chandraraj S 1987 Failure of articular process (zygapophysial) joint development as a cause of vertebral fusion (blocked vertebrae). Journal of Anatomy 153: 55–62.

Case 39   Cerebellar tonsil ectopia

COMMENT
Always remember that the arterial blood supply to the anterior inferior cerebellar arteries, the basilar artery and the superior cerebellar arteries may be compromised by pressure upon the vertebral arteries.

PROFILE

A 45-year-old woman who does not smoke or drink alcohol.

PAST HISTORY

She had a hysterectomy some years ago.

PRESENTING COMPLAINT (Fig. 39.1)

Constant bilateral neck pain that radiates to the lower cervical spine and into the cervico-shoulder regions, particularly on the right side, since a motor vehicle accident 3 years ago. The neck pain varies in intensity causing occasional occipital headaches. The neck pain worsens with activity, especially lifting objects and flexing her cervical spine. Because of the neck pain, she can only sit for short periods of time. On looking up she feels slight 'dizziness'.

The neck pain and headaches are made worse with coughing and sneezing but settle with rest. Considerable doses of NSAIDs and analgesics provide only temporary relief. She wanted a diagnosis to be made as she was concerned about her hitherto unexplained symptoms.

AETIOLOGY

Motor vehicle accident 3 years ago.

EXAMINATION

Cervical spine flexion and extension were limited due to neck pain with a minor degree of 'dizziness'; extension being very limited, i.e. to only approximately 10°. All other ranges of movement elicited neck pain but were not limited by it. There was generalized tenderness in the paraspinal cervical muscles on deep palpation. Her blood pressure was normal, at 120/80 in the seated position.

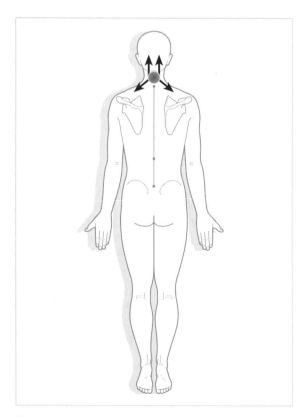

Figure 39.1

IMAGING REVIEW

Plain X-ray films of her neck showed a loss of normal lordosis with a kyphosis above the C5 vertebra. On cervical spine flexion, there was a slight anterolisthesis of C4 on C5. There were osteophytes at the antero-inferior margins of the C4 and C5 vertebral bodies.

CLINICAL IMPRESSION

Possible vertebral artery compression in certain positions of the neck and head causing vertigo.

WHAT ACTION SHOULD BE TAKEN?

A cervical spine MRI was ordered and this showed: 'Minimal uncovertebral joint hypertrophy in the lower cervical spine with no significant exit foramen encroachment. C5–6 shallow central lateral disc protrusion extending to the right with early disc narrowing and loss of cervical lordosis' (Fig. 39.2A and B). However, the report did not mention the ectopia of the cerebellar tonsils amouting to approximately 10 mm of cerebellar ectopia, a mild form of Chiari I malformation. (A Chiari I malformation is usually

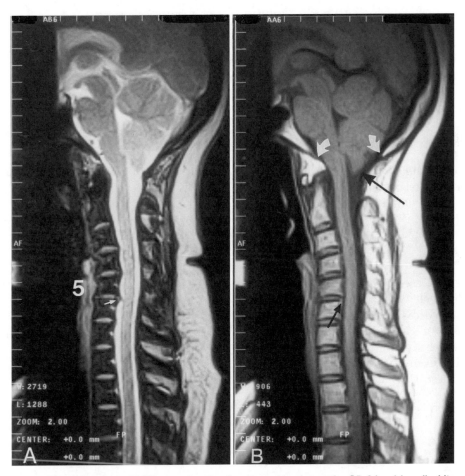

Figure 39.2 (A) A sagittal T2-weighted MRI scan showing the disc protrusion at the C5–6 level (small white arrow) and loss of the normal cervical lordosis with a mild kyphosis at the C5 level. (B) A sagittal T1-weighted MRI scan showing loss of the normal cervical lordosis with a mild kyphosis at the C5 level and disc material at the C5–6 level posteriorly (small black arrow). The cerebellar tonsil ectopia is seen more clearly on the T1-weighted image and the anterior and posterior margins of the foramen magnum are shown by the small white curved arrows. Note the cerebellar tonsil ectopia projecting below the foramen magnum (large black arrow); this woman had a mild form of Chiari I malformation.

not associated with other brain anomalies although spinal cord, skull base and spine lesions are common in this disorder (Osborn 1994).)

TREATMENT

This woman was told that she had a loss of the normal cervical lordosis with a C5–6 shallow central to lateral disc protrusion with the latter most probably causing most of her bilateral neck and cervico-shoulder pains. She was told that the slight dizziness experienced on looking up may well be due to compression of blood vessels within the foramen magnum (particularly the vertebral arteries) due to the tonsillar ectopia causing a stenotic effect upon soft tissue structures within the foramen magnum during certain neck movements. She was told that she could obtain a surgical opinion regarding the C5–6 disc protrusion but, as she did not have radicular symptoms, she decided not to proceed with a referral. She was advised not to extend her cervical spine as this precipitates the episodes of dizziness. As she was taking considerable doses of non-steroidal and analgesic medication, she was offered a trial course of needle acupuncture to see if this would help her neck pain; she agreed to this.

RESULTS

She was very pleased to have a diagnosis made and she did well with acupuncture treatment apart from one occasion when a locum acupuncturist, instead of giving her acupuncture treatment while she sat in a chair, asked her to lie prone on the examination table with a pillow under her chest; this introduced cervical spine

extension and she became very 'dizzy'. She was then asked to sit for a few minutes and the dizziness passed. The acupuncture treatment provided significant relief and enabled her to lessen her medication. (When performing acupuncture in the seated position, ensure that the patient cannot fall of the chair.)

Key point(s)

1. When a patient feels 'dizzy' on performing certain neck movements, the possibility of arterial compromise should be considered as one likely factor. The probable area of compromise would be of the vertebral arteries.
2. Consider the possibility of a previously asymptomatic Chiari I malformation when a person is involved in a motor vehicle accident (or other neck injury) and experiences neurological symptoms such as vertigo.

REFERENCE

Osborn AG 1994 Diagnostic neuroradiology. Mosby, St Louis, p 15.

FURTHER READING

Bunc G, Vorsic M 2001 Presentation of a previously asymptomatic Chiari I malformation by a flexion injury to the neck. Journal of Neurotrauma 18: 645–648.
Gamache F W 1997 Diagnosis and treatment of congenital neurologic abnormalities affecting the cervical spine. In: Frymoyer JW (ed.) The adult spine: principles and practice, 2nd edn. Lippincott-Raven, Philadelphia, pp 1223–1231.
Strayer A 2001 Chiari I malformation: clinical presentation and management. Journal of Neuroscience Nursing 33: 90–96, 104.

Thoracic spine cases

INTRODUCTION

Before presenting the thoracic spine cases it is important to consider the following summary of some possible causes of thoracic spine pain, with or without radiculopathy (Table viii).

PHYSICAL EXAMINATION

The physical examination should be orderly and systematic and should include the following thoracic examinations as indicated by the patient's presenting complaint(s) (Table ix).

Table viii   Some possible causes of thoracic spine pain

Acute spinal pain
  Febrile disorders
  Injury
Chronic spinal pain
1. *Traumatic, mechanical or degenerative*
- Thoracic spine strain; fatigue, obesity, pregnancy causing altered biomechanics, avulsion fracture of T1 spinous process (clay shoveller's fracture)
- Injuries of bone, joint, intervertebral disc or ligaments
- Degenerative or traumatic changes of the spine (osteoarthrosis; spondylosis)
- Scoliosis: primary and secondary; kyphoscoliosis
- Spinal or intervertebral canal stenosis
- Spinal origin – cervical spine osteoarthrosis and disc herniation (especially C4–C7), cervicothoracic junction injury, thoracic spine osteoarthrosis including joints (e.g. costovertebral, zygapophysial, intervertebral with disc), thoracolumbar junction injury
- Other thoracic joints – sternoclavicular, manubriosternal, costochondral, sternocostal
- Disorders of ribs (including 12th rib syndrome, rib tip syndrome, slipping rib syndrome), muscles, ligaments, e.g. ossified ligamenta flava
- Other – costochondrites, Tietze's syndrome, xiphoidalgia, myofascial syndrome, thoracic outlet syndrome, intercostal neuralgia. Post-nephrectomy syndromes with entrapment of 12th thoracic intercostal nerve in the scar tissue. Serratus anterior nerve palsy
- Subscapular bursitis
2. *Joint dysfunction*
- Zygapophysial
- Intervertebral disc
- Costochondral
3. *Metabolic*
- Osteoporosis
- Osteomalacia
- Hyper- and hypo-parathyroidism
- Ochronosis
- Fluorosis
- Hypophosphataemic rickets
4. *Unknown causes*
- Inflammatory arthropathies of the spine, such as ankylosing spondylitis, the spondylitis of Reiter's (Brodie's) disease, psoriasis, ulcerative colitis, Whipple's and Crohn's diseases; diffuse idiopathic skeletal hyperostosis
- Rarely polymyositis and polymyalgia rheumatica
- Paget's disease of bone
- Scheuermann's 'disease'
5. *Infective conditions of bone, joint and theca of the spine*
- Osteomyelitis
- Tuberculosis
- Melioidosis
- Undulant fever (abortus and melitensis)
- Typhoid and paratyphoid fever and other *Salmonella* infections
- Syphilis
- Yaws
- Very rarely Weil's disease (leptospirosis icterohaemorrhagica)
- Spinal pachymeningitis
- Chronic meningitis
- Subarachnoid or spinal abscess

- Herpes zoster
- Post-herpetic neuralgia
6. *Psychogenic*
- Anxiety
- Depression
- Hysteria
- 'Compensation neurosis'
- Malingering
7. *Neoplastic – benign or malignant, primary or secondary*
- Osteoid osteoma
- Eosinophilic granuloma
- Metastatic carcinomatosis
- Bronchial carcinoma
- Oesophageal carcinoma
- Sarcoma
- Myeloma
- Primary and secondary tumours of spinal canal and nerve roots: ependymoma; neurofibroma; glioma; angioma; meningioma; lipoma; rarely cordoma
- Reticuloses, e.g. Hodgkin's disease
- Neoplasms of the chest wall and pleura
8. *Cardiac and vascular*
- Myocardial infarction
- Coronary insufficiency
- Pericarditis
- Pulmonary embolism
- Subacute bacterial endocarditis
- Grossly enlarged left atrium in mitral valve disease
- Luetic or dissecting thoracic aorta aneurysm; aneurysm with thoracic vertebral involvement
- Enlarged thoracic aortic aneurysm
- Subarachnoid or spinal haemorrhage
9. *Pulmonary*
- Embolus
- Pneumothorax
- Pneumonia
- Pleurisy
- Pleurodynia (Bornholm's disease)
10. *Oesophageal*
- Spasm
- Rupture
- Oesophagitis
- Aerophagy
- Hiatus hernia
11. *Acute subdiaphragmatic*
- Stomach disorders, e.g. peptic ulcer, carcinoma
- Biliary, renal, duodenal, pancreatic and subphrenic disorders
12. *Blood disorders*
- Acute haemolytic states
13. *Drugs*
- Corticosteroids
- Methysergide
- Compound analgesic tablets

Modified from Hart (1985) and Bland (2000).

Table ix Some elements of the thoracic spine physical examination

Erect posture examination

Observe for
Fluidity of movement
Body build
Skin markings – café-au-lait spots, lipomata, melanoma
Posture
Deformities
Scoliosis
  Idiopathic
  Postural with pelvic obliquity
Spine alignment

Test spinal column motion for
Flexion
Extension
Side bending
Rotation

Compression of rib cage

Intercostal expansion at nipple line
(a) 5–7.6 cm (normal)
(b) <2.6 cm (ankylosing spondylitis)

Palpate for
Muscle spasm
Myofascial trigger points
Supraspinous and interspinous ligament tenderness
Adjacent muscle tenderness
Relative motion between adjacent vertebrae (by motion
  palpation) in an attempt to find restricted movement

Observe gait
Steady or unsteady

Seated

Neurological tests
Knee jerk, ankle jerk
Pinprick sensation on torso and lower limbs
Vibration sensation at ankles
Straight leg raising

Measure
Thigh circumference bilaterally
Calf circumference bilaterally

Supine
Kernig test (spinal cord stretch)*
Tests to increase intrathecal pressure:
  Naffziger test*
  Valsalva manoeuvre*
Superficial abdominal reflexes (upper T7–10; lower T10–L1)
Test sensation and motor power
Palpation of chest
Auscultation

Prone – Palpate thoracic spine, over related joints,
  and trigger points

Adapted from Hoppenfeld (1976), Keim & Kirkaldy-Willis (1987), Hart (1985) and Mackenzie (1985).

The symptoms and signs caused by a herniated thoracic disc depend on the location of the herniation:

• Figure ix shows the clinical features of a *posterolateral* thoracic disc herniation that may cause nerve root impingement, as summarized in the figure.

• *Midline* herniation may cause symptoms in the arm, thoracic spine and/or in the legs as well as sensory loss, bladder incontinence and upper motor neuron lesion signs.

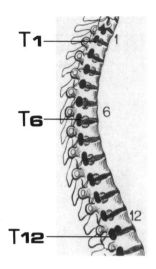

HERNIATION	T1-2	T2-3	T3-4	T4-5	T5-6, T6-7	T7-9/10	T10-12
NERVE ROOT	T1	T2	T3	T4	T5, T6	T7-9/10	T10-12
SENSORY SUPPLY							
				Nipple line level		T7 at xiphoid process level, T10 at umbilicus level	T10 at umbilicus level; T12 at groin level
PAIN	Medial arm and shoulder (deep ache)	Axilla	Intercostal dermatome	Intercostal dermatome; T4 syndrome: vague pain & paraesthesiae in upper limbs, not dermatomal, diffuse & vague head & posterior neck pain (may also involve upper thoracic vertebrae)	Intercostal dermatome	Intercostal dermatome	Intercostal (T10 & T11) dermatomes; Thoraco-lumbar T12 & L1 ventral rami (subcostal and iliohypogastric nerves respectively) ▶ lower abdominal wall, skin of groin, lateral iliac crest (as the lateral cutaneous branch)
MOTOR WEAKNESS	All small muscles of hand	-	The intercostal muscles are segmentally innervated and are difficult to evaluate individually				
SCREENING EXAM	Thumb abduction, Finger Abduction	-	-	T4 syndrome: spinal tenderness & joint stiffness (T4-T5)	Beevor's sign (T5-12) to test rectus abdominis muscle's segmental innervation integrity (umbilicus should not move when patient does a quarter sit-up)		
REFLEXES	-	-	-	-	-	Superficial upper abdominal	Superficial lower abdominal

Figure ix   The clinical features of a posterolateral thoracic disc herniation that may cause nerve root impingement. Adapted from: Hoppenfeld (1976, 1977), Wilkinson (1986), Kenna & Murtagh (1989), McGuckin (1986), Maigne (2000), Lawrence & Bukkum (2000), Pauchet & Dupret (1937) and Chusid (1985).

REFERENCES

Bland J H 2000 Diagnosis of thoracic pain syndromes. In: Giles LGF, Singer KP (eds) Clinical anatomy and management of thoracic spine pain. Butterworth-Heinemann, Oxford, pp 145–156.

Chusid J G 1985 Correlative neuroanatomy and functional neurology. Lange Medical Publications, Los Altos, p 241.

Hart F D 1985 Back, pain in. In: Hart FD (ed.) French's Index of Differential Diagnosis, 12th edn. Butterworth & Co. Ltd, Oxford, pp 72–73.

Hoppenfeld S 1976 Physical examination of the spine and extremities. Appleton-Century-Crofts, New York, p 262.

Hoppenfeld S 1977 Orthopaedic neurology: A diagnostic guide to neurologic levels. J. B. Lippincott, Philadelphia, p 45.

Keim H A, Kirkaldy-Willis W H 1987 Clinical symposia. Low back pain 39. Ciba-Geigy, Jersey.

Kenna C, Murtagh J 1989 Back pain and spinal manipulation. Butterworths, Sydney, p 168.

Lawrence D J, Bukkum B 2000 Chiropractic management of thoracic spine pain of mechanical origin. In: Giles LGF, Singer KP (eds) Clinical anatomy and management of thoracic spine pain. Butterworth-Heinemann, Oxford, pp 244–256.

Mackenzie I 1985 Spine, tenderness of. In: Hart FD (ed.) French's index of differential diagnosis, 12th edn. Butterworth & Co. Ltd, Oxford, p 788.

Maigne J -Y 2000 Cervicothoracic and thoracolumbar spinal pain syndromes. In: Giles LGF, Singer KP (eds) Clinical anatomy and management of thoracic spine pain. Butterworth-Heinemann, Oxford, pp 157–168.

McGuckin N 1986 The T4 syndrome. In: Grieve GD (ed.) Modern manual therapy of the vertebral column. Churchill Livingstone, London, pp 370–376.

Pauchet V, Dupret S 1937 Pocket atlas of anatomy, 3rd edn. Oxford University Press, London.

Wilkinson J L 1986 Neuroanatomy for medical students. Bristol, John Wright and Sons, p 29.

Case 40 Intervertebral disc herniation

COMMENT
This lady was considered a malingerer due to her various complaints.

PROFILE

A 40-year-old married woman.

PAST HISTORY

She had her tonsils removed at approximately 27 years of age. She had a fall 10 years ago and 'banged' her head on the floor.

PRESENTING COMPLAINT (Fig. 40.1)

Thoracic spine pain in the vicinity of T9–10, particulary on the right side, i.e. in the region in which a laminectomy was performed approximately 4 years ago. This pain has worsened in the last 3–4 weeks and now radiates, intermittently, from the T9–10 level along the adjacent right intercostal nerve to the front of her chest, at approximately the lower region of the sternum and below her right breast. This pain can last for about 45 minutes during which period she takes very 'shallow breaths' until the pain passes. She also complains of some 'hypersensitivity' of the right anterolateral part of her upper chest; this sensation extends as far as approximately the second rib level.

   She is frustrated because she has been labelled a 'malingerer' and wants to know why she has debilitating symptoms in spite of having had surgery at the T9–10 level.

AETIOLOGY

She fell heavily onto her buttocks and back when she slipped and fell 6 years ago.

EXAMINATION

Deep reflexes in the upper extremities were normal but it was difficult to elicit the knee jerks (L2,3,4), although these were elicited using a reinforced patella reflex test; the reflexes bilaterally were only one plus (two plus being normal).

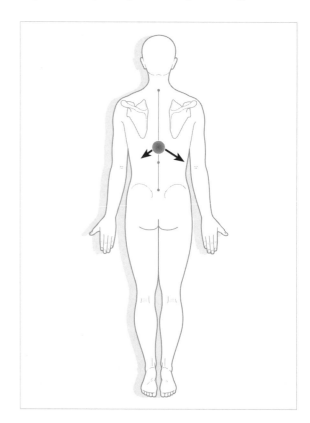

Figure 40.1

The ankle jerks (S1) were normal as was vibration sensation to a tuning fork applied to her left and right ankles. Pinprick sensation of the arms and hands was normal, as was the case in all parts of the legs and feet, apart from a feeling of hypoaesthesia on the lateral aspect (L2) of her right thigh. The circumference of her thighs was the same on the left and right sides. Percussion of her spine elicited considerable tenderness at approximately T4–5 and particularly at T9–10 where the laminectomy was performed approximately 4 years ago. Power in the lower extremities was normal. Coughing did not cause any pain and the Naffziger test (compression of the jugular veins for 15 seconds before the patient was asked to cough) did not cause any pain.

Active thoracic spine ranges of movement in the seated position were as follows:

1. Flexion – limited by approximately 15% due to pain on the right side of T9–10.
2. Extension – approximately of full range but caused pain on the right side of T9–10.
3. Left rotation – limited to approximately 15% due to pain on the right of T9–10.
4. Right rotation – limited to approximately 15% due to pain on the right side of T9–10.

Auscultation of the heart and lungs was within normal limits. The blood pressure in the right arm was 134/88 and in the left arm 132/82, in the seated position, indicating no coarctation of the aorta.

IMAGING REVIEW

The report of a CT scan of her abdomen and pelvis before and after intravenous contrast (Fig. 40.2A) made no reference to the central to left-sided calcified extruded disc material in the spinal canal at the T9–10 level. As her symptoms persisted, further thoracic spine plain X-ray films had been taken five months later and these showed a small area of calcification posterior to the T9–10 disc space within the intervertebral foramen (Fig. 40.2B). This finding led to a thoracic myelogram where dye

was introduced by a lumbar puncture and clear CSF was obtained. This myelogram showed a 'minimal hold-up of the contrast at the T9–10 level' due to an extradural indentation (Fig. 40.2C). This was followed by a CT thoracic spine scan which showed a central to left-sided calcified extradural mass at the T9–10 level; this represented calcified extruded disc material (Fig. 40.2D).

The patient had then undergone a laminectomy for removal of the T9–10 disc material.

CLINICAL IMPRESSION

Possibly residual or recurrent disc at the T9–10 level.

WHAT ACTION SHOULD BE TAKEN?

As she still had a thoracic spine pain syndrome at presentation, a post-surgery CT thoracic spine scan was ordered; this showed that there was still 'a prominent piece of ossification centrally and anteriorly in the spinal canal', thought to be causing some degree of cord compression at this level (Fig. 40.2E). An MRI of the thoracic spine showed 'residual calcified disc material at the T9–10 level which indents the anterior thecal sac and abuts and mildly flattens the

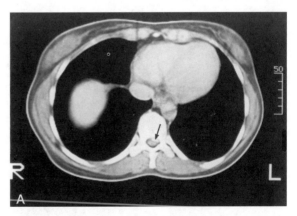

Figure 40.2 (A) A CT scan at the T9–10 level after intravenous contrast. Note the central to left-sided calcified extruded disc material in the spinal canal (black arrow). R & L = right and left sides, respectively, of the patient.

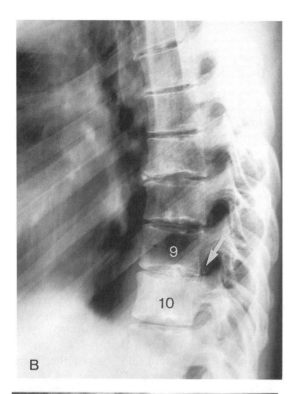

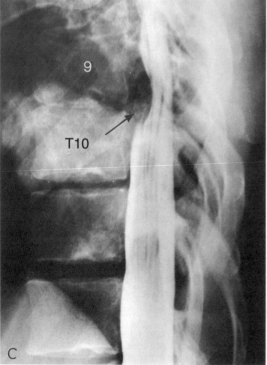

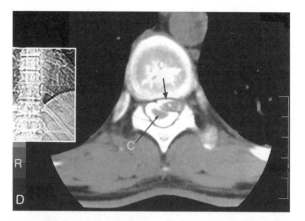

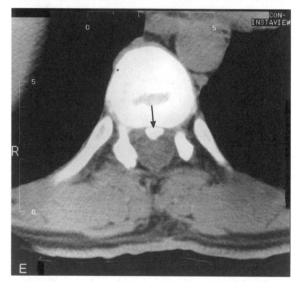

Figure 40.2 (B) A lateral thoracic spine plain X-ray film taken 5 months after the CT scan shows a small area of calcification posterior to the T9–10 disc space within the intervertebral foramen (white arrow). 9 = ninth thoracic vertebra; 10 = tenth thoracic vertebra. (C) A thoracic spine myelogram showing a 'minimal hold-up of the contrast at the T9–10 level' due to an extradural indentation (black arrow). 9 = ninth thoracic vertebra; 10 = tenth thoracic vertebra. (D) A post-contrast CT thoracic spine scan showing a central to left-sided calcified extra-dural mass at the T9–10 level (arrow), i.e. a calcified disc protrusion. C = spinal cord within the cerebrospinal fluid. Note that the cord is somewhat displaced. T = right side of patient. (E) A post-surgery CT thoracic spine scan showing that there was still 'a prominent piece of ossification centrally and anteriorly in the spinal canal' thought to be causing some degree of cord compression at this level (arrow). R = right of patient.

Figure 40.2

anterior cord, with some narrowing of the cord at this level'.

In order to understand the significance of this finding, Fig. 40.3 shows a horizontal histology section through a thoracic vertebra. This shows the vertebral body, the spinal canal, the left and right intervertebral foramina, the left and right zygapophysial joints with their facet cartilage, the lamina and the spinous process.

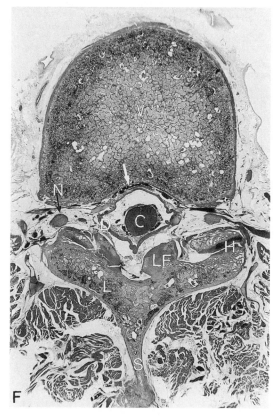

Figure 40.3 Superior to inferior view of a 200-micron thick post-mortem histological section through the T10–11 level of the thoracic spine of a 40-year-old male. N = spinal nerve ganglion; LF = ligamentum flavum; L = lamina; D = dural tube (thecal sac); C = spinal cord; H = hyaline articular cartilage on the facet surfaces of the zygapophysial joints; S = spinous process; V = vertebral body. The small space between the anterior part of the dural tube and the posterior part of the vertebral body, or intervertebral disc, has small blood vessels in it (white arrow). In addition, there is a recurrent meningeal nerve from each side (not visible at this magnification). Protruded disc material could press on the blood vessels causing pain of ischaemic origin (Jayson 1997), the recurrent meningeal nerve, and the pain-sensitive anterior part of the dural tube causing pain. See also colour plate section.

Figure iv (General Introduction) shows the complex innervation of the nerve supply of the thoracic ventral compartment at the level of the vertebral body and intervertebral disc.

TREATMENT

The findings of the post-surgical CT and MRI scans were explained to the patient, as were the possible pain mechanisms such as: (i) pain resulting from irritation of the small blood vessels being compressed between the residual calcified disc material and the dural tube; (ii) compression of the recurrent meningeal nerves between the calcified disc material and the dural tube; and (iii) direct pressure upon the pain-sensitive anterior part of the dural tube. She was advised not to undergo further surgery unless her symptoms deteriorated and she was also advised to avoid movements that irritated her symptoms. She was told that it would be prudent to keep fit and to take part in exercise, such as walking, that did not aggravate her symptoms. She was particularly pleased to know why she still had residual symptoms following surgery and that her condition was real and not imagined.

RESULTS

She accepted her post-surgical condition and heeds the advice provided as a result of a thorough reappraisal of her symptoms. The conservative approach to her pain syndrome with a detailed explanation of her condition, which was indeed 'real', made her feel very much better.

Note

It should be noted that dural sympathetic innervation, if irritated at one particular level, e.g. T9, which has led to nociceptive stimulation, may enter the spinal cord at many levels (up to about 9, i.e. from T5 to L1) (Groen & Stolker 2000).

Key point(s)

1. Thoracic disc herniation has long been a difficult entity to diagnose and treat and there is no typical presentation (Errico et al 1997).
2. Never label a patient as being a malingerer unless you have made a thorough appraisal of all facts – not many patients wish to be invalids!

REFERENCES

Errico J E, Stecker S, Kostuik J P 1997 Thoracic pain syndrome. In: Frymoyer JW (ed.) The adult spine: principles and practice, 2nd edn. Lippincott-Raven, Philadelphia, pp 1623–1637.
Giles L G F 2000 Diagnosis of thoracic spine pain and contraindications to spinal mobilization and manipulation. In: Giles LGF, Singer KP (eds) Clinical anatomy and management of thoracic spine pain. Butterworth-Heinemann, Oxford, pp 283–297.

Groen G J, Stolker R J 2000 Thoracic neural anatomy. In: Giles LGF, Singer KP (eds) Clinical anatomy and management of thoracic spine pain. Butterworth-Heinemann, Oxford, pp 114–141.
Jayson M I V 1997 Why does acute back pain become chronic? Spine 22(10): 1053–1056.

FURTHER READING

Awwad E E, Martin D S, Smith K R, Baker B K 1991 Asymptomatic versus symptomatic herniated thoracic discs: their frequency and characteristics as detected by computed tomography after myelography. Neurosurgery 28: 180–186.
Frymoyer J W 1997 The adult spine: principles and practice, 2nd edn. Lippincott-Raven, Philadelphia.
Groen G J, Baljet B, Drukker J 1990 Nerves and nerve plexuses of the human vertebral column. American Journal of Anatomy 188: 282–296.

Case 41   Zygapophysial joint facet fracture

COMMENT
Always carefully look at the imaging and not at just the report.

PROFILE

A 43-year-old man of muscular build.

PAST HISTORY

He had always been healthy and fit and he had no recollection of trauma apart from a motor bike accident approximately 10 years ago following which he was not immediately aware of this pain.

PRESENTING COMPLAINT (Fig. 41.1)

A 10-year history of chronic mid to lower thoracic spine pain that radiates to the left side of his chest as far as the mid-clavicular line, often associated with paraesthesiae and occasional pain referral to his left arm. He initially felt pain and 'pins and needles' at approximately the T8 level, then the left-sided chest pain occurred during long drives in the car. The pain intensity varies depending on what he does. He now experiences recurrences of the pain after short drives in the car and he finds this very frustrating.

He was referred with an extensive background of investigations including MRI studies of the thoracic spine. He had also had stress tests performed to rule out a cardiac problem; there was no indication of heart problems. He had also been investigated for an oesophageal/gastric cause and a pulmonary cause, all to no avail. There was no night pain. Coughing and sneezing were painless. He was frustrated and depressed as the cause of his pain could not be found.

AETIOLOGY

Possible motor bike injury approximately 10 years ago.

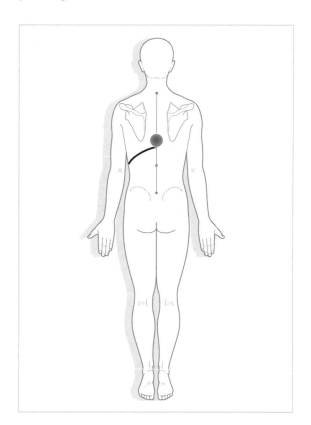

Figure 41.1

EXAMINATION

On deep palpation of the paraspinal muscles he was tender over the T6–10 level and there was increased tone of the paraspinal muscles. The deep reflexes in the upper and lower extremities were normal, as was the case with pinprick sensation. Vibration sensation at the ankles and elbows was normal. Active ranges of thoracic spine movement were limited by approximately 20% in forward bending and in left and right lateral bending.

IMAGING REVIEW

Plain X-ray films showed minor degenerative lipping at the T6–9 vertebral bodies anteriorly. The MRI thoracic spine was non-contributory.

CLINICAL IMPRESSION

'Mechanical' spinal pain as the pain is reproducible on thoracic spine flexion and left and right lateral bending. There is no night pain to suggest a serious pathology and MRI had not shown any disease process or space occupying lesion.

WHAT ACTION SHOULD BE TAKEN?

Bearing in mind that a MRI study can be less useful than a CT scan for looking at bones, a CT scan from T3 to T10 was ordered; this was reported as showing 'minimal degenerative change in the rib articulations at T8 and T9 with small anterior vertebral osteophytic change at the T8–9 level'. However, on carefully reviewing the CT slice images, it was noted that the left zygapophysial synovial joint facet at the T8–9 level was abnormal and probably represented a fracture of the superior articular facet of T9 (Fig. 41.2). As a result, an isotope bone scan was performed of the thoracic spine and this showed 'mildly increased isotope accumulation in the region of the left T8–9 facets, typical of degenerative or post-traumatic changes'.

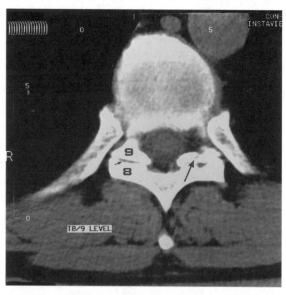

Figure 41.2 A CT axial thoracic spine view at the T8–9 level clearly shows the fracture (large black arrow) of the superior articular facet of the T9 vertebra. (For comparison with 'normal' histology, please see Fig. 40.3.) The inferior articular process of the T8 vertebra is shown by the numeral 8 and the superior articular process of the T9 vertebra is shown by the numeral 9. On the right side (R) there is a normal zygapophysial (facet) joint with hyaline articular cartilage (small arrow) between the facet surfaces.

TREATMENT

He was greatly relieved to find that the cause of his problem was benign and that there was not an underlying more sinister pathological reason for his chronic pain syndrome. Because it was considered that the left T8–9 zygapophysial joint was probably irritating the intercostal nerve root on the left side, he was sent for an orthopaedic opinion. The orthopaedic surgeon agreed with the diagnosis and suggested a facet block injection.

RESULTS

The facet block injection gave considerable pain relief. He was left with a painful 'trigger point' in the mid-axillary line after prolonged sitting, so an anaesthetic with steroid injection into the trigger point was performed; this gave him dramatic relief. He later required a further facet block injection for the left T8–9 zygapophysial joint and he was very satisfied with the result.

Gronblad M, Korkala O, Liesi P, Korarju E 1985 Innervation of synovial membrane and meniscus. Acta Orthopaedica Scandinavica 56: 484–486.

Gronblad M, Weinstein J N, Santavirta S 1991 Immunohisto-chemical observations on spinal tissue innervation. Acta Orthopaedica Scandinavica 62: 614–622.

Manchikanti L 1999 Facet joint pain and the role of neural blockade in its management. Current Review of Pain 3: 348–358.

Stolker R J, Groen G J 2000 Medical and invasive manage-ment of thoracic spinal pain. In: Giles LGF, Singer KP (eds) Clinical anatomy and management of thoracic spine pain. Butterworth-Heinemann, Oxford, pp 205–222.

Stolker R J, Vervest A C, Groen G J 1993 Percutaneous facet denervation in chronic thoracic spine pain. Acta Neurochirugica (Wien) 122: 82–90.

Stolker R J, Vervest A C, Groen G J 1994 Parameters in electrode positioning in thoracic percutaneous facet denervation: an anatomical study. Acta Neurochirugica (Wien) 128: 32–39.

Key point(s)

1. Zygapophysial (facet) joint pain can occur due to injury of these joints as various structures, such as the joint capsule and the synovial folds, have noci-ceptors in them.
2. Inflammation of these joints may cause joint cap-sule distension resulting in pressure on the adjacent nerve root or the spinal nerve itself.
3. Be wary of pain that appears to be mechanical in nature but is actually due to osseous spinal injury.

FURTHER READING

Bogduk N, Schwarzer A 1995 Facet joint pain. Australian Family Physician 23: 924.

Giles L G F, Harvey A R 1987 Immunohistochemical demon-stration of nociceptors in the capsule and synovial folds of human zygapophysial joints. British Journal of Rheumatology 26: 362–364.

Case 42   Osteoporosis

COMMENT
Repeat imaging, when dictated by the history, symptoms and signs, should be considered even when previous images are relatively recent.

PROFILE

A 68-year-old overweight man who was perspiring at consultation.

PAST HISTORY

His past medical history included an 11-year history of low back pain for which he had undergone decompressive L4–5 laminectomy that failed to give him relief and exacerbated his symptoms. Therefore, he underwent a coccygectomy but this did not help his symptoms either. He had had a spinal cord stimulator (epidural catheter) implanted in an attempt to control his chronic low back pain but this did not produce any worthwhile pain relief. Therefore, the electrodes were repositioned, with the most superior tip being placed around the thoracolumbar junction. He also has a 14-year history of Crohn's disease, hypertension and chronic, stable angina.

PRESENTING COMPLAINT (Fig. 42.1)

His consultation was specifically only for constant and severe chronic mid to lower thoracic spine pain which is not associated with any upper limb symptoms. Approximately 12 months ago he suddenly experienced acute thoracic pain that lasted for approximately 4 months then recurred, prompting his consultation.

Movement aggravates his thoracic spine pain but the pain does not awaken him at night. Coughing aggravates his pain, as does changing position. He had tried narcotic analgesia but this

apparently 'caused memory loss' so he stopped taking it.

AETIOLOGY

Unknown.

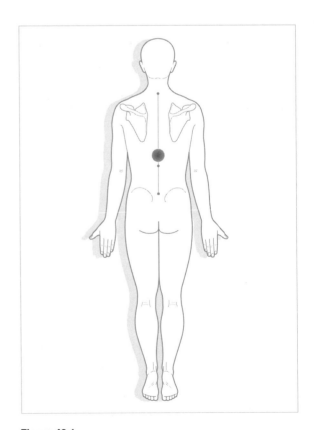

Figure 42.1

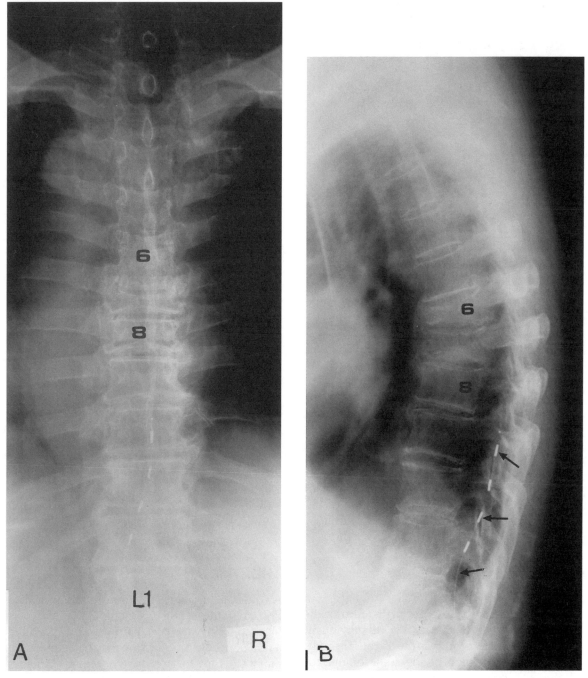

Figure 42.2 Plain film radiographs of the thoracic spine in (A) the anteroposterior and (B) lateral projections. Note the osteoporosis within associated significant vertebral body crush fractures at the T6 and T7 levels. Also note the gas in the T7–8 disc and the epidural spinal cord catheter terminating at the level of T9 (see arrows).

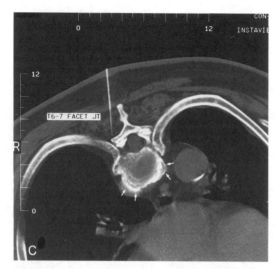

Figure 42.2 (C) Thoracic spine CT scan at the T6–7 zygapophysial 'facet' level showing needle placement for the facet block injection. R = right side of patient. Note the marginal osteophyte formation on the vertebral body (small white arrows). The thecal sac shows an abnormally narrowed configuration behind both the T6 and T7 vertebral bodies but the cause is not evident and there is generous fat around the thecal sac within the bony spinal canal.

EXAMINATION

He is considerably overweight and somewhat hypertensive with a blood pressure of 170/90. Examination of the cardiovascular system was otherwise unremarkable. The deep reflexes in the lower extremities were normal apart from an absent right knee jerk. Pinprick sensation of the lower limbs was unremarkable. There was slight tenderness on palpation from the lower thoracic region to the sacrum.

IMAGING REVIEW

Thoracic and lumbar spine plain film radiographs taken approximately 3 years previously showed moderate compression of the T6 body and some compression of the superior margin of the T12 body, both being consistent with past trauma. Slight degenerative osteoarthritic changes were present in the mid-thoracic spine. The spinal cord stimulator was noted from the

T9 level down; this had been inserted in an attempt to control his low back pain.

CLINICAL IMPRESSION

? Mid-thoracic spine vertebral body compression fractures due to osteoporosis. Differential diagnosis to include bone lytic disease.

WHAT ACTION SHOULD BE TAKEN?

New plain film thoracic spine radiographs were ordered and showed 'osteoporosis with severe loss of height in the T6 and T7 vertebral bodies and associated degeneration of the T7–8 disc as evidenced by gas in this disc space. The upper margin of a spinal cord stimulator is noted at the T9 level (Fig. 42.2A and B). A CT thoracic spine scan was ordered from T5 to T9. This showed:

Loss of T6 and T7 vertebral body height is associated with marginal osteophyte formation and on the bone windows the cortex of these bones remains intact suggesting that these changes are due to previous trauma rather than to an infiltrative and destructive bone process.

A three-phase bone scan was ordered as a precaution to exclude lytic disease and this showed 'diffusely increased tracer uptake in the mid-thoracic spine at approximately T6–8 but the plain X-ray films suggest that this is not due to metastatic disease'.

Laboratory tests were performed as a precaution (ESR, serum alkaline phosphatase and serum calcium) and were within normal limits.

TREATMENT

As the patient had tried various types of medication, and the spinal cord stimulator had been inserted for his low back pain, it was decided that a trial of needle acupuncture may be helpful as an initial attempt to stop his chronic mid-thoracic spine pain but this was of no help. Therefore, a right T6–7 'facet' joint block injection was arranged under CT control (Fig. 42.2C) as this was the main level for his pain on deep palpation.

RESULTS

The facet joint block injection resulted in a good response for his thoracic spine pain. He was advised to try taking paracetamol if symptoms dictated the need for analgesic medication periodically. The right T6–7 facet block injection accurately localized the source of his mid-thoracic spine pain and was useful as a diagnostic and therapeutic procedure. This injection gave relief for approximately 2 years then he returned for a further evaluation. At this time he was advised to lose a considerable amount of weight and to have a further facet block injection at the same level. On that occasion, he received less effective pain control so he decided to take paracetamol periodically for pain relief.

Key point(s)
1. Osteoporosis is a clinical condition characterized by decreased skeletal bone mass in which the bone is otherwise normal (Kostuik & Heggeness 1997).
2. Common fracture sites in patients over 60 years of age are in the hip, proximal tibia, wrist and the thoracic and lumbar spines (Kostuik & Heggeness 1997).

REFERENCE

Kostuik J P, Heggeness M H 1997 Surgery of the osteoporotic spine. In: Frymoyer JW (ed.) The adult spine: principles and practice, 2nd edn. Lippincott-Raven, Philadelphia, pp 1639–1664.

FURTHER READING

Lawson M T 2001 Evaluating and managing osteoporosis in men. Nursing Practice 26: 26–36.
Perry III H M, Morley J E 2001 Osteoporosis in men: are we ready to diagnose and treat? Current Rheumatology Reports 3: 240–244.
Tobias F H 1996 Metabolic bone disease. In: Axford J (ed.) Medicine. Blackwell Science, Oxford, pp 4.1–4.29.

Case 43 Pancoast's tumour

COMMENT
Beware of joint pain that cannot be reproduced or aggravated by joint movements designed to strain the joint.

PROFILE

A 72-year-old unmarried man of short stature. He smokes approximately 25 cigarettes per day and drinks beer.

PAST HISTORY

No unusual conditions and he said he had 'always been fit and healthy' until being knocked over by a motor vehicle 1 year ago.

PRESENTING COMPLAINT (Fig. 43.1)

Pain on the left side of his neck with radiation to behind the left eye causing 'dull and constant' headaches with intermittent 'acute' headache episodes. Pain at the cervicothoracic junction extending to approximately the T4 level. Pain in the right shoulder that is only slightly aggravated when he moves his right arm across his chest; the shoulder was not painful on any other active movements of the shoulder joint.

On turning his head to the left side he feels 'dizzy', although he does not feel he will lose his balance but rather that 'objects move in front of the eyes'.

AETIOLOGY

He was knocked over by a motor car 1 year ago but did not require hospitalization.

EXAMINATION

The deep reflexes in the upper and lower extremities were normal as was the case with pinprick sensation. Vibration sensation at the ankles and elbows was normal. Cervical spine left rotation was limited by approximately

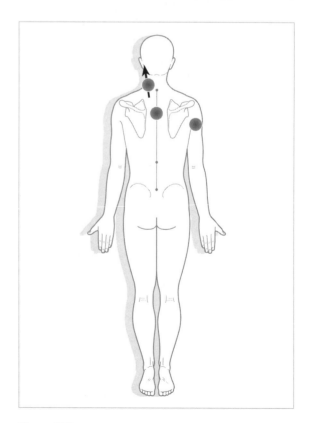

Figure 43.1

50% due to left cervical and cervico-shoulder pain and 'dizziness'. Passive right shoulder movements were of full range and painless; there was minor pain on active right arm internal rotation.

IMAGING REVIEW

The patient did not have any previous imaging.

CLINICAL IMPRESSION

Cervical spine spondylosis. Referred pain in the right shoulder – query Pancoast's tumour in right lung.

WHAT ACTION SHOULD BE TAKEN?

In view of his symptoms a series of cervical and thoracic spine films was ordered as well as chest posteroanterior (P-A) and lateral films. The cervical spine films showed 'extensive spondylitic changes throughout the cervical spine with disc narrowing and marginal osteophyte formation; disc narrowing is most severe at the C3–4 and the C6–7 levels and the marginal osteophyte formation is also most prominent at these levels (Fig. 43.2A)'. The thoracic spine X-ray report read: 'No destructive bone lesions are identified. There are minor degenerative osteophytes forming at all thoracic levels. The disc spaces appear satisfactory' (Fig. 43.2B). The chest P-A film (Fig. 43.2C) and lateral film showed 'A Pancoast's tumour in the right lung apex extending down to the right superior mediastinum, widening the mediastinum slightly with pleural thickening and a small effusion at the base of the right lung.' A CT scan of the chest, to better assess the right apical lung mass, was immediately ordered (Fig. 43.2D). A plain X-ray was taken to look at his ribs but there was no radiological evidence of metastatic disease. However, a whole body bone scan was performed (Fig. 43.2E) and this showed increased tracer uptake at the following sites: T10 vertebral body, left 5th and 6th ribs at the costochondral junction, the right 6th rib anteriorly, the right wrist and increased tracer activity in the lumbar spine.

The conclusion was:

Increased activity at T10 is non-specific. It could represent bony metastasis or an osteoporotic crush fracture. Plain film correlation in the first instance is recommended. Increased rib activity is most likely metastatic; however in this location it could be traumatic. The right wrist activity is most likely degenerative. Plain film correlation is recommended.

TREATMENT

This man was referred to the oncology department where biopsy confirmed the diagnosis of a Pancoast's tumour. He had radiotherapy but it was not successful and his symptoms became worse with the development of severe pain in his right shoulder and upper arm, particularly on the medial aspect, and he complained of

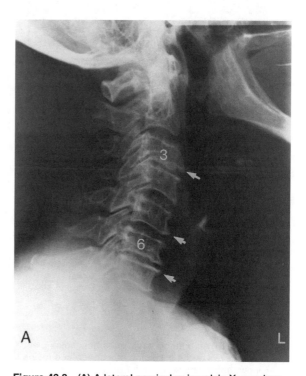

Figure 43.2 (A) A lateral cervical spine plain X-ray view showing 'extensive spondylitic changes throughout the cervical spine with disc narrowing and marginal osteophyte formation. The disc narrowing is most severe at the C3–4 and the C6–7 levels and the marginal osteophyte formation is also most prominent at these levels' (e.g. white arrows).

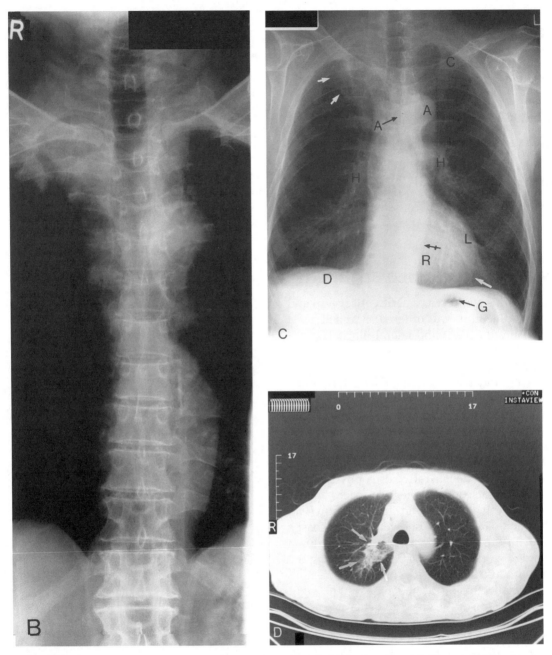

Figure 43.2 (B) An anteroposterior thoracic spine plain X-ray view showing minor degenerative osteophytes forming at all thoracic levels and a suspicion of a space-occupying lesion in the right lung apex. (C) A chest posteroanterior plain X-ray view that clearly shows the Pancoast's tumour (white arrows show the approximate border) in the apex of the right lung. A = aortic knuckle; D = dome of right diaphragm; A arrow = aortic arch; L = left ventricle; H = hilar shadow; C = clavicle; single white arrow = apex of the heart; tailed black arrow = descending thoracic aorta; G = gas in the upper part of the stomach ('megenblase'). (D) A CT scan of the chest showing the Pancoast's tumour on the right side (arrows).

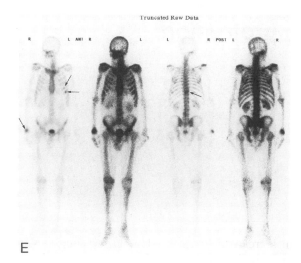

Truncated Raw Data

Figure 43.2 (E) Whole body bone scan truncated raw data. Arrows show areas of increased tracer uptake.

allodynia (pain resulting from a non-noxious stimulus to normal skin) and hyperpathia (abnormally exaggerated subjective response to painful stimuli) which made it very difficult for him to sleep at night. The neuropathic pain that he developed was most likely related to the involvement of his T1 nerve root and perhaps sympathetic chain at the apex of his right lung. He remained in hospital on various analgesics that were given in an attempt to relieve his symptoms. However, the result was that, when he was actually pain free, he was completely asleep.

RESULTS

Chemotherapy was not helpful and he passed away within 3 months of the original diagnosis.

REFERENCES

Clark C R 1997 Differential diagnosis and nonoperative management. In: Frymoyer JW (ed.) The adult spine: principles and practice, 2nd edn. Lippincott-Raven, Philadelphia, pp 1323–1347.
Patten J 1996 Neurological differential diagnosis, 2nd edn. Springer-Verlag, Berlin.

FURTHER READING

Kim P, Hains F, Wallace M C, Mior S A 1993 Pancoast tumour: a case report. Journal of the Canadian Chiropractic Association 37: 214–220.
Shaw R A 1984 Pancoast's tumor. Annals of Thoracic Surgery 37: 343–345.

Case 44   Intervertebral disc protrusion

COMMENT

It is a fallacy to believe that, once a patient receives a significant cash settlement following litigation for a work-related injury, the patient's symptoms will automatically disappear. This case is just one of many examples of symptoms persisting following settlement of a work-related claim.

PROFILE

A 43-year-old, somewhat overweight, married man who has worked as an electrician for approximately 28 years. He does not smoke cigarettes and only drinks alcohol socially.

PAST HISTORY

He had a tonsillectomy at approximately 6–7 years of age. He broke the right tibia at approximately 12 years of age. As an adult, he injured his right knee while playing basketball and required two surgical procedures to rectify this problem. Seven years ago he suffered some transient cervical and upper thoracic spine strain while carrying a heavy electrical object. His general medical practitioner sent him for cervical and thoracic spine X-ray films but they did not indicate any skeletal abnormality.

Six years ago he was working in a ceiling, in a twisted position, when the ladder on which he was standing slipped, causing him to become jammed in the ceiling. This incident caused some transient bruising in the thoracic spine and around his ribs but no long-lasting sequelae.

PRESENTING COMPLAINT (Fig. 44.1)

Constant pain in the lower thoracic spine at approximately the T10 level which varies in intensity depending on activity. He experiences some radiation to the ribs bilaterally from T10; sometimes this will go to the front of the ribcage when severe.

Coughing, sneezing or bearing down increase the pain at T10. If he rakes the yard, he experiences an increase in his pain. He can no longer play basketball, golf or cricket because of his pain. On getting into a motor vehicle, the twisting action can aggravate the T10 level pain.

The pain does not wake him up at a particular time during the night and it is not a deep-seated

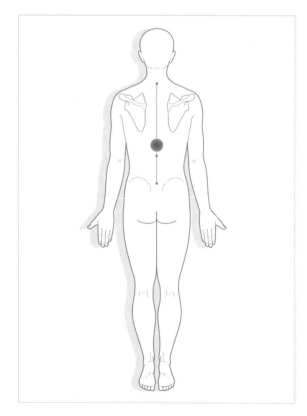

Figure 44.1

bone pain. However, he does wake up in the early hours and has to move around periodically during the night to obtain some relief. Heat from the hot shower gives temporary relief. When he arises in the morning, the pain is more noticeable.

He has tried anti-inflammatory medication, physiotherapy and local anaesthetic and cortisone injections with no relief.

AETIOLOGY

Six years ago he moved a heavy (approximately 65 kg) battery for a locomotive from the back of a utility vehicle. As he slid the battery forward with his left arm stretched forwards, while trying to keep the trolley still with one foot, the battery slid off the back of the utility and caught the top edge of the trolley with the result that it fell. He instinctively grabbed it as he had previously seen a battery explode when someone dropped it. He immediately felt pain in the T10 region and some pain in the right buttock and leg.

EXAMINATION

In the erect posture, there was no evidence of pelvic obliquity or scoliosis. Percussion of the spine elicited some tenderness at approximately the T10 level. The sacroiliac joint strain test did not cause any sacroiliac joint pain. Deep palpation of the paraspinal muscles elicited pain at the T10 level. Toe walking power (S1) and heel walking power (L5) were normal but the latter caused some 'jarring' at approximately T10. Deep reflexes in the upper and lower extremities were normal. Pinwheel sensation of the upper and lower extremities, as well as the posterior aspect of the torso, was normal. Vibration sensation at the elbows and ankles was normal.

Active ranges of spinal movement were as follows.

Thoracic spine

1. Flexion – full range and painless.
2. Extension caused some pain at approximately T10 at full range.

3. Left lateral bending caused some pain at T10 at full range.
4. Right lateral bending caused pain at T10 with approximately 20% restriction of mobility.
5. Left rotation – limited by approximately 10% due to T10 pain.
6. Right rotation – limited by approximately 30% due to T10 pain.

Cervical spine

1. Flexion – at full range caused some pain and 'tightness' at approximately T10.
2. Extension – full range and painless.
3. Left and right lateral bending caused pain at approximately T10 at full range.
4. Left and right rotation – full range and painless.

Lumbar spine

1. Flexion – finger tips reached to within 5 cm of the floor.
2. Extension caused some pain at T10 at full range.
3. Left lateral bending – full range but caused T10 pain.
4. Right lateral bending – limited by approximately 20% due to T10 pain.
5. Left rotation – limited by approximately 10% due to T10 pain.
6. Right rotation – limited by approximately 30% due to T10 pain.

The Valsalva manoeuvre (bearing down) caused an increase in pain at the T10 level.

IMAGING REVIEW

Original plain thoracic spine X-rays reported: 'No skeletal abnormality is demonstrated'. Plain thoracic spine X-rays taken 2 years later reported: 'Minor degenerative spurring at one or two levels' of the thoracic spine with 'minimal early spurring' in the lumbar spine. A further thoracic spine plain X-ray film examination taken 4 years later reported: 'Mild degenerative changes are present in the thoracic spine with marginal

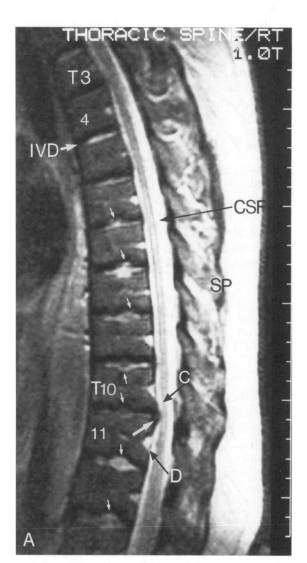

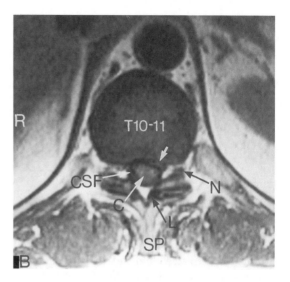

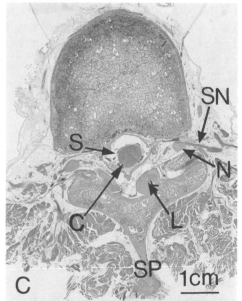

Figure 44.2 (A) A sagittal T2-weighted thoracic MRI scan which shows the Schmorl's nodes from T6 to T12 (small white arrows). Note the T10–11 disc protrusion compressing the anterior part of the dural tube (D) and apparently touching the spinal cord (C) which lies within the dural tube surrounded by cerebrospinal fluid (CSF) that is white on the T2-weighted MRI image. IVD = disc with normal hydration (as compared to the T3–4 disc that shows desiccation (blackening); SP = spinous process. The numerals 3, 4, 10 and 11 indicate thoracic vertebral bodies. (B) An axial T1-weighted thoracic MRI scan through the T10–11 intervertebral disc showing the left-sided disc protrusion (small white arrow) that impresses upon the dural tube with some distortion of the spinal cord itself (C) as it lies within the cerebrospinal fluid (CSF) that appears as a dark area around the cord on this T1-weighted image. L = ligamentum flavum; N = spinal ganglion within the intervertebral foramen; SP = spinous process. (C) A 200-micron thick horizontal histological section from autopsy material through a T10–11 vertebral body that helps to demonstrate the histological anatomy; compare with (B). C = spinal cord; L = ligamentum flavum; N = spinal ganglion within the intervertebral foramen; S = subarachnoid space for the cerebrospinal fluid; SN = spinal nerve leaving the intervertebral foramen; SP = spinous process.

osteophytosis and loss of disc height at multiple levels. Focal loss of disc height seems most marked at the T10–11 level . . .'.

A thoracic spine CT scan reported: 'Some minor degenerative changes . . . with vertebral body anterior osteophytosis and some minor degenerative changes at the costovertebral joints. A Schmorl's node is present in the superior end-plate of T8'.

A MRI thoracic spine scan showed Schmorl's nodes from T6 to L1 (Fig. 44.2A); because of their frequency it was considered that they may be associated with a congenital developmental anomaly known as persistent notochord (which can remain asymptomatic unless injury is superimposed). It also showed 'some encroachment upon the thoracic canal, slightly eccentrically towards the left side at T10–11, by a disc protrusion' (Fig. 44.2B).

CLINICAL IMPRESSION

T10–11 disc protrusion.

WHAT ACTION SHOULD BE TAKEN?

No further imaging was necessary. The patient was reassured that his pain was genuine and he was greatly relieved to find out that there was indeed a reason for his spinal symptoms. He was advised not to lift heavy weights or bend his spine into awkward positions during work and he was advised to perform only light duties. He was referred for an orthopaedic opinion, which confirmed the T10–11 disc protrusion and associated symptoms but surgery was not considered as an option at that time.

TREATMENT

He was informed that he may require surgery, in due course, in spite of doing sedentary work, but that this should not be undertaken lightly as this type of surgery has a high risk. It was suggested that it would be better for him to keep fit by going to a gymnasium and to spend

time swimming, to see if this would help him to maintain his present levels of activity As Panadeine Forte caused side effects, such as constipation, he was referred back to his general medical practitioner to consider a simple analgesic such as paracetamol instead.

RESULTS

The advice provided gave considerable relief but, as symptoms still persisted 5 years after settlement of his work injury claim, he returned for a further consultation. That consultation led to the MRI scan seen in Fig. 44.3, which clearly showed that he still had a T10–11 disc protrusion pressing upon the dural tube and touching the spinal cord.

He was referred for a neurosurgical opinion with the result that his condition was confirmed but, again, surgery was not contemplated due to risk factors. He manages his pain with paracetamol, exercise and by performing only light duties.

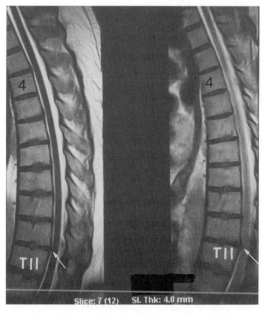

Figure 44.3 These two T2-weighted sagittal MRI images of the thoracic spine were taken 5 years after the scan shown in Fig. 44.2A. Note that the T10–11 disc protrusion is still present (arrows).

Note

This is only one of many cases where a patient went through the process of litigation for a work-related injury, but his symptoms persisted after a significant cash settlement.

Key point(s)

1. Thoracic spine disc protrusions are notoriously difficult to diagnose.
2. Unfortunately, it is often thought that individuals with work-related disability exaggerate their complaints and suffer from psychiatric disorders such as depression and neuroticism only until they receive a 'curative' financial settlement, at which time they are able to return to work (Margoshes & Webster 2000), even though recent studies have refuted this concept (Burns et al 1995, Mendelson 1982).

REFERENCES

Burns J W, Sherman M L, Devine J, Mahoney N, Pawl R 1995 Association between workers' compensation and outcome following multidisciplinary treatment for chronic pain: roles of mediators and moderators. Clinical Journal of Pain 11: 94–102.

Margoshes B G, Webster B S 2000 Why do occupational injuries have different health outomes? In: Mayer TG, Gatchel RJ, Polatin PB (eds) Occupational Musculoskeletal Disorders. Lippincott Williams & Wilkins, Philadelphia, pp 47–61.

Mendelson G 1982 Not 'cured by a verdict:' effect of legal settlement on compensation claiments. Medical Journal of Australia 2: 132–134.

FURTHER READING

Flynn T W 1996 The thoracic spine and rib cage. Butterworth-Heinemann, Oxford.

Giles L G F, Singer K P 2000 Clinical anatomy and management of thoracic spine pain. Butterworth-Heinemann, Oxford.

Hoppenfeld S 1977 Orthopaedic neurology: A diagnostic guide to neurologic levels. J. B. Lippincott, Philadelphia.

Case 45 Burst fracture

COMMENT
Beware of patients who apparently sustain a seemingly simple vertebral body compression fracture.

PROFILE

A 41-year-old man who currently does not work, as a result of a motorbike accident. He is a person of muscular build who does not smoke and only drinks alcohol socially.

PAST HISTORY

He said he had not suffered from any unusual childhood illnesses or unusual adult illnesses and had experienced 'perfect health all [his] life' prior to a motorbike accident that occurred 12 months ago. He said he had always kept active and that this had kept his muscles well toned.

PRESENTING COMPLAINT (Fig. 45.1)

Constant pain, that varies in intensity, at approximately the T12 area; this pain can go 'up and down' a few segments and it radiates bilaterally around the rib cage to the lower sternum.

Coughing and sneezing significantly increase his pain, which is activity related. Bearing down also increases this pain. He says he has great difficulty sleeping at night as his thoracolumbar region is very painful and he finds this is distressing as he has to 'toss and turn all night'. He says he has some pain intermittently that radiates into the right lower abdomen and then into the right testicle; he believes this pain comes from the thoracolumbar region.

He had never had any of the above pains before the motorbike accident. He does not take medication as he is wary of possible side-effects.

AETIOLOGY

He was riding his motorbike toward a roundabout when he was knocked off the motorbike when a car hit him at speed. During the accident, he bounced off the bonnet of the car

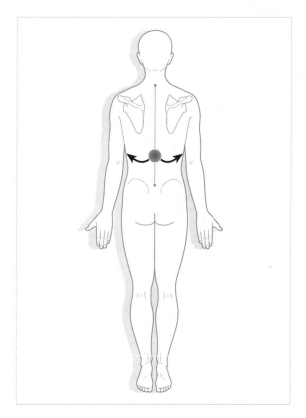

Figure 45.1

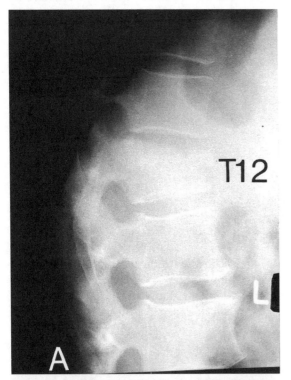

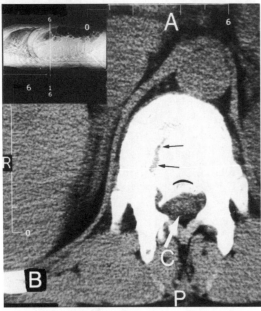

Figure 45.2 (A) A lateral thoracic spine plain film X-ray showing the compression fracture of the T12 vertebral body with anterior wedging. (B) Axial CT thoracic spine scan through the T12 vertebral body that shows the burst fracture of the body of the T12 vertebra, with considerable retropulsion of a posterior bony fragment into the spinal canal causing a reduction of cross-sectional area of approximately 35%. Small arrows show part of the fracture line. The retropulsed posterior fragment in the spinal canal lies posterior to the semicircular black line that represents the approximate area at which the anterior part of the spinal canal would normally be seen. A = anterior; C = spinal cord; P = posterior; R = right side of patient. The insert shows the level of the axial scan slice.

and over the windscreen then ended up lying in the street.

EXAMINATION

In the erect posture, there was no clinical evidence of pelvic obliquity or of scoliosis. Percussion of the thoracic and lumbar spines did not indicate any particular tenderness. Deep palpation of the paraspinal muscles elicited pain bilaterally in the cervical spine at the C4–7 level and at the thoracolumbar junction region.

The deep reflexes in the upper and lower extremities were normal, as was the case with vibration sensation at the elbows and ankles. Pinprick sensation over the arms, hands and legs was normal but there was some hypoaesthesia on the medial aspect of his left foot (L5). Motor power in the upper and lower extremities was normal, as was the case with the foot pulses. The temperature of both feet appeared to be equal and normal on palpation. The superficial upper abdominal reflexes (T7–10) and lower abdominal reflexes T10–L1 appeared to be normal.

Active thoracic spine ranges of movement were all limited by 50% due to 'stiffness' and, on flexion, he moved with a lumbar 'flat back' due to protective muscle splinting.

IMAGING REVIEW

Plain X-ray films showed what appeared to be a simple uncomplicated compression fracture of the T12 vertebral body (Fig. 45.2A) with anterior wedging.

CLINICAL IMPRESSION

? T12 burst fracture.

WHAT ACTION SHOULD BE TAKEN?

A thoracic spine CT scan was performed. This showed that the fracture was much more serious, with a burst fracture of the body of T12 vertebra with considerable retropulsion of a posterior bony fragment into the spinal canal causing a reduction of cross-sectional area of approximately 35% (Fig. 45.2B).

He saw an orthopaedic surgeon who advised him not to undergo surgery and, as he was coping well with his condition, this view was supported.

TREATMENT

He was advised not to take part in any excessively flexed, extended or rotated spine activities that would place heavy loads on his spine. He was also advised to swim as much as possible to maintain muscle tone as he already had a good physique. In addition he was told to seek immediate orthopaedic or neurosurgical advice should he experience any symptoms such as leg pain or weakness, bowel or bladder dysfunction, or any increase in his current symptoms. A MRI scan was considered but was declined at this time as surgery was not planned.

RESULTS

He continues to remain fit and active and has managed to adapt to his injury with resulting impairment.

Key point(s)

1. The thoracolumbar junction (T11–L2) is the commonest site for spinal fractures (El-Khoury & Brandser 1997).
2. When a vertebral body compression fracture appears uncomplicated on lateral plain X-ray films, remember that a burst fracture may be present with bony fragment(s) in the spinal canal.

REFERENCE

El-Khoury G Y, Brandser E A 1997 Radiography of spinal disorders. In: Frymoyer JW (ed.) The adult spine, principles and practice, 2nd edition. Lippincott-Raven, Philadelphia, pp 413–442.

FURTHER READING

Hitchon P W, Torner J C, Haddad S F, Follett K A 1998 Management options in thoracolumbar burst fractures. Surgical Neurology 49: 619–626.
Isomi T, Panjabi M M, Kato Y, Wang J L 2000 Radiographic parameters for evaluating the neurological spaces in experimental thoracolumbar burst fractures. Journal of Spinal Disorders 13: 404–411.
Panjabi M M, Kifune M, Wen L, Arand M, Oxland T R, Lin R M, Yoon W S, Vasavada A 1995 Dynamic canal encroachment during thoracolumbar burst fractures. Journal of Spinal Disorders 8: 39–48.
Petersilge C A, Pathria M N, Emery S E, Masaryk T J 1995 Thoracolumbar burst fractures: evaluation with MR imaging. Radiology 194: 49–54.

Case 46   Intervertebral disc protrusion

COMMENT
Thoracic spine disc bulges and protrusions may cause straight forward symptoms and signs, as in this case, or they may present as a complex group of symptoms and signs as presented in previous cases.

PROFILE

A 39-year-old man who does not smoke or drink alcohol and is physically very fit.

PAST HISTORY

At approximately 15 years of age he injured his mid-thoracic spine while playing football, but he recovered over a period of time. He then fell off a horse and caused an aggravation of his mid-thoracic spine pain. This pain usually resolves itself within a few days after seeing a chiropractor who treats him with heat packs and massage.

PRESENTING COMPLAINT (Fig. 46.1)

Acute or chronic mid-thoracic spine pain that does not radiate to either side. He pointed to approximately the T6–7 level.

Coughing, sneezing and bearing down markedly increase the mid-thoracic spine pain. He is not awakened at a particular time during the night, i.e. there is no night pain. Bowel and bladder function appear to be normal, although he wonders if bowel motions are affected when the pain is severe. He cannot take a deep breath because this aggravates his pain. He also has to be careful with lifting, sitting and bending his spine forward, backward and laterally, as these movements increase his pain.

He does not like to take medication as he found than a NSAID was of no help, but caused gastric pain. He said he had seen four or five

general medical practitioners and each time he was given a NSAID, which he did not take after realizing that the first one had caused gastric pain.

His chiropractor referred him for a further evaluation because of a clinical suspicion of a

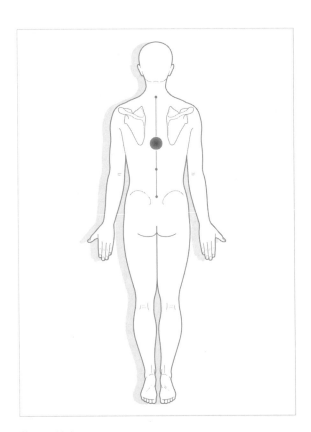

Figure 46.1

216

disc lesion and wanted to have a thoracic spine MRI performed and also requested that treatment be provided as deemed appropriate.

AETIOLOGY

He has had remissions and exacerbations for some 20 years and his current acute mid-thoracic spine pain was due to bending forwards two days prior to consultation to pick up, from the floor, a light object; he felt a 'stabbing pain' in the mid-thoracic spine with radiation to both scapulae and 'stiffness' in the thoracic spine.

EXAMINATION

The deep reflexes in the arms and legs were normal as was pinprick sensation. Power and muscle tone in the legs and feet were normal and the plantar response was normal, i.e. downward. The pulses and the temperature of both feet were normal and equal. Percussion of the thoracic spine did not elicit any pain but deep palpation of the paraspinal muscles elicited pain at approximately the T6–7 level. Vibration sensation was normal.

Active thoracic spine ranges of movement were as follows:

1. Flexion caused pain in the mid-thoracic spine when his fingers reached to his knees.
2. Extension – limited by approximately 50% due to mid-thoracic spine pain.
3. Lateral bending – limited by approximately 30% to each side due to mid-thoracic spine pain.
4. Rotation to the left and right sides – full and painless.

Ribcage compression elicited the following:

1. In the anteroposterior plane, there was an increase in mid-thoracic spine pain.
2. In the left to right coronal plane there was no pain.
3. On oblique compression from the left anterior to the right posterior side of the ribcage there was an increase in mid-thoracic spine pain.

In the seated and slumped forward position there was an increase in mid-thoracic spine pain; the addition of left and right SLR, respectively, caused a further increase in mid-thoracic spine pain. Supine SLR was of full range and painless. Supine cervical spine flexion caused an increase in mid-thoracic spine pain.

IMAGING REVIEW

Thoracic spine plain film anteroposterior and lateral views were unremarkable.

CLINICAL IMPRESSION

Disc protrusion at the T6–7 level.

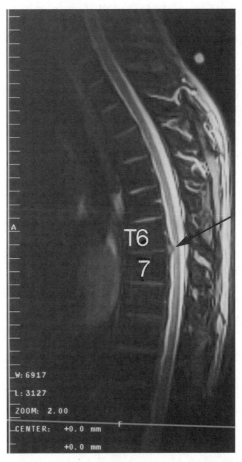

Figure 46.2 A sagittal T2-weighted thoracic spine MRI scan showing a focal posterior disc protrusion at T6–7 with impression on the thoracic cord.

WHAT ACTION SHOULD BE TAKEN?

A thoracic spine MRI was ordered in view of his symptoms and the clinical findings to determine whether there was a disc bulge or protrusion in the mid-thoracic spine. The MRI showed:

A focal centrolateral disc protrusion at the T6–7 level, extending to the left of the midline. There is efface-ment of the CSF and early impression on the anterior aspect of the thoracic cord (Fig. 46.2). There is minimal disc narrowing at this level. No bony abnormality. The remainder of the cord appears intact.

TREATMENT

The patient was advised not to perform any heavy lifting or activities where he would have to hyperflex or hyperextend his thoracic spine. He was offered the option of seeing an orthopaedic surgeon or of trying needle acupuncture treatment. He chose the acupunc-ture treatment.

RESULTS

At the third acupuncture treatment session he reported that he now had only a 'low-grade dull awareness' of mid-thoracic spine pain, so he was advised to return if further treatment was indi-cated. He has subsequently been well and not needed further treatment 3 years following his acupuncture treatment.

Key point(s)

1. The symptom of increased pain on coughing, sneezing and bearing down strongly suggests a disc protrusion if there is no night pain to suggest an overt pathological process.
2. A central disc protrusion is suspected if the pain is centrally located with no radiation of pain affecting the nerve roots.

FURTHER READING

Errico T J, Stecker S, Kostuik J P 1997 Thoracic pain syndromes. In: Frymoyer JW (ed.) The adult spine: principles and practice, 2nd edn. Lippincott-Raven, Philadelphia, pp 1623–1637.
Longworth W, McCarthy P W 1997 A review of research on acupuncture for the treatment of lumbar disk protrusions and associated neurological symptomatology. Journal of Alternative and Complementary Medicine 3: 55–76.

Case 47   Spinal cord syrinx

COMMENT
If the cervicothoracic spine is subjected to forceful trauma and symptoms and signs consistent with a spinal cord injury develop, a complete diagnostic work-up, including a MRI study, is warranted.

PROFILE

A 39-year-old somewhat overweight married man who does not smoke and only drinks alcohol socially.

PAST HISTORY

He has an allergy to Digesic that causes 'blurring of vision and nausea'. He had osteomyelitis in the left 'hip' region at approximately 6–8 years of age from which he made a complete recovery following surgery.

PRESENTING COMPLAINT (Fig. 47.1)

A 'burning' sensation from approximately the T5 level 'down to the feet'. When lying in bed he may get 'spasms in the legs which shake a lot', usually one leg being affected at a time; the symptoms may then affect the other leg. He cannot sit or stand for more than a few minutes without moving because of the mid-thoracic spine pain. He also experiences a 'stabbing' sensation at approximately the T5 level which can radiate around his torso. He periodically experiences headaches which begin in the lower cervical spine and radiate up over the occipital and temporal regions of his skull without any definite time interval or frequency.

He walks with a slightly spastic gait and says the injury has resulted in some sexual disturbance in that he cannot maintain an erection. He also has a bowel problem in that he sometimes has 'soiling' on his underpants due to a lack of bowel control. He has to empty his bladder regularly, i.e. by timing, rather than by urge, otherwise he cannot control his bladder.

AETIOLOGY

Two and a quarter years ago he was working late at night in a mine; he had 'fired' the rock

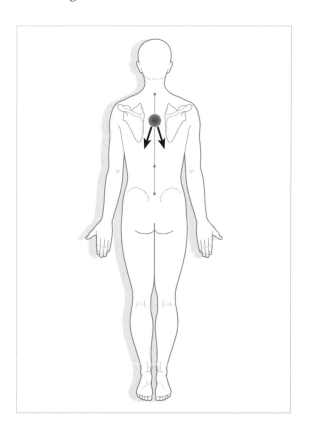

Figure 47.1

face before hosing it down to settle the dust. He looked up and saw a large rock slab falling towards him, so he turned and started to run away from it but it hit his upper thoracic spine, knocking him face down onto other rocks. He immediately felt 'numbness' from approximately his 'nipple level down'. His legs felt 'paralysed', particularly his right leg but he gradually recovered and was then able to walk again but he gradually developed the above presenting symptoms.

EXAMINATION

In the erect posture there was no obvious clinical evidence of pelvic obliquity or of scoliosis. Percussion of his spine at the T4–6 level elicited local pain with a sensation of 'numbness' lower in his thoracic spine. Deep palpation of the paraspinal muscles elicited considerable tenderness over the T4–6 level. Toe walking power (S1) and heel walking power (L5) were somewhat weak. The deep reflexes in the upper extremities were normal but the knee jerks (L4) were considerably hyper-reflexive bilaterally, suggesting an upper motor neuron lesion. The ankle jerks appeared to be approximately normal. The plantar response (Babinski test) was strongly upward turning on the right and, to a lesser degree, on the left (indicating a pathological response, i.e. an upper-motor neuron lesion). The upper (T7–10) and lower (T10–L1) superficial abdominal reflexes could not be elicited.

Light touch and pinprick sensation of the cervico-shoulder region (C4, C5, T1–2 dermatomes), the arms and hands was normal. Pinprick sensation below the nipple line on the front and back of the torso was diminished; on the lateral aspect of his left thigh (L2) he expressed pinpricking as feeling like a 'burning' sensation but on the medial aspect of his left thigh (L3) there was a subjective 'numbness'. Pinprick on the left and right calves, laterally, elicited a 'burning' sensation and the same sensation was reported for light touch using cotton wool over the same area. His feet were particularly hypersensitive to pinpricking

and he reported the pinpricking as feeling as if his feet were 'strongly burning' on the lateral (S1) and medial aspects (L5). There was a patchy distribution of sensation in his legs and feet. (These findings most likely indicate injury to his spinal cord.) Applying a vibrating tuning fork to the left ankle gave an approximately normal response but there was considerable subjective diminution in sensation when the tuning fork was placed on the right ankle. (This suggests an injury to the posterior columns of his spinal cord.) Power in the upper and lower limbs appeared to be normal, apart from difficulty with toe and heel walking. The pulses in his feet appeared normal. The temperature of his feet was equal on palpation, apart from his toes which felt cold on each foot; both feet had a bluish colour (suggesting some possible difficulty with his circulation).

In the supine position, cervical spine flexion elicited pain at approximately the T5 level. Supine left and right SLR, respectively, elicited some mid-thoracic spine pain, as did SLR plus foot dorsiflexion. Bilateral knee flexion caused mid-thoracic spine pain. (All these tests suggested that tractioning the spinal cord was causing pain in the upper to midthoracic spine).

Active thoracic spine movements in the seated position were as follows:

1. Flexion caused pain at approximately T5.
2. Extension caused similar pain but also an ache at the thoracolumbar region.
3. Left and right rotation did not cause any thoracic spine pain but caused some thoracolumbar junction 'ache'.
4. Lateral bending did not cause any thoracic spine pain but caused some thoracolumbar junction 'ache'.

The blood pressure in the left arm was 112/80 in the seated position.

IMAGING REVIEW

Plain film radiographs of his cervical and thoracic spines were non-contributory.

CLINICAL IMPRESSION

Upper thoracic cord injury.

WHAT ACTION SHOULD BE TAKEN?

A thoracic spine MRI scan. This showed 'post-traumatic cord abnormality at T1 with syrinx and posterior spinal stenosis' with effacement of the posterior aspect of the thecal sac and perhaps the thoracic spinal cord at this level (Fig. 47.2A and B).

In order to determine whether decompression of the spinal cord was necessary a neurological opinion was sought.

TREATMENT

He was advised not to perform any heavy manual work. In addition, he was advised not to work underground as this could be dangerous to him and to his work colleagues. The neurosurgeon advised the patient that, if there were any suggestion of neurological deterioration, he should immediately present for review.

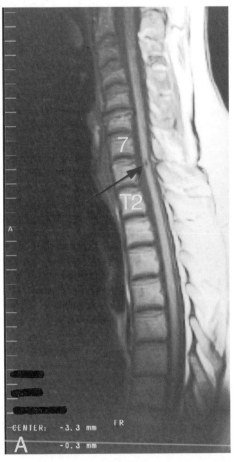 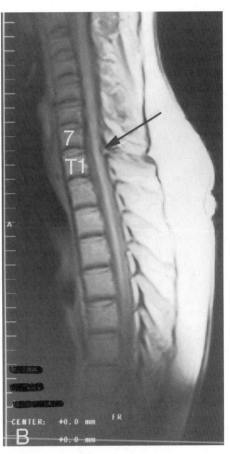

Figure 47.2   (A) A sagittal T1-weighted thoracic spine MRI scan showing the small post-traumatic syrinx at the T1 level (arrow) which indicates an injury to the spinal cord itself. A = anterior; T2 = second thoracic vertebra; 7 = seventh cervical vertebra. (B) Sagittal T1-weighted thoracic spine MRI scan showing the effacement of the posterior aspect of the thecal sac and the thoracic spinal cord at this level (arrow). A = anterior; T1 = first thoracic vertebra; 7 = seventh cervical vertebra.

Key point(s)

1. It is important to consider the possible development of a post-traumatic syrinx in patients with various symptoms and signs following a spinal injury.
2. Note that the presentation of a post-traumatic syrinx may be quite subtle (Zdeblick & Ducker 1997).
3. Note that the onset of symptoms from a post-traumatic syrinx can be quite delayed from the time of injury with delays from 6 months to 16 years having been reported (Barnett et al 1971, Marshall et al 1987, Shannon et al 1981).
4. It is interesting to note that the symptoms were mainly felt at approximately the T5 level, whereas the syrinx and posterior spinal stenosis were at the T1 level. Therefore, in complex cases it is wise to perform imaging that extends above and below the symptomatic area.

REFERENCES

Barnett H J, Jousse A T, Morley T P, Lougheed W M 1971 Posttraumatic syringomyelia. Paraplegia 9: 33–37.

Marshall L F, Knowlton S, Garfin S R et al 1987 Deterioration following spinal cord injury: a multicenter study. Journal of Neurosurgery 66: 400–404.

Shannon N, Symon L, Logue V, Cull D, Kang J, Kendall B 1981 Clinical features, investigation and treatment of post-traumatic syringomyelia. Journal of Neurology, Neurosurgery and Psychiatry 44: 35.

Zdeblick T A, Ducker T B 1997 Posttraumatic syringomyelia. In: Frymoyer JW (ed.) The adult spine: principles and practice, 2nd edn. Lippincott-Raven, Philadelphia, pp 1317–1320.

FURTHER READING

el Masry W S, Biyani A 1996 Incidence, management and outcome of post-traumatic syringomyelia. In memory of Mr Bernard Williams. Journal of Neurology, Neurosurgery and Psychiatry 60: 141–146.

Kramer K M, Levine A M 1997 Posttraumatic syringomyelia: a review of 21 cases. Clinical Orthopedics 334: 190–199.

Perrouin-Vervbe B, Lenne-Auier K, Robert R, Auffray-Calvier E, Richard I, Mauduyt de la reve I, Mathe J F 1998 Post-traumatic syringomyelia and post-traumatic spinal cord stenosis: a direct relationship: review of 75 patients with a spinal cord injury. Spinal Cord 35: 137–143.

Perrouin-Verbe B, Robert R, Lefort M, Agakhani N, Tadie M, Mathe J F 1999 Syringomyelie post-traumatique. Neurochirurgie 45 Suppl 1: 58–66.

Case 48   Extradural cystic lesion

COMMENT
Be suspicious of spinal pain that cannot be aggravated by mechanically stressing the spine on performing various movements.

PROFILE
A 57-year-old housewife.

PAST HISTORY
She had kept fit and healthy during her busy life.

PRESENTING COMPLAINT (Fig. 48.1)
Chronic mid-thoracic spine pain. Coughing sometimes aggravates the symptoms as does sneezing. Plain X-ray films had been non-contributory.

AETIOLOGY
Unknown.

EXAMINATION
There was no clinical evidence of pelvic obliquity or of postural scoliosis. Deep palpation of the paraspinal muscles elicited pain over the T4–6 level of the thoracic spine. The deep reflexes in the upper and lower extremities were normal, as was pinprick sensation. Active ranges of thoracic spine movement were of full range and did not cause any increase in pain. The Valsalva manoeuvre caused a slight increase in her pain (suggesting a space-occupying lesion). Bowel and bladder function were normal.

IMAGING REVIEW
There was no previous imaging.

CLINICAL IMPRESSION
A space-occupying lesion within the spinal canal. Intervertebral disc bulge/protrusion. Benign or malignant intraspinal lesion.

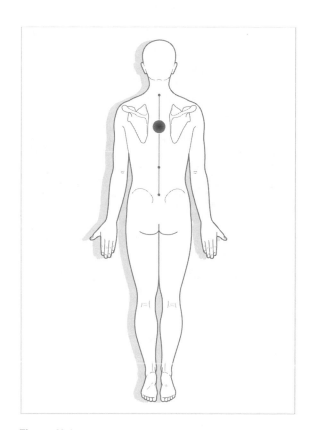

Figure 48.1

WHAT ACTION SHOULD BE TAKEN?

A thoracic spine MRI. This found:

'There is a small area located posterior to the thecal sac at the level of T5 that measures approximately 5 × 10 mm. It is oval in shape, behaves like spinal fluid and it does not enhance. It probably represents a small arachnoid cyst abutting the posterior aspect of the thecal sac but it does not appear to put pressure on the thecal sac' (Fig. 48.2A,B,C).

In view of the imaging findings, the following blood tests were performed as a precaution (Box 48.1). These results were within normal limits.

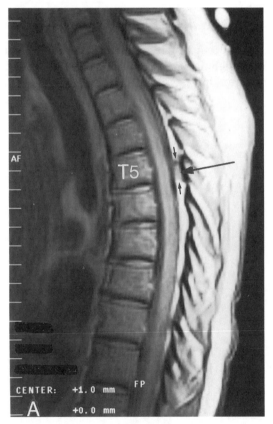

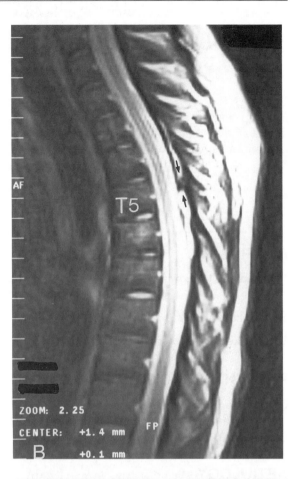

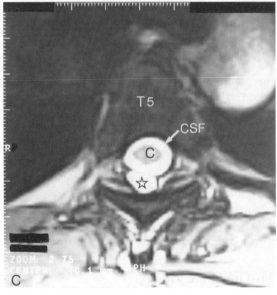

Figure 48.2 (A) A sagittal T1-weighted thoracic spine MRI scan that shows the small cystic lesion (arrows) lying posterior to the thecal sac at the T5 level. There is no obvious mass effect on the thecal sac or spinal cord. (B) A sagittal T2-weighted thoracic spine MRI scan that shows the small cystic lesion (arrows) lying posterior to the thecal sac at the T5 level. (C) An axial T2-weighted thoracic spine MRI scan through the small cystic lesion showing the cross-sectional area of the lesion (star). C = spinal cord lying within the cerebrospinal fluid (CSF). T5 = fifth thoracic vertebral body.

Box 48.1

Specimen type		Units	Reference range
Haemoglobin	127	g/l	(115–160)
Red cell count	4.39	$\times 10^{12}$/l	(3.90–5.60)
Red blood count dist width	13		(12–15)
Haematocrit	0.39		(0.37–0.47)
MCV (mean corpuscular volume)	88	fl	(75–95)
MCH (mean corpuscular haemoglobin)	28.9	pg	(27.0–32.0)
MCHC (mean corpuscular haemoglobin concentration)	330	g/l	(310–350)
Platelet count	240	$\times 10^9$/l	(150–400)
White cell count	8.1	$\times 10^9$/l	(3.5–10.0)
Neutrophils	35.7	$\times 10^9$/l	(2.0–7.5)
Lymphocytes	1.7	$\times 10^9$/l	(1.0–4.0)
Monocytes	0.7	$\times 10^9$/l	(0.0–0.8)
Eosinophils	0.1	$\times 10^9$/l	(0.0–0.4)
Basophils	0.0	$\times 10^9$/l	(0.0–0.1)
ESR (erythrocyte sedimentation rate)	12	mm/hr	(5–15)

In view of the previous MRI findings, a further MRI was taken 6 months later. This reported:

The small cystic lesion lying posterior to the thecal sac at the T5 level remains unchanged in size and signal characteristics since the previous MRI examination. There is no pressure on the thecal sac, spinal cord or on the adjacent nerves of the T5–6 intervertebral foramina.

TREATMENT

The patient was reassured that the thoracic spine lesion was benign and harmless. She was seen by a spinal surgeon at which time the option of surgery was discussed and it was decided that the lesion should be left as it was unless her symptoms increased.

RESULTS

Some years later she still had no increase in symptomatology.

Key point

Small extradural (epidural) benign cystic lesions initially cause uncharacteristic spinal pain (Rickenbacher et al 1982). Therefore, be wary of thoracic spine pain that cannot be reproduced by mechanical stressing of spinal joints, particularly when the Valsalva manoeuvre causes a slight increase in pain.

REFERENCE

Rickenbacher J, Landolt A M, Theiler K 1982 Applied anatomy of the back. Springer-Verlag, Berlin, p 294.

FURTHER READING

Kochan J P, Quencer R M 1991 Imaging of cystic and cavitary lesions of the spinal cord and canal. The value of MR and intraoperative sonography. Radiology Clinics of North America 29: 867–911.
Netter F H 1962 The Ciba collection of medical illustrations, Vol 1, Nervous system. Ciba Pharmaceutical Co, USA, p 99.
Rimmelin A, Clouet P L, Salatino S, Kehrli P, Maitrot D, Stephan M, Dietemann J L 1997 Imaging of thoracic and lumbar spinal extradural arachnoid cysts: report of two cases. Neuroradiology 39: 203–206.

Case 49 Post-traumatic anterior longitudinal ligament calcification

COMMENT

Remember the possible role of the sympathetic nervous system when patients present with autonomic type symptoms.

PROFILE

A 51-year-old married man who does not smoke cigarettes or drink alcohol.

PAST HISTORY

He had not had any unusual childhood or adult illnesses, apart from some lower sternal pain since an injury approximately 2 years ago; he had been told that this pain was due to 'indigestion'.

PRESENTING COMPLAINT (Fig. 49.1)

Lower thoracic spine pain that radiates to the right side as far as the subscapular region. When this pain is severe, he feels 'breathless'.

Medication, spinal manipulation, physiotherapy, and acupuncture treatment have all been of no help.

AETIOLOGY

He was assaulted by a large person who hit his head with such force that he was propelled backwards and hit the lower back part of his thoracic spine against a fixed shelf. His thoracic spine arched backwards and 'twisted over the shelf', and he 'felt and heard a tearing sensation' in the lower thoracic spine. He thought his shirt had been torn but later found it had not. He fell to the floor unconscious for a few seconds; upon regaining consciousness, he felt 'breathless' and dazed but apparently managed to defend himself. He felt he could not breathe

properly, so his general medical practitioner sent him for thoracic spine radiographs and gave him cortisone medication followed by physiotherapy treatment. He never had any lower thoracic spine pain before the injury described above.

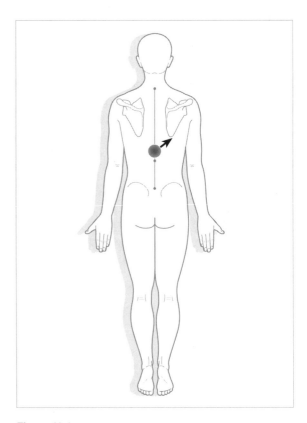

Figure 49.1

EXAMINATION

Deep reflexes in the upper and lower extremities were normal. Pinprick sensation was normal for the arms and legs except for diminished sensation (hypoaesthesia) in the right big toe (L5). Light touch was normal over the extremities and torso. Auscultation of the heart and lungs was normal. Vibration sensation at the ankles and elbows was normal. Percussion of the lower thoracic and upper lumbar spines caused an increase in local pain at the T7–10 level. Deep palpation over the paraspinal muscles elicited pain at the T7–10 level bilaterally. The Valsalva manoeuvre (bearing down) did not increase his pain, so a space-occupying lesion was considered to be unlikely. Hand grip strength was normal. Power in the lower limbs was normal. Plantar responses were normal.

Passive left lateral bending was limited by approximately 10% due to some T10–L1 pain. Right lateral bending was limited by approximately 10% due to pain at approximately the T8 level that radiated to below the right scapula. Left and right rotation were limited by approximately 20% due to pain in the T7–8 region. Thoracic spine active ranges of movement were as follows:

1. Flexion – limited by approximately 10% due to a feeling of 'shortness of breath'.
2. Extension – limited by approximately 50% due to pain at approximately the T7–8 level.

IMAGING REVIEW

Plain X-ray films of the thoracic spine were reported as showing 'idiopathic calcification in the T6–7 disc with early calcification appearing in the T7–8 disc. Tiny ostophytes at the vertebral body margins at the T7–8, T8–9 and T9–10 levels'. A very important finding was overlooked, i.e. the slight calcification, probably in the anterior longitudinal ligament, as seen on the lateral thoracic spine X-ray film (Fig. 49.2A). A further thoracic spine plain X-ray examination had reported on the T6–7 disc calcification and 'some aortic calcification'.

CLINICAL IMPRESSION

Mechanical spinal pain due to soft tissue injuries associated with the lower thoracic spine. ? Autonomic nervous system involvement in view of his 'shortness of breath' at times.

WHAT ACTION SHOULD BE TAKEN?

In order to further investigate the apparent calcification in the anterior longitudinal lig ment, a thoracic CT scan was performed through the mid T9 to mid T12 levels. The CT report stated:

There are very minor degenerative changes noted with small osteophytes beginning to form at the vertebral body margins at all levels examined. No evidence of fractures is seen. There are no paravertebral soft tissue masses to suggest adjacent haematomas. The spinal canal is not compromised. The exiting foramina are all satisfactory.

Unfortunately, the calcification in the anterior longitudinal ligament, that probably indicates

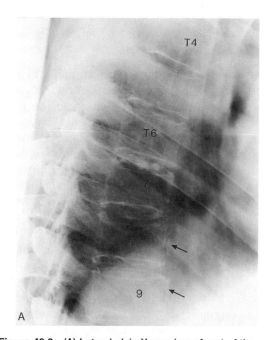

Figure 49.2 (A) Lateral plain X-ray view of part of the thoracic spine (T4–T9) showing the 'idiopathic calcification in the T6–7 disc with early calcification appearing in the T7–8 disc'. Also note the slight calcification probably located within the anterior longitudinal ligament (arrows). T4 = fourth thoracic vertebra; T6 = sixth thoracic vertebra; T9 = ninth thoracic vertebra.

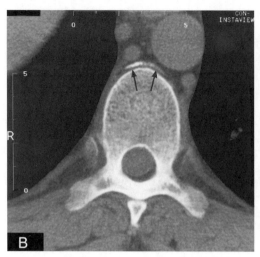 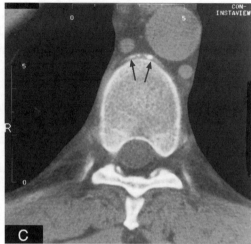

Figure 49.2 (B, C) CT thoracic spine scan through the 8th thoracic vertebra showing the calcification in the anterior longitudinal ligament (arrows).

tearing of the anterior longitudinal ligament with subsequent calcification, was not reported (Fig. 49.2B and C).

TREATMENT

The patient was reassured that he had a benign condition causing his symptoms of mid to lower thoracic spine pain with radiation to the right subscapular region. He was told that the innervation of the spine is very complex and that it was likely that he had injured the sympathetic plexus on the vertebral bodies at the time that the anterior longitudinal ligament and possibly other adjacent soft tissues, were injured when his thoracic spine was hyperextended and that this may be the cause of his periodic shortness of breath when he experiences exacerbations of his thoracolumbar pain. As mentioned in Case 40, Groen and Stolker (2000) have stated that injuries to the thoracic spine may refer pain sensation up and down several segments, so this neurological mechanism may be involved in his shortness of breath.

RESULTS

He responded well to the explanation of his soft tissue injuries and possible sequelae and was

pleased to know that an organic cause for his condition had been found as he had been told to stop malingering. He has now learned to live with his condition.

Key point

Hyperextension of the thoracic spine can cause tearing of the anterior longitudinal ligament and probable injury to the autonomic sympathetic plexus adjacent to the vertebral bodies and discs.

REFERENCE

Groen G J, Stolker R J 2000 Thoracic neural anatomy. In: Giles LGF, Singer KP (eds) Clinical anatomy and management of thoracic spine pain. Butterworth-Heinemann, Oxford, pp 114–141.

FURTHER READING

Burke D C 1971 Hyperextension injuries of the spine. Journal of Bone and Joint Surgery 53: 3–12.
Terk M R, Hume-Neal M, Fraipont M, Ahmadi J, Colletti J 1997 Injury of the posterior ligament complex in patients with acute spinal trauma: evaluation by MR imaging. American Journal of Roentgenology 168: 1481–1486.

Case 50   Osteophyte

COMMENT
When patients describe unusual symptoms, look
to the spine as one possible source.

PROFILE

A 32-year-old married woman.

PAST HISTORY

She had undergone a gastroscopy for her ongoing
and unexplained symptoms; this procedure
revealed slight oesophagitis but there was nothing
else of relevance in her history.

PRESENTING COMPLAINT (Fig. 50.1)

For one year she has suffered from intermittent
severe 'stabbing pains' in the upper thoracic
spine that radiate to the left side and to under
the left breast; sometimes the pain radiates into
the left arm.

Standing erect relieves the pain and sleeping
with one pillow is better than using more than
one pillow. There is no increase in pain on
coughing or sneezing.

She is not aware of what precipitates the
symptoms that may occur at any time during
the day or night. There is no night pain *per se*
but she may feel pain on turning over during
the night. She thinks that picking up her small
child is an aggravating factor. She is very
concerned that she may have a serious pathological condition.

AETIOLOGY

She could not recall having had any injuries to
her upper thoracic spine or neck.

EXAMINATION

Deep palpation over the paraspinal muscles in
the upper thoracic spine (particularly T2–4)
elicited local pain. The deep reflexes in the
upper and lower extremities were normal, as
was the case with vibration sensation at the

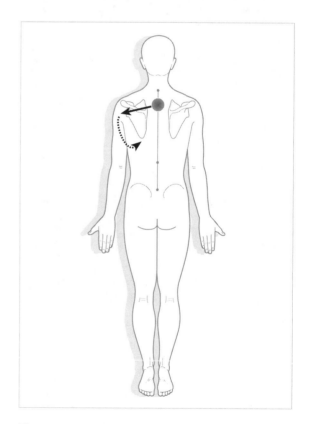

Figure 50.1

229

elbows and ankles. Power in the upper and lower extremities was normal. Pinprick sensation did not elicit any areas of altered sensation. Bending forwards caused an increase in her symptoms.

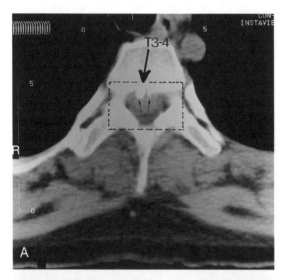

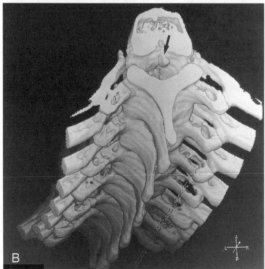

Figure 50.2 (A) Axial CT thoracic spine scan at the T3–4 level showing the posterior central osteophytes projecting from the disc–vertebral body junction. Note how the osteophytes encroach upon the pain-sensitive anterior part of the dural tube (small arrows). The area in the rectangle is represented in an essentially normal thoracic spine by the histological section in Fig. 50.3. (B) Thoracic spine three-dimensional reconstruction oblique tunnel view looking from above. Note the midline posterior osteophyte (arrow) at the T3–4 level.

IMAGING REVIEW

Plain film cervical spine and chest films, respectively, showed mild straightening of the upper cervical lordosis and slight old post-traumatic deformity of the C5 vertebral body. No other changes were noted.

CLINICAL IMPRESSION

Upper thoracic spine disc protrusion. Differential diagnosis – spinal canal space-occupying lesion or bone pathology (considered less likely as there is no pattern of night pain).

WHAT ACTION SHOULD BE TAKEN?

A CT thoracic spine was ordered from the T2 to T7 levels. This showed 'Midline T3–4 disc level small posterior osteophyte beginning to encroach upon the spinal canal' (Fig. 50.2A). In order to better visualize the midline posterior osteophyte, a three-dimensional reconstruction oblique tunnel view, looking from above, was also obtained (Fig. 50.2B). This more clearly defined the extent of the osteophyte.

TREATMENT

The patient was told that the midline posterior osteophyte was most likely the cause of her symptoms and she was reassured that there was no more significant pathology. She was advised to sleep on her side using only one pillow to fill the gap between her shoulder and the side of her head and neck and she was told that it would be best to avoid all movements where she might bend forwards and cause the osteophyte to further impinge upon the pain-sensitive thecal sac and associated blood vessels and the recurrent meningeal nerves.

The issue of whether surgery should be performed was discussed and it was decided that, unless her symptoms deteriorated, then it would be more appropriate to control them by avoiding postures that aggravate her symptoms, to which she agreed now that she had been reassured that there was no 'dangerous' pathology.

RESULTS

She responded well to the above advice.

To better understand the anatomy of the thoracic spinal canal and related structures, see the cadaveric histopathology section in Fig. 50.3.

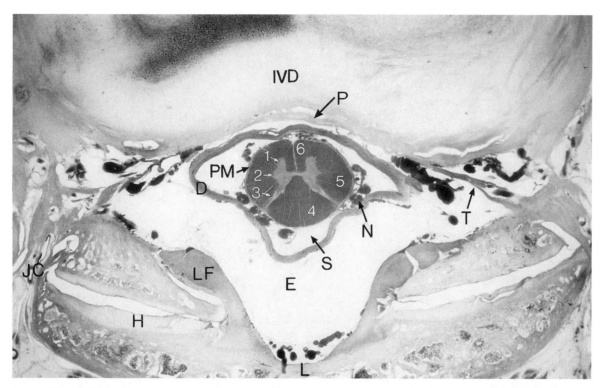

Figure 50.3   A 200-micron thick horizontal (axial) histological section through the thoracic spine of a 40-year-old male cadaver representing the approximate area in the rectangle in Fig. 50.2A. This shows the anatomy of the spinal canal and related structures at this level but without osteophytes. D = dural tube (thecal sac); E = extra dural (epidural) space; H = hyaline articular cartilage on the inferior articular process facet of the vertebra above; IVD = intervertebral disc; JC = zygapophysial (facet) joint capsule; L = lamina junction; LF = ligamentum flavum; N = dorsal (posterior) nerve root; P = posterior longitudinal ligament; PM = pia mater; S = subarachnoid space; T = transforaminal ligament crossing the intervertebral foramen; 1 = anterior grey column; 2 = lateral grey column; 3 = posterior grey column; 4 = posterior funiculus; 5 = lateral funiculus; 6 = anterior funiculus. (Erhlich's haematoxylin and light green counter stain.)

Key point

When a patient is concerned about a serious pathology possibly causing the symptoms, a CT scan or a MRI scan can be used not only as a diagnostic test, but also as a therapeutic measure which can allay patient fears of a serious pathology being present.

FURTHER READING

Daita G, Marino K, Gotoh S, Ueno K, Takamura H 1975 The protrusion of thoracic intervertebral disc-thoracic spondylosis. No Shinkei Geka 3: 509–515.
O'Neill T W, McCloskey E V, Kanis J A, Bhalla A K, Reeve J, Reid D M, Todd C, Woolf A D, Silman A J 1999 The distribution, determinants, and clinical correlates of vertebral osteophytosis: a population based survey. Journal of Rheumatology 26: 842–848.
Smith D E, Godersky J C 1987 Thoracic spondylosis: an unusual cause of myelopathy. Neurosurgery 20: 589–593.

Conclusion

The reader will have realized the value of taking a thorough history and performing an appropriate physical examination and carefully looking at available or new imaging in an attempt to help the patient.

Patients do not normally like to be unwell. In my experience, there are very few malingerers, so one should be on one's guard not to be suspicious of a patient's motives without evidence to substantiate an impression of malingering.

Most clinicians are decent ethical practitioners but clearly errors occur in many fields of health care. We all make diagnostic or treatment errors from time to time but these errors should readily be acknowledged so that aggrieved patients can get a fair deal.

Patients appearing for medicolegal consultation and examination following a work-related injury or a motor vehicle injury, should not be arbitrarily classified as having a 'zero percent permanent incapacity' awarded when workers sustain a serious injury such as a moderately large disc prolapse (Giles 2001).

It must be remembered that it is a privilege to care for patients and that every endeavour should be made to make an appropriate diagnosis and to alleviate the physical pain and any psychological distress that many patients endure.

It is essential to perform an appropriate and thorough diagnostic work up on which to base efficient best practice management. Patient management should include obtaining a signed informed consent form once treatment options and risks have been discussed. In addition, patient cooperation should be sought regarding patient involvement in, for example, a healthy lifestyle and performing exercises.

Finally, a detailed understanding of the spine requires intimate knowledge of the gross and histological anatomy of this complex organ. The gross anatomical and histological and histopathological examples used in this text would not have been available were it not for the tremendous gift made by so many individuals when they bequeath their bodies to university institutions where anatomical and histological studies can be performed. Students of anatomy should remember the privilege associated with working on human material in order to better comprehend the human body.

REFERENCE

Giles L G F 2001 Medicolegal reporting for spinal injuries. Plaintiff 44: 21–23.

Definitions and abbreviations

Antalgic posture a posture assumed by patients experiencing acute low back pain, with or without leg pain, in which they lean away from the painful area.

Anteroposterior (A-P) the *position* of patients when an X-ray beam is directed to their anterior surface and an X-ray plate is positioned behind them. In this text, the A-P radiographs are *viewed* from behind the patient; the patient's right side is indicated by a right marker (R).

Cloward procedure Cloward (1958) used an anterior interbody fusion operation for treating affected protruding discs and/or osteophyte complexes in the region of C4 to C7.

Coarctation of aorta a fibrous constriction in the aorta: 98% are distal to the origin of the left sub-clavian artery, but 2% may be abdominal or in the lower thoracic aorta. Usually presents as proximal hypertension due to mechanical obstruction and a low renal perfusion pressure. It is associated with congenital berry aneurysms in the cerebral circulation, and 60% of patients have a bicuspid aortic valve. Patients are often asymptomatic, but may experience leg fatigue or claudication (Pumphrey 1996). Coarctation causes systolic and diastolic hypertension in the upper extremities (Verrier 1994).

Cobb's method (1948) method for measuring the angle of scoliotic spinal curvature. The angle of curvature is measured by drawing lines parallel to the superior surface of the most upper vertebral body of the curvature and to the inferior surface of the lowest vertebra of the curvature (Fig. x).

Degenerative spondylolisthesis (Pseudospondylolisthesis) is secondary to longstanding degenerative arthrosis of the lumbar zygapophysial

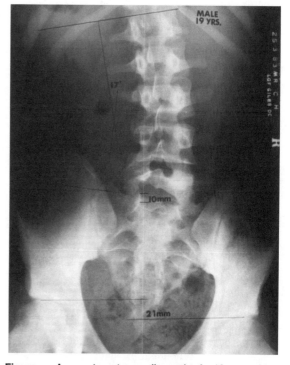

Figure x An erect posture radiograph of a 19-year-old male showing a right leg length deficiency of 21 mm, sacral base obliquity and postural scoliosis with a 17° angle of curvature. R = right side of the patient. Note the vertical plumb-line shadow which is used for measuring leg lengths by drawing a horizontal line from the top of each femur head to meet the plumb-line at right angles. Sacral base obliquity is measured by drawing a horizontal line from each superior sacral notch to meet the plumb-line at right angles. The vertical difference between paired horizontal lines gives the difference in leg lengths and the difference in height between the superior sacral notches. (Reproduced with permission from Giles L G F 1989 Anatomical basis of low back pain. Williams & Wilkins, Baltimore.)

joints and discovertebral articulations, without a pars separation (Yochum et al 1996).

Disability an alteration of an individual's capacity to meet personal, social, or occupational demands because of an impairment (American Medical Association 1993). Disability refers to an activity or task the individual cannot accomplish (Luck & Florence 1988).

Haemangioma general term denoting a benign or malignant vascular tumour that resembles the classic type of haemangioma but occurs at any age (*Dorland's Illustrated Medical Dictionary* 1994).

Impairment an alteration of an individual's health status (American Medical Association 1993) or any loss or abnormality of psychological, physiological, or anatomical structure or function (WHO 1980).

Intervertebral disc conditions

Anular bulge refers to a concentric extension of the margins of the disc circumferentially beyond the vertebral margins (Hodges et al 1999).

Broad-based protrusion refers to protrusion of disc material extending beyond the outer edges of the vertebral body apophyses over an area greater than 25% (90°) and less than 50% (180°) of the circumference of the disc (Fardon & Milette 2001).

Contained herniation is when nuclear material does not escape from the confines of the anular fibres.

Extrusion is the extension of the nucleus completely through the outer anulus into the epidural space (Hodges et al 1999).

Herniation is defined as a localized displacement of disc material beyond the limits of the intervertebral disc space (Fardon & Milette 2001).

Protrusion is a focal area of extension of the nucleus beyond the vertebral margin that remains beneath the outer anular and posterior longitudinal ligament complex (Hodges et al 1999).

Sequestration is a specific type of extrusion in which there is a free disc fragment (Hodges et al 1999).

Intra-articular synovial fold a fibrous or highly vascular fat-filled zygapophysial joint synovial fold which is covered by the synovial lining membrane.

Intranuclear cleft a hypointense linear signal on a T2-weighted MRI image within the centre of the intervertebral disc.

'Leg length' inequality the absolute inequality in length of the lower limbs. In this text a 'significant leg length inequality' is referred to when an inequality of 9 mm or more is found using an accurate method for erect posture radiography (Fig. x).

Manipulation (Cassidy & Kirkaldy-Willis 1988) The definition given by Sandoz (1976, 1981) is both clear and concise. A manipulation or lumbar intervertebral joint 'adjustment' is a passive manual manoeuvre during which the three-joint complex is suddenly carried beyond the normal physiological range of movement without exceeding the boundaries of anatomical integrity. The usual characteristic is a thrust – a brief, sudden, and carefully administered 'impulsion' that is given at the end of the normal passive range of movement. It is usually accompanied by a cracking noise.

Neuro-orthopaedic tests

Adson's test – used to determine the state of the subclavian artery, which may be compressed by an extra cervical rib or by tightened scalenus anticus and scalenus medius muscles, which can compress the artery where it passes between them on its way to the upper extremity.

Take the patient's radial pulse at the wrist and while continuing to feel the pulse, abduct, extend, and externally rotate the arm; then instruct the patient to take a deep breath and to turn the head toward the arm being tested. If there is compression of the subclavian artery, a marked diminution or absence of the radial pulse will be felt (Hoppenfeld 1976).

Babinski test – run a pointed instrument across the plantar surface of the foot from the calcaneus along the lateral border to the forefoot. In a negative reaction, the toes either do not move at all or bunch up uniformly or turn down. If there is a positive reaction, the great toe extends while the other toes plantar flex and splay. A positive Babinski reflex indicates an upper motor neuron lesion. In the new born, a positive Babinski is normal; however, the reflex should disappear soon after birth (Hoppenfeld 1976).

Cervical spine compression test – narrowing of the neural foramen, pressure on the facet joints, or muscle spasm can cause increased pain upon compression. In addition, the compression test may faithfully reproduce pain referred to the upper extremity from the cervical spine, and, in doing so, may help locate the neurological level of any existing pathology. Press down upon the top of the seated patient's head. If there is an increase in pain in either the cervical spine or the extremity, note its exact distribution and whether it follows any previously described dermatome (Hoppenfeld 1976).

Gaenslen's sign – the patient lies supine on the table, and is asked to draw both legs up to the chest; the patient is then shifted to the side of the table to enable one buttock to extend over the edge of the table. Allow the unsupported leg to drop over the edge, while the opposite leg remains flexed. Complaints of subsequent pain in the sacroiliac joint area gives an indication of pathology in that area.

Hoffman's sign – briefly pinch the nail of the middle finger; normally there should be no reaction at all. A positive reaction produces flexion of the terminal phalanx of the thumb and of the second and third phalanx of another finger. If present, this is an indication of an upper motor neuron lesion (Hoppenfeld 1977).

Hoover test – this test helps to determine whether the patient is malingering when stating that the leg cannot be raised. The examiner's hands are put under the patient's heels and, as the patient tries to raise one leg, the opposite heel is used to gain leverage; this causes downward pressure to be felt on the examiner's hand in genuine cases. If the patient does not bear down while attempting to raise one leg, the patient is probably not really trying.

Kernig test – this procedure applies tension to the spinal cord and can reproduce pain. Ask the patient to lie supine, then to place both hands behind the head and to forcibly flex the head onto the chest. The patient may complain of pain in the cervical spine, and, occasionally, in the low back or down the legs, an indication of meningeal irritation, nerve root involvement, or irritation of the dural coverings of the nerve roots. Ask the patient to locate the area from which the pain originates.

Lasegue's sign – flex the hip with the knee flexed, followed by the knee being gradually straightened.

Milgram test – the patient lies supine on the examining table with legs straight, then actively raises them to a position about 5 cm from the table and holds this position for as long as possible.

This manoeuvre stretches the iliopsoas muscle, the anterior abdominal muscles, and increases the intrathecal pressure. If the patient can maintain this position for 30 seconds without pain, intrathecal pathology may be ruled out. If the patient cannot hold the position, or cannot lift the legs at all, or experiences pain in the attempt, there may be intrathecal or extrathecal pathology (e.g. herniated disc).

Naffziger test – a compression test designed to increase intrathecal pressure by increasing the intraspinal fluid pressure. The jugular veins are gently compressed for about 10 seconds until the patient's face begins to flush. The patient is asked to cough; if coughing causes pain, there is probably pathology pressing upon the theca. The patient is asked to locate the painful area.

Patrick or Fabere test – a test for detecting pathology in the hip, as well as in the sacroiliac joint. The patient lies supine on the table and places the foot of the painful side on the opposite knee. This causes the hip joint to be flexed, abducted, and externally rotated. In this position, inguinal pain gives a general indication of pathology in the hip joint or the surrounding muscles. At full ranges of flexion, abduction, and external rotation, the femur is fixed in relation to the pelvis. To stress the sacroiliac joint, place one hand on the flexed knee joint and the other hand on the opposite anterior superior iliac spine. Press down on each of these points and if the patient complains of increased pain, there may be sacroiliac joint pathology.

Slump test – the patient sits with the back straight and the legs hanging over the edge of the examination table then slumps the cervical and thoracic spines forward; then straighten one leg at a time to traction the dura. If further dural traction is necessary, dorsiflex the foot. Ask the patient to extend the neck and, if low back or leg pain is relieved, the pain arises from the spine (Kenna & Murtagh 1989).

Swallow test – difficulty or pain upon swallowing can sometimes be caused by cervical spine pathology such as bony protuberances, bony osteophytes, or by soft tissue swelling due to haematomas, infection, or tumour in the anterior portion of the cervical spine (Hoppenfeld 1976).

Valsalva manoeuvre – the patient is asked to bear down as if trying to move the bowels; this increases the intrathecal pressure. If bearing down causes pain in the spine, or radiating pain, there is probably pathology either causing intrathecal pressure or involving the theca itself.

Obliquity

Pelvic obliquity – this is a lateral inclination of the pelvis which is tilted downward to the short leg side (Fig. x).

Sacral base obliquity – a lateral inclination of the sacral base (Fig. x).

Osteoarthritis (degenerative joint disease, degenerative arthritis, hypertrophic arthritis) – characterized by degeneration of articular cartilage, hypertrophy of bone at joint margins, and synovial membrane changes; usually associated with pain and stiffness (Hellmann 1992).

Osteoarthrosis Chronic non-inflammatory arthritis.

Persistent notochord in rare instances the notochord, instead of being entirely confined to the intervertebral discs, persists in whole or in part (Diethelm 1974, Tondury 1958). The result may be an unossified central canal in the vertebral body or conical depressions in the upper and lower endplates (Rickenbacher et al 1982).

Scoliosis

Angle of curvature – the angle between lines drawn parallel to the superior surface of the upper vertebra of the curvature and to the inferior surface of the lowest vertebra of the curvature.

Postural (compensatory) – this is a lumbar or thoracolumbar scoliosis (lateral curvature) which is an adaptation of the vertebral column to pelvic obliquity and which is convex on the short leg side. The intervertebral discs are wedged from the concave to the convex sides on the A-P radiograph with the discs being wider on the convex side of the scoliosis (Fig. x).

Structural idiopathic – a lateral curvature with fixed rotational deformity of the spine.

Shoe-raise therapy the provision of a shoe-raise on the side of the short leg. The raise on the heel is equal to the difference in leg lengths and the raise on the sole can be 5 mm less.

Spinal pain

Acute spinal pain refers to severe pain of recent onset (less than 4 weeks) with marked limitation of spinal movements (Skoven et al 2002).

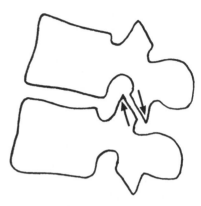

Figure xi Note the subluxation (imbrications telescoping) of the zygapophysial joint facet surfaces as indicated by the arrows. (Reproduced with permission from Giles L G F 1989 Anatomical basis of low back pain. Williams & Wilkins, Baltimore.)

Chronic spinal pain refers to pain of long duration (13 weeks or more) without marked limitation of spinal movements.

Sub-acute spinal pain refers to pain of greater than 4 weeks and less than 13 weeks.

Spondylosis osteophytosis secondary to degenerative intervertebral disc disease (Weinstein et al 1977).

Subluxation in this text, the term is used when apposing facet surfaces of the zygapophysial joint are no longer congruous, as demonstrated by imbrication (telescoping) of the zygapophysial joint facet surfaces (Hadley 1964) (Fig. xi).

Tropism asymmetry in the horizontal plane of paired left and right zygapophysial joints.

Zygapophysial joint the diarthrodial synovial joint between adjacent vertebral arches (apophyseal joint, 'facetal' joint, interlaminar joint).

Zygapophysial joint cartilage according to Hadley (1964) this is of the hyaline articular cartilage variety and it lines the facet surfaces; extensions of cartilage beyond the facet surface, known as 'bumper-fibrocartilage', are not composed of hyaline cartilage (Hadley 1964).

REFERENCES

American Medical Association (1993) Guides to the evaluation of permanent impairment, 4th edn. American Medical Association, Illinois, p 2.

Cassidy J D, Kirkaldy-Willis W H 1988 Manipulation. In: Kirkaldy-Willis WH (ed.) Managing back pain, 2nd edn. Churchill Livingstone, New York, pp 287–296.

Cloward R B 1958 The anterior approach for removal of ruptured cervical disks. Journal of Neurosurgery 15: 602–617.

Cobb J R 1948 Outline for the study of scoliosis. Instructional course lectures. American Academy of Orthopedic Surgeons 5: 261–275.

Diethelm L 1974 Fehlbildungen des Corpus vertebrale. In: Diethelm L et al (eds) Handbuch der medizinischen Radiologie, Bd 6, Teil 1: Rontgendiagnostik der Wirbelsaule, 1. Teil. Berlin, Heidelberg, New York, Springer, pp 190–263.

Dorland's illustrated medical dictionary, 28th edn. W.B. Saunders Co, Philadelphia.

Fardon D F, Milette P C 2001 Nomenclature and classification of lumbar disc pathology. Spine 26: E93–E113.

Giles L G F 1989 Anatomical basis of low back pain. Williams & Wilkins, Baltimore.

Hadley L A 1964 Anatomico-roentgenographic studies of the spine. Charles C. Thomas, Springfield, IL, pp 178, 183.

Hellmann D B 1992 Arthritis and musculoskeletal disorders. In: Schroeder SA et al (eds) Current medical diagnosis and treatment. Appleton & Lange, Norwalk, CT.

Hodges S D, Humphreys C, Eck J C, Covington L A 1999 Posterior extradural lumbar disk fragment. Journal of the Southern Orthopaedic Association 8: 222–228.

Hoppenfeld S 1976 Physical examination of the spine and extremities. Appleton-Century-Crofts, New York.

Hoppenfeld S 1977 Orthopaedic neurology: A diagnostic guide to neurologic levels. J B Lippincott, Philadelphia.

Kenna C, Murtagh J 1989 Back pain and spinal manipulation: A practical guide. Butterworth-Heinemann, Oxford, pp 98–101.

Luck J V Jr., Florence D W 1988 A brief history and comparative analysis of disability systems and impairment rating guides. Orthopedic Clinics of North America 19: 839–844.

Pumphrey C W 1996 Heart disease. In: Axford JS (ed.) Medicine. Blackwell Science Ltd, Oxford, p 5.80.

Rickenbacher J, Landolt A M, Theiler K 1982 Applied anatomy of the back. Springer-Verlag, Berlin, p 44.

Sandoz R 1976 Some physical mechanisms and effects of spinal adjustments. Annals of the Swiss Chiropractic Association 6: 91.

Sandoz R 1981 Some reflex phenomena associated with spinal derangements and adjustments. Annals of the Swiss Chiropractic Association 7: 45.

Skoven J S, Grasdal A L, Haldorsen E M H 2002 Relative cost-effectiveness of extensive and light multidisciplinary treatment programs versus treatment as usual for patients with chronic low back pain on long-term sick leave. Spine 27: 901–910.

Tondury G 1958 Entwicklungsgeschichte und Fehlbildungen der Wirbelsaule. In: Junghans H (ed.) Die Wirbelsaule in Forschung und Praxis, Bd 7. Hippokrates, Stuttgart.

Verrier E D 1994 The heart: II. Congenital diseases. In: Way LW (ed.) Current surgical diagnosis and treatment. Appleton and Lange, Norwalk, CT, pp 383–410.

Yochum T R, Rowe L J, Barry M S 1996 Natural history of spondylolysis and spondylolisthesis. In: Yochum TR, Rowe LJ (eds) Essentials of skeletal radiology, 2nd edn. Williams & Wilkins, Baltimore, pp 327–372.

Weinstein P R, Ehni G, Wilson C B 1977 Clinical features of lumbar spondylosis and stenosis. In: Weinstein PR, Ehni G, Wilson CB (eds) Lumbar spondylosis, diagnosis, management and surgical treatment. Year Book Medical Publishers, Chicago, pp 115–133.

World Health Organization 1980 International classification of impairments, disabilities and handicaps. World Health Organization, Geneva, Switzerland.

Index